Advanced Techniques of Endoscopic Lumbar Spine Surgery

Hyeun Sung Kim • Michael Mayer
Dong Hwa Heo • Cheol Woong Park
Editors

Advanced Techniques of Endoscopic Lumbar Spine Surgery

Springer

Editors
Hyeun Sung Kim
Department of Neurosurgery
Nanoori Hospital Gangnam
Seoul
South Korea

Dong Hwa Heo
Department of Neurosurgery
Seoul Bumin Hospital
Seoul
South Korea

Michael Mayer
Institute for Spinal Research
Schön Klinik München Harlaching
Paracelsus Medical University
Munich
Germany

Cheol Woong Park
Department of Neurosurgery
Daejeon Woori Hospital
Daejeon
South Korea

ISBN 978-981-15-8252-3 ISBN 978-981-15-8253-0 (eBook)
https://doi.org/10.1007/978-981-15-8253-0

This Springer imprint is published by the registered company Springer Nature Singapore Pte Ltd.
The registered company address is: 152 Beach Road, #21-01/04 Gateway East, Singapore 189721, Singapore

Foreword

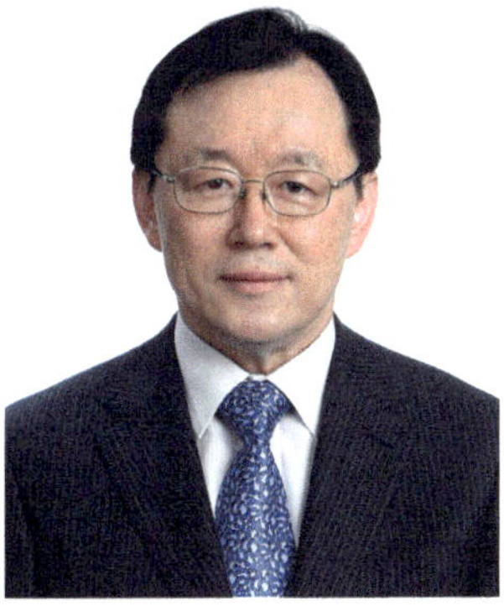

First of all, it would be congratulatory to the current and former presidents of KOSESS, the editorial staffs, and all the authors that are publishing a contemporary book of endoscopic spine surgery (ESS). What impressed us the most was that the youngest spine group in Korea, KOSESS inaugurated only less than 3 years ago, made the textbook of spinal endoscopy. Nowadays, the development of ESS had been so rapid that a traditional textbook cannot contain the newest issue in a specific clinical field. It takes more than two years to complete a traditional textbook. In this regard, a contemporary textbook could be a solution and medium to keep a reader updated with the qualified new subjects of ESS.

As a strong supporter during Dr. G Choi's inauguration preparation of KOSESS, one must be proud that publishing the contemporary textbook of ESS was done by such a young age group. In KOMISS, particularly in KOSESS, there are many globally leading personalities in the frontier spirit, by whom KOSESS could make this textbook without significant difficulty in such a short period. The book would be made smaller in size than an ordinary textbook for a user to carry in a pocket, perhaps as a matter of efficiency. Hopefully, this would become a handbook of ESS for beginners and trainees of ESS, and also for any endoscopic spine surgeon who needs to be updated feeding their ESS procedure into the text. It would be recommendable for all the readers not to understand the handbook as a low-quality one. The editor should have wanted the book to be useful for a surgeon who is practically at the front line.

Finally, it should be our hope that the contemporary textbook must be published annually in line with the role of this book although the contents are fewer than this textbook to keep the surgeons not to drop out of line.

Chun Kun Park
The Catholic University of Korea
Seoul, South Korea

Foreword

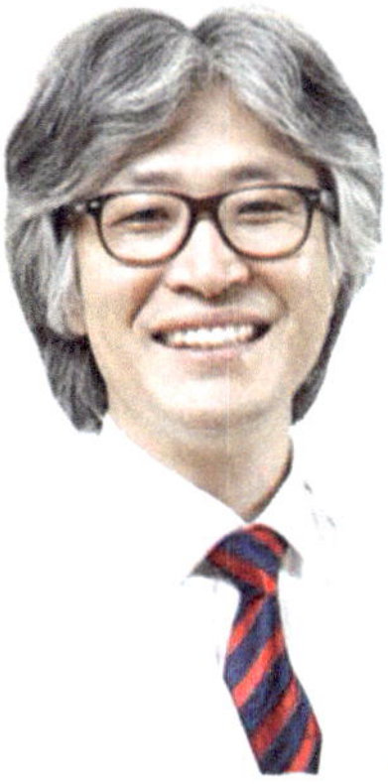

The history of spine surgery goes back at least 5,000 years with the first evidence of spinal surgery in Egyptian mummies from 3000 BC. In the nineteenth century, the meaningful modern spinal surgery was born, and the last few decades have been a period of rapid technological advancement. The speed of medical advancement is ever so fast that it is significant for the spine surgeons to keep updated. It may make us feel overwhelmed and inundated with massive amount of new literatures and technologies to master.

The Korean Research Society of Endoscopic Spine Surgery (KOSESS) is on the front line of the field of endoscopic spine surgery, working closely with the members to help the colleagues be up-to-date with the most recent and innovative skills and knowledge. I am honored to be part of the first textbook ever published by the KOSESS. There are many endoscopic spine surgery books, but I am very proud of this book for its innovative nature that may help the surgeons to be at the cutting-edge of the endoscopic spine surgery.

I would like to give a special thanks to the former presidents of the KOSESS, Dr.Yong Ahn and Dr.Gun Choi, who had made this project possible. I also would like to thank all the 24 authors who have burned the midnight oil in making this book. I also express how thankful I am to Dr.Dong Hwa Heo, a coordinator and one of the authors. He made this book possible to come as one. All of them are the best spine surgeons in the nation, and I am proud that we have worked together to create this master project.

I was given an opportunity as the third president of the KOSESS, and I am honored to be able to be part of this noble project that may be a guiding light to many. In my practice of endoscopic spine surgery for 20years, my team and I have performed more than 23,000 cases. I humbly can say that I am fortunate to be trained to do traditional open surgery, microscopic surgery, small and large channel uniportal endoscopic spine surgery, and biportal endoscopic surgery. The wide range of experience I have had in different types of surgeries has given me an insight and different perspectives.

This book shows you how to treat the most common spine disorders that we see in the clinic such as lumbar central stenosis, lumbar foramina stenosis, lumbar disc herniation, lumbar interbody fusion which makes this book very practical. This book will help you to get acquainted with the endoscopic instruments and terms, different surgical categories, namely samll working channel uniportal endoscopy, large working channel uniportal endoscopy, and biportal endoscopy. It also covers different surgical approaches such as transforaminal, interlaminar, paraspinal, translaminar, contralateral, and one level above approach. Not a single endoscopy or an approach works for every case that it is essential for a spine surgeon to understand each instrument and approach to deliver the best outcome. This book could be of great help to the residents undergoing a training, to young spine surgeons, and also to those who are actively practicing in the field.

Some may still question the needs for the endoscopic surgery opposed to the traditional open surgery. "Why do endoscopic surgery when the traditional open surgery still has a great outcome with less financial restraint on the patient?" Some believe that they are conservative and old-schooled and I agree that may be just Ok. But why do we settle for just fine when we can go the extra mile? In the history of mankind, there were always some who would take risk and try new technologies. I believe that is what drove us to evolve into what we are today. And I do hope that this book is one of the steps that has meaningful effect on the history of the spine surgery in the time to come.

Cheol Woong Park
Department of Neurosurgery
Nanoori Hospital
Seoul, South Korea

Foreword

Prepare for a happy and healthy life!

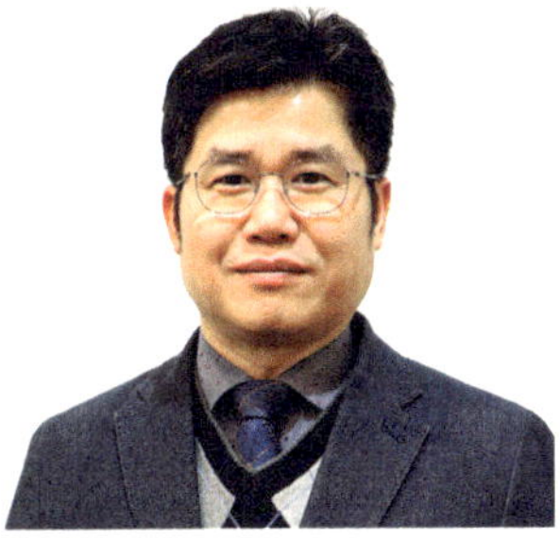

To live a happy and healthy life is the most basic desire of man, and the development of medicine has made steady progress for this purpose. Conquest of degenerative spinal disease is a very important field for providing a happy and healthy life for older patients, and spinal surgery has been steadily developed for the conquest of degenerative spinal disease.

Spinal endoscopic surgery started with a transforaminal approach, but with steady progress with the interlaminar approach, it is now expanding to almost all areas of degenerative spinal disease.

However, there is still a need for further development and a process that can make it universal. The Korean Research Society of Endoscopic Spine Surgery (KOSESS) has prepared a textbook that can be used to learn spinal endoscopic surgery for this purpose.

KOSESS will further develop and organize endoscopic spine surgery through studies and discussions, and through textbooks, spine surgeons will make it easier for them to learn endoscopic spine surgery and provide them with safety.

Hyeun Sung Kim
Department of Neurosurgery
Nanoori Hospital Gangnam
Seoul, South Korea

Preface

Why a contemporary book with the latest knowledge and trends of spinal endoscopy is necessary.

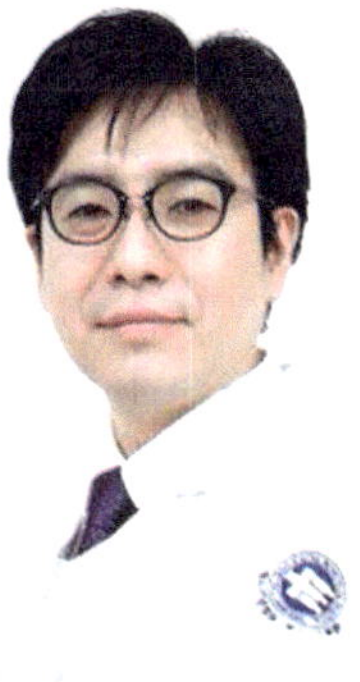

In the past, spinal endoscopic surgeries have been performed mainly in the treatment of lumbar disc herniation.

Recently, the indications for spinal endoscopic surgery have been further expanded due to the breakthrough of surgical methods and surgical instruments. The performance of endoscopic surgery has been greatly improved.

Currently, spinal endoscopic surgery can be applied from the cervical spine to the sacrum, and the indications for central stenosis, lateral recess stenosis, foraminal stenosis, cystic disease, and migrated disc herniation are widely available as well as for disc prolapse. Now, spinal endoscopic approaches are being tried from disc removal to laminectomy and lumbar interbody fusion.

In the past, vertebral endoscopic surgery was mainly performed with the percutaneous transforaminal approach, but now various approaches including the posterior approach, paraspinal approach, the transpedicular approach, and contralateral approach have been attempted.

In addition, uniportal endoscopic approach with a single channel has been performed previously, but the biportal endoscopic approach using two channels has been tried and developed rapidly.

Currently, the trend of spinal endoscopic surgery is changing and developing rapidly, and many articles about new surgical methods are published. However, there are very few cases of spinal endoscopic textbooks that reflect the latest trends. Therefore, we would like to publish a contemporary book on spinal endoscopy that contains the latest knowledge of spinal endoscopic surgery.

I have invited expert spinal endoscopy surgeons who have a lot of practical experience and excellent academic achievement as the author of this book. We will publish not only text-oriented textbooks, but also surgery-related photographs, pictures, and surgical videos, so that readers can learn about surgery and apply them to real surgery. We will do our best to publish the contemporary book of spinal endoscopic surgery which shows the latest trend of the rapidly developing spinal endoscopic approaches and promise to update continuously, not this version.

Seoul, South Korea
25 February 2020

Dong Hwa Heo

Acknowledgement

This textbook was produced with the support of the Korean Minimally Invasive Spine Surgery Society (KOMISS) and the Korea Research Society of Endoscopic Spine Surgery (KOSESS).

Congratulatory Address

Fundamental progress has to do with the reinterpretation of basic ideas.
Alfred North Whitehead
English Mathematician and Philosopher
1861–1947

The development of endoscopic spine surgery in the last 45 years is a history of trial and error, success and failure, brilliant ideas and technical advancements, and finally the triumph of a true, disruptive, minimally invasive surgical technique.

Since Hijikata inaugurated the first "percutaneous nucleotomy" in 1975, pioneers such as Yoshinori Suezawa (first endoscopic discectomy), Parviz Kambin (Kambin triangle), Tony Yeung (first transforaminal approach), Sebastian Ruetten (first interlaminar approach), and lately Jin Sung Kim (endoscopic interbody fusion) and Hyeun Sung Kim (endoscopic decompressions) (just to mention a few) have driven this technology to high-level standard minimally invasive procedures.

Interestingly, full-endoscopic decompression of lumbar of thoracic spinal stenosis or removal of lumbar disc herniations has been most successfully developed and implemented in clinical routine, in countries where microsurgical techniques have not been very popular. Even though the technological step from "open" decompression or discectomy to full-endoscopic techniques is big, the acceptance by the young generation of surgeons has been high, and even in countries with "microsurgical tradition" full-endoscopic techniques are about to "cannibalize" microsurgical techniques.

The advantages of less "collateral damage," less blood loss, less peri- and post-op morbidity, and faster rehab times are obvious. These advantages even supersede longer technical learning curves.

In this contemporary book of endoscopic spine surgery edited by members of the Korean Society of Endoscopic Spine Surgery (KOSESS), all current endoscopic techniques for the treatment of lumbar spinal stenosis, lumbar foraminal stenosis, lumbar disc herniations, and for lumbar fusion are presented by world-class top experts.

If you consider that more than 75% of all spine pathologies as well as surgical techniques fall into these categories, this book is like a contemporary up-to-date "cookbook" for every surgeon who is interested in improving his minimally invasive surgical armamentarium. All current surgical approaches for various pathologies are described in detail and with a tremendous value of experience.

The editors and authors should be congratulated for gathering the pioneers and peers to share their experience with us all.

Salzburg, Austria
March 2020

Michael Mayer

Contents

Part I

Special Issue of Endoscopic Spine Surgery

Paradigm Shifting of Endoscopic Spine Surgery

Dong Hwa Heo, Michael Mayer, Hyeun Sung Kim, and Chun Kun Park

Introduction

Recently, the new concept of spine surgeries has been introduced such as virtual reality, biomaterials, robotics, navigation, and endoscopic surgery. We suggest that the mainstream of minimally invasive spine surgery may be endoscopic spine surgeries.

As you all know, laparoscopic approaches of abdominal surgeries or gynecological surgeries and arthroscopic approaches of joint surgeries were common and ordinary surgical procedures. Moreover, endoscopic approaches of the brain also have been attempted for brain tumor surgeries including skull base surgery. In the present, endoscopic spine surgeries have been vigorously developed, and indications of endoscopic spine surgeries have been extended from disc herniation to stenosis and instability and from lumbosacral to cervical area [1, 2].

Generations of Endoscopic Spine Surgery

Full endoscopic transforaminal approaches were firstly tried for lumbar disc herniation without bone work [3]. This is the first generation of endoscopic spine surgery of lumbar lesion (Fig. 1, Table 1). Followed second generation of endoscopic spine surgery is the posterior interlaminar approach without bone work for the removal of rupture disc herniation of lumbosacral area. Interlaminar endoscopic lumbar approach was firstly attempted in lumbosacral disc herniation rather than transforaminal approach. After trial of posterior interlaminar approach, it was able to perform posterior endoscopic decompressive procedures including laminectomy and laminotomy. New endoscopic specialized instruments such as endoscopic drill systems, reaming systems of foraminoplasty, and endoscopic Kerrison rongeur were developed. As a result, endoscopic decompressive laminectomy, endoscopic laminotomy, lateral foraminotomy (paraspinal approach), and foraminoplasty were possible. Therefore, indications of endoscopic surgeries have been extended from disc herniation to lumbar central stenosis and foraminal stenosis (Fig. 1, Table 1) [4].

D. H. Heo
Department of Neurosurgery, Seoul Bumin Hospital, Seoul, South Korea

M. Mayer (✉)
Institute for Spinal Research, Schön Klinik München Harlaching, Paracelsus Medical University, Munich, Germany
e-mail: mmayer@schoen-kliniken.de

H. S. Kim
Department of Neurosurgery, Gangnam Nanoori Hospital, Seoul, South Korea

C. K. Park
Department of Neurosurgery, Good doctor Teun-Teun Hospital, Anyang, South Korea
e-mail: ckpmd@catholic.ac.kr

H. S. Kim et al. (eds.), *Advanced Techniques of Endoscopic Lumbar Spine Surgery*,
https://doi.org/10.1007/978-981-15-8253-0_1

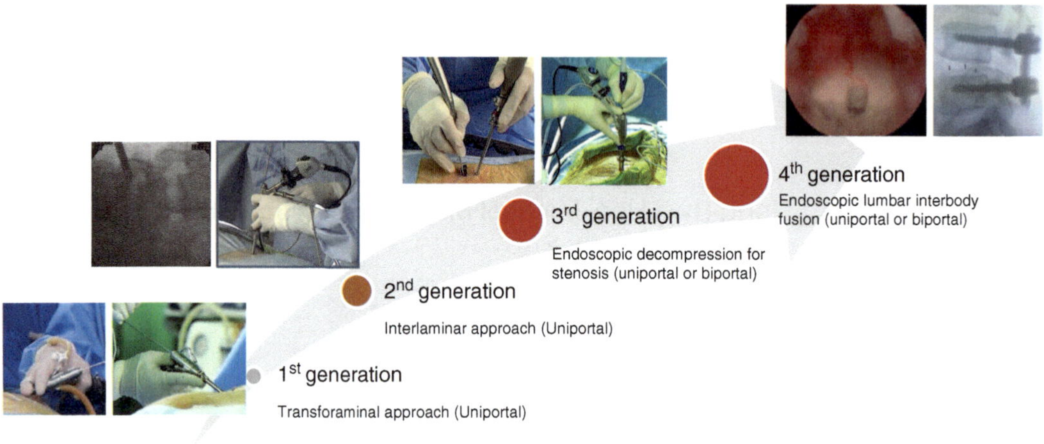

Fig. 1 Paradigm shifting of endoscopic spine surgery from first to fourth generation in lumbar area

Table 1 Generation of endoscopic spine surgery in lumbar lesion

	1st generation	2nd generation	3rd generation	4th generation
Endoscopy systems	Uniportal	Uniportal	Uniportal and biportal	Uniportal and biportal
Approach	Transforaminal approach	Interlaminar approach	Endoscopic laminectomy Endoscopic foraminotomy	Endoscopic lumbar interbody fusion
Indications	Lumbar disc herniation	Lumbar disc herniation	Central or lateral recess stenosis Foraminal stenosis	Spondylolisthesis Instability Combined lesion

Also, modified interlaminar endoscopic systems with a large working channel was developed for the treatment of lumbar stenosis. And biportal endoscopic surgeries have been re-emerged and developed in South Korea. Now, lumbar stenosis is able to be fully decompressed by large working channel interlaminar endoscopic systems or biportal endoscopic approaches [5]. The third generation of endoscopic spine surgery is endoscopic decompressive procedure for lumbar stenotic lesion by uniportal or biportal [5]. Especially, compared to uniportal endoscopic approach, biportal endoscopic surgery has different characteristics; there were two portals including endoscopic channel and working channel. Biportal endoscopic surgery was well known as abbreviation name of UBE (unilateral biportal endoscopy) in South Korea. This biportal endoscopic approach was advantage of decompressive surgical procedure [4].

Another recent issue of endoscopic spine surgery may be endoscopic lumbar interbody fusion (Fig. 1, Table 1) [2]. There were three approaches of endoscopic lumbar interbody fusion: first is the trans-Kambin triangle approach, second is the endoscopy-assisted transforaminal lumbar interbody fusion, and third is the endoscopy-assisted lateral lumbar interbody fusion [2]. Although early clinical results of endoscopic lumbar interbody fusion surgeries may be relatively favorable, we need to investigate long-term outcome and comparative study

The paradigm of endoscopic spine surgeries is still moving, and surgical techniques and instruments of endoscopic spine surgeries are still developing. Finally, the boundary and indications between conventional surgery and endoscopic surgery seem to be narrow or to disappear. We should make an effort to learn a new technique of endoscopic spine surgeries (Fig. 1).

References

1. Kim M, Kim H, Adsul NM, et al. Evolution of spinal endoscopic surgery. Neurospine. 2019;16(1):6–14.
2. Heo DH, Son SK, Eum JH, Park CK. Fully endoscopic lumbar interbody fusion using a percutaneous unilateral biportal endoscopic technique: technical note and preliminary clinical results. Neurosurg Focus. 2017;43(2):E8.
3. Mayer HM. A history of endoscopic lumbar spine surgery: what have we learnt? Biomed Res Int. 2019;2019:4583943.
4. Heo DH, Lee DC, Park CK. Comparative analysis of three types of minimally invasive decompressive surgery for lumbar central stenosis: biportal endoscopy, uniportal endoscopy, and microsurgery. Neurosurg Focus. 2019;46(5):E9.
5. Lee C, Choi M, Ryu DS, et al. Efficacy and safety of full-endoscopic decompression via Interlaminar approach for central or lateral recess spinal stenosis of the lumbar spine: a meta-analysis. Spine. 2018;43(24):1756–64.

Nomenclature of Endoscopic Spine Surgery

Choi Il, Jin-Sung Kim, and Yong Ahn

Introduction (Key Point and Purpose) of Approach

Endoscopic spine surgery was introduced a few decades ago and has rapidly progressed since then, owing to the development of various types of drills and instruments (scope, punch, and dissector). Besides, highly skilled surgeons have created a variety of endoscopic surgical methods. Even though the overall history of endoscopic spine surgery is quite long, the procedure has various names, causing a lack of standard terminology in the literature and spinal societies. It has also disturbed the communication of concerns between surgeons, patients, and hospitals.

To date, international community meetings have not yet defined nomenclature for endoscopic spine procedures. In this chapter, we will introduce the nomenclature, as suggested by the AOSpine minimally invasive spine surgery curriculum task force (MISTFT) (1). Moreover, we will add recently updated procedures and concepts of the AOSpine MISTFT nomenclature. We hope that this chapter can provide a common sense to spine surgeons, nurses, radiologists, and students that are involved with endoscope spinal procedures.

AOSpine minimally invasive spine surgery curriculum task force (MISTFT) suggested nomenclature.

This method was defined by them and key opinion leaders of endoscopic spine surgery. They searched for the terms "spine, full endoscopic, working channel endoscope, spine endoscopy, and percutaneous" in PubMed, reviewed the results, and classified the following principles. The previously utilized nomenclature was searched and compared with each other, and the outcomes of surgery were analyzed. It was integrated into a systematic nomenclature system: (1) approach corridor, (2) mode of visualization, (3) spinal segment, and (4) type of procedure. Then, a new nomenclature was proposed with the above system. The rationale of the nomenclature was described. That data was sent to 30 key opinion leaders of the entire endoscopic spine surgery societies. Finally, 24 key opinions were reviewed, discussed, and accepted in the current form. Finally, they took the nomenclature system.

For understanding this nomenclature system, at first, the term "endoscopic spine procedure" should be analyzed and defined. Endoscopy is defined as the medical examination of a hollow

C. Il
Department of Neurological Surgery, Dongtan Sacred Heart Hospital, University of Hallym University, Hwaseong, South Korea

J.-S. Kim (✉)
Department of Neurosurgery, Seoul St. Mary's Hospital, The Catholic University of Korea, Seoul, South Korea

Y. Ahn
Department of Neurosurgery, Gil Medical Center, Gachon University College of Medicine, Incheon, South Korea

H. S. Kim et al. (eds.), *Advanced Techniques of Endoscopic Lumbar Spine Surgery*,
https://doi.org/10.1007/978-981-15-8253-0_2

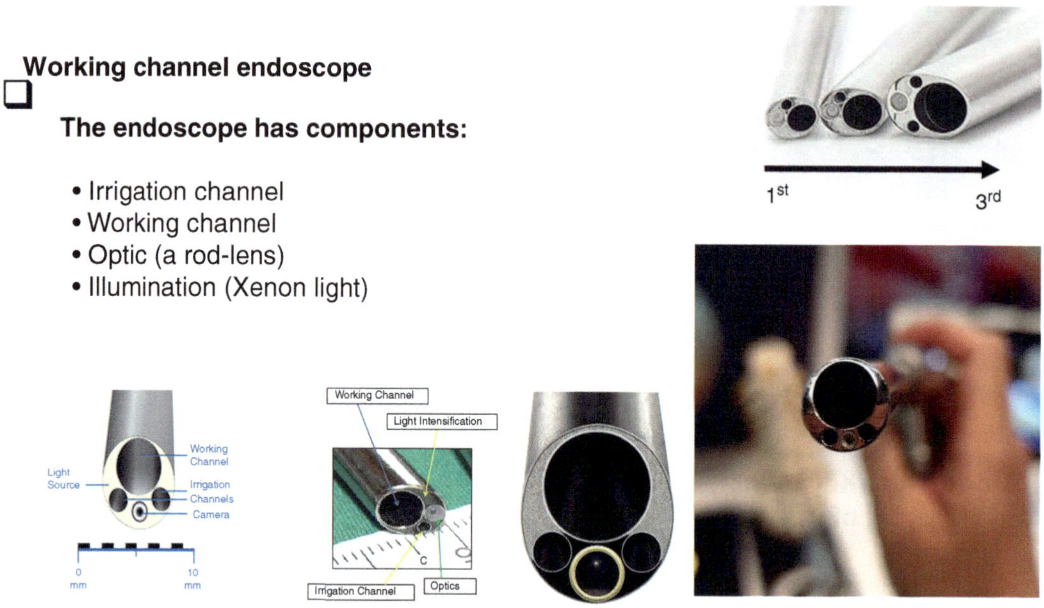

Fig. 1 The working channel endoscopy should have the four components in one scope

organ of the body in the dictionary. **The working channel endoscopy should the four components in one scope**: (1) irrigation channel, (2) working channel, (3) optic (a rod-lens system), and (4) illumination (xenon light) (Fig. 1).

Many endoscopic armamentaria and procedures include the means to manipulate, ablate, resect, and remove pathologic lesions via the surgical corridor of the endoscope. Historically, before the year 2000, the term "percutaneous" was used. After the year 2000, the term "full endoscope" was introduced. They proposed the term "full endoscopic" to describe procedures performed with a working channel endoscope, which is different from endoscopic-assisted surgery that requires another pathway for the surgical working procedure.

Endoscopic spine surgery is described in Fig. 2 and has been subdivided into "full-endoscopic surgery" and endoscopic-assisted surgery

Understanding and Unifying the Nomenclature

This uniform system is divided into four parts as follows: (1) approach corridor (anterior, posterior, interlaminar, and transforaminal), (2) visualization of the lesion (endoscopic), (3) segment (cervical, thoracic, and lumbar), and (4) procedure (discectomy, foraminotomy, and decompression).

It is named in the following order: working channel endoscopy (full endoscopic), approach corridor (anterior, posterior, interlaminar, transforaminal), spinal segment (cervical, thoracic, and lumbar), and procedure performed (discectomy and foraminotomy, lateral recess decompression, and unilateral laminotomy for bilateral decompression).

The approach corridor is divided into the "anterior" and "posterior" approach in cervical spine surgery. In thoracolumbar surgery, the "transforaminal" and "interlaminar" approach is the commonly used method. The interlaminar approach includes the "interlaminar contralateral approach." In the paper, the most mentioned term for the working channel is "full endoscopic" or "percutaneous," and either can be used. "Full endoscopic" or "percutaneous" can be omitted as they are considered redundant expressions. It can be termed as "endoscopic." The spine segment is classified as cervical, thoracic, and lumbar. The procedures include discectomy, foraminotomy, lateral

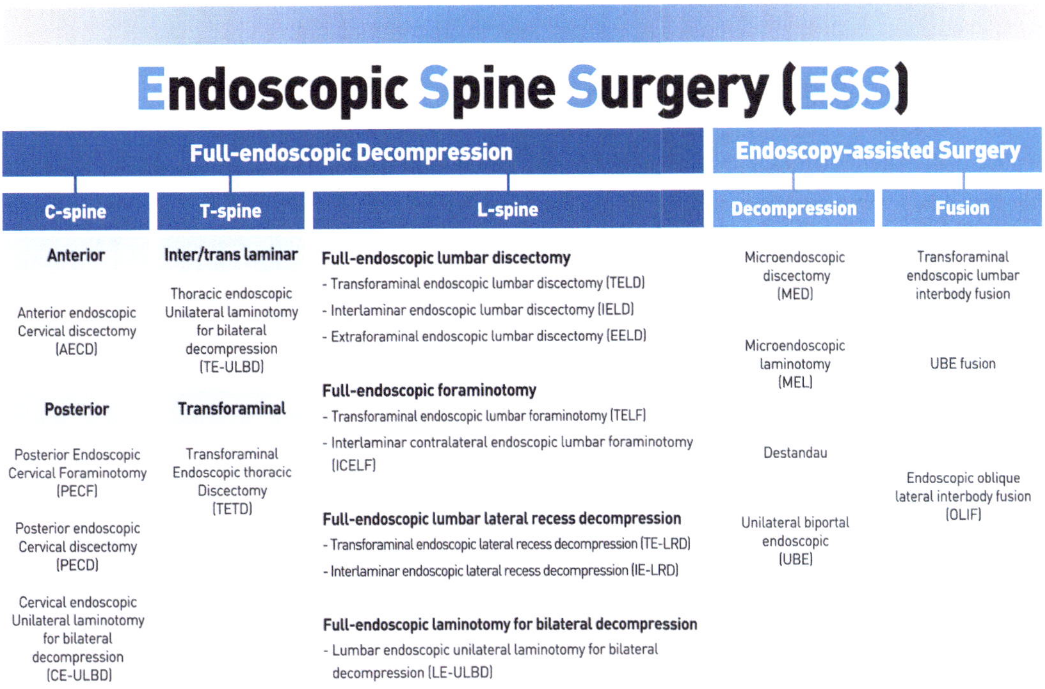

Fig. 2 Summary of current spinal procedures using endoscopic visualization in the literature and article (courtesy of the AOSpine MISTFT) [41]

Fig. 3 The system of the AOSpine MISTFT

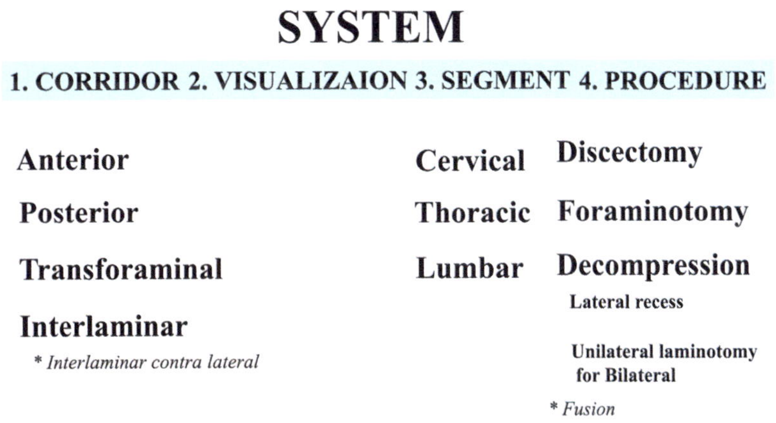

recess decompression, and unilateral laminotomy and bilateral decompression.

We can label the samples by the nomenclature system (Fig. 3).

They reviewed the background, previously used nomenclature, goal of surgery, and proposed nomenclature. They then suggested and summarized the nomenclature (Fig. 4).

Among these surgeries, the most popular endoscopic spine procedures are posterior endoscopic cervical discectomy (PECD) or foraminotomy (PECF), transforaminal endoscopic lumbar discectomy (TELD), and interlaminar endoscopic lumbar discectomy (IELD). Among many endoscopic spine procedures, six techniques were described as follows with case illustrations:

AOSpine Endoscopic Spine Surgery Nomenclature system

Approach corridor / visualization / segment of spine / procedure

Full-endoscopic discectomy

Full-endoscopic discectomy
- Anterior endoscopic cervical discectomy (AECD)
- Posterior endoscopic cervical discectomy (PECD)

Full-endoscopic thoracic discectomy
- Transforaminal endoscopic thoracic discectomy (TETD)

Full-endoscopic lumbar discectomy
- Transforaminal endoscopic lumbar discectomy (TELD)
- Interlaminar endoscopic lumbar discectomy (IELD)
- Extraforaminal endoscopic lumbar discectomy (EELD)

Full-endoscopic foraminotomy
- Posterior endoscopic cervical foraminotomy (PECF)
- Transforaminal endoscopic lumbar foraminotomy (TELF)
- Interlaminar contralateral endoscopic lumbar foraminotomy (ICELF)

Full-endoscopic lumbar lateral recess decompression
- Transforaminal endoscopic lateral recess decompression (TE-LRD)
- Interlaminar endoscopic lateral recess decompression (IE-LRD)

Full-endoscopic laminotomy for bilateral decompression
- Cervical endoscopic unilateral laminotomy for bilateral decompression (CE-ULBD)
- Thoracic endoscopic unilateral laminotomy for bilateral decompression (TE-ULBD)
- Lumbar endoscopic unilateral laminotomy for bilateral decompression (LE-ULBD)

Fig. 4 Suggested new nomenclature for endoscopic spinal procedures (courtesy of the AOSpine MISTFT) [41]

Posterior Endoscopic Cervical Discectomy (PECD) or Foraminotomy (PECF)

Traditionally, this procedure was termed "posterior cervical laminoforaminotomy" or "cervical foraminotomy" or "keyhole foraminotomy" [1–4]. Ruetten and colleagues initially introduced this procedure [5]. It was published under various names in the paper. The purpose of this procedure is direct visualization and decompression of the exiting nerve root from its origin to the lateral margin of the caudal pedicle. In the literature, it is called "full-endoscopic posterior cervical foraminotomy" (FPCF) [5, 6]. Posterior cervical endoscopic discectomy [7], posterior full-endoscopic cervical discectomy (PFECD) [8], posterior percutaneous endoscopic cervical foraminotomy and discectomy (PPECD) [9], posterior percutaneous endoscopic cervical discectomy (PPECD) [10, 11], and endoscopic posterior cervical foraminotomy (EPCF) [12] 49.

"They proposed the nomenclature for" posterior endoscopic cervical foraminotomy (PECF) or discectomy (PECD).

Herein, we present a typical case (Fig. 5).

A 56-year-old taxi driver visited our clinic for both Rt. tingling sensation for 2 years.

A preoperative magnetic resonance imaging (MRI) scan showed a left-sided protruded disc at C6/7 level with C7 root compression. We performed a "full-endoscopic" posterior (corridor), cervical (segment) discectomy (procedure).

Transforaminal Endoscopic Lumbar Discectomy (TELD)

The approach to the disc through the "triangle of Kambin" is the beginning of endoscopic surgery. With this safe entry pass way, Yeung developed YESS endoscopy and related equipment. It makes safe and efficient pathologic disc removal

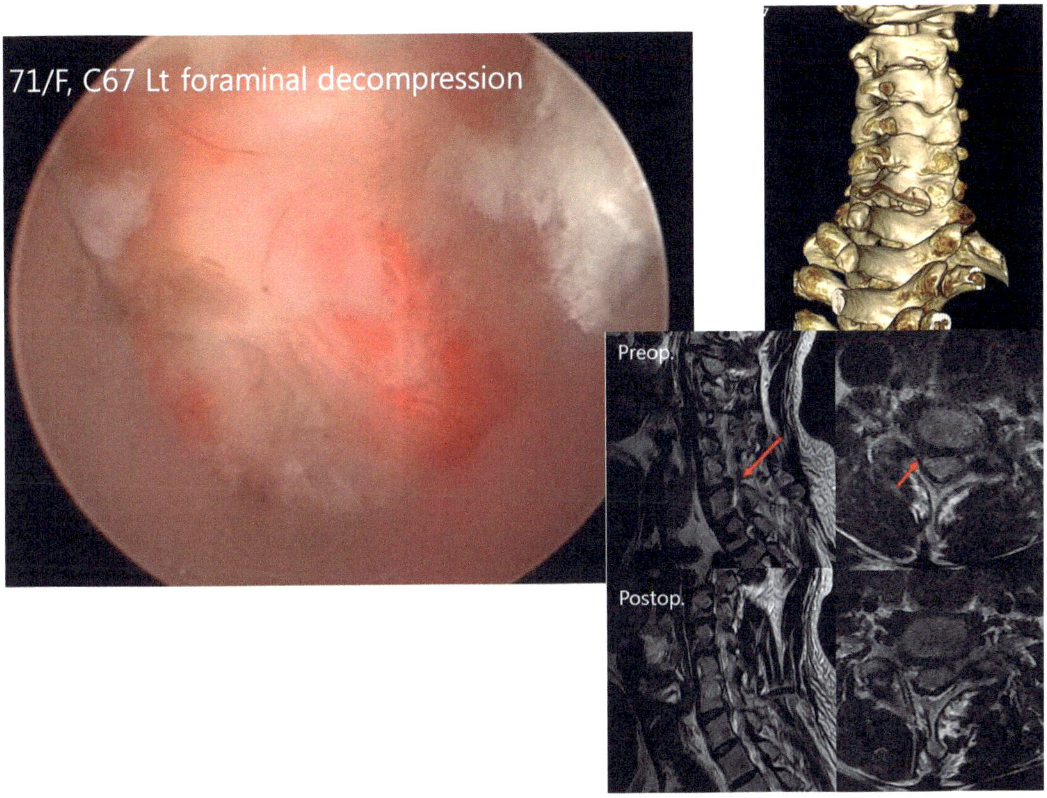

Fig. 5 Clinical case of posterior (corridor) endoscopic cervical (segment) discectomy (procedure) (the use of this picture was permitted by Dr. CW Lee)

possible.possible. Recently, the use of drills and reamers enabled foraminotomy for decompressing the compressed root in the intervertebral cavity. The goal of this procedure is resection of any disc herniation by visualizing the segmentally decompressed nerve roots. In the literature, arthroscopic microdiscectomy [13], minimally invasive disc surgery [14], posterolateral endoscopic excision for lumbar disc herniation [15], transforaminal posterolateral endoscopic discectomy [16], full-endoscopic transforaminal lumbar discectomy [17], transforaminal endoscopic discectomy [18], and percutaneous transforaminal endoscopic discectomy [19, 20] were named. They suggested "transforaminal endoscopic lumbar discectomy" for this procedure (Fig. 6).

Interlaminar Endoscopic Lumbar Discectomy (IELD)

The traditional approach window for resection of any disc herniation and visualization of decompressed nerve roots is the interlaminar space. The interlaminar area was used from the era of classic open surgery until tubular, microscopic surgery. The first endoscopic trial for this window was the interlaminar endoscopic discectomy of L5/S1. Device development permits access to no other lesion except L5/S1. For the terms full-endoscopic interlaminar access (FEIL) [21, 22], full-endoscopic interlaminar approach (FEIA) [23], interlaminar access (ILA) for percutaneous endoscopic lumbar discectomy

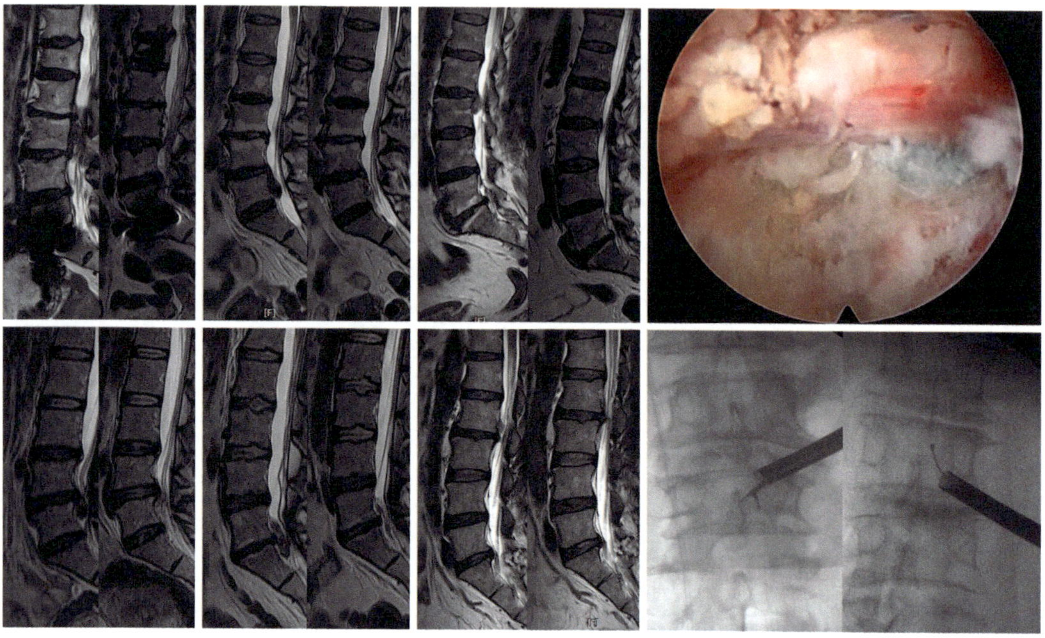

Fig. 6 Conventional transforaminal (corridor) endoscopic lumbar (segment) discectomy (procedure). Transforaminal (corridor) endoscopic lumbar (segment) discectomy (procedure). The use of this picture was permitted by Dr. CW Lee

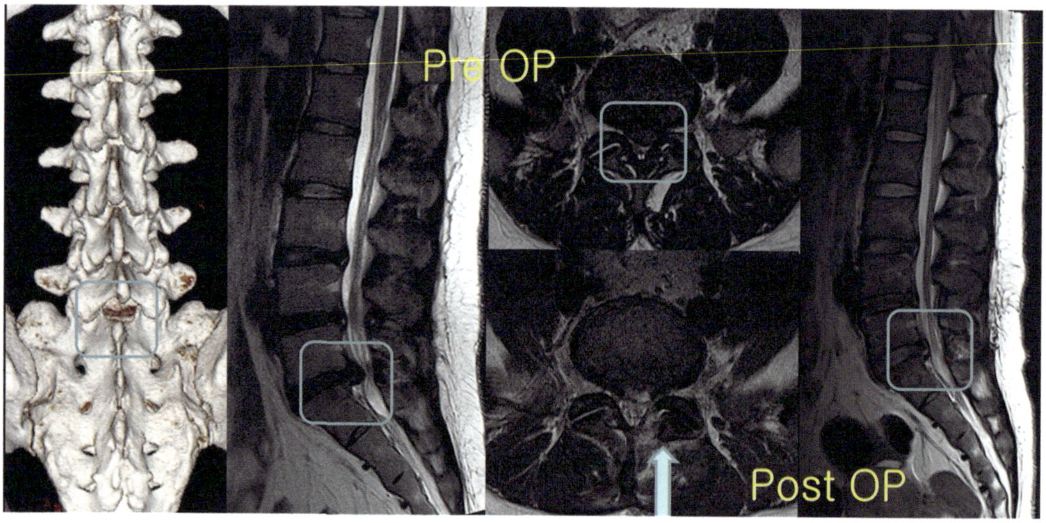

Fig. 7 Interlaminar (corridor) endoscopic lumbar (segment) discectomy (procedure)

(PELD) [24], percutaneous endoscopic interlaminar discectomy (PEID) [25–28], percutaneous endoscopic discectomy (PED) [26, 29], microendoscopic discectomy via interlaminar approach [30], and endoscopic lumbar discectomy [30], they suggested interlaminar endoscopic lumbar discectomy (IELD) (Fig. 7).

Lumbar Endoscopic Unilateral Laminotomy for Bilateral Decompression (LE-ULBD)

Unilateral approach bilateral decompression (ULBD) is a safe and efficacious treatment option for spinal stenosis [31]. Compared to conven-

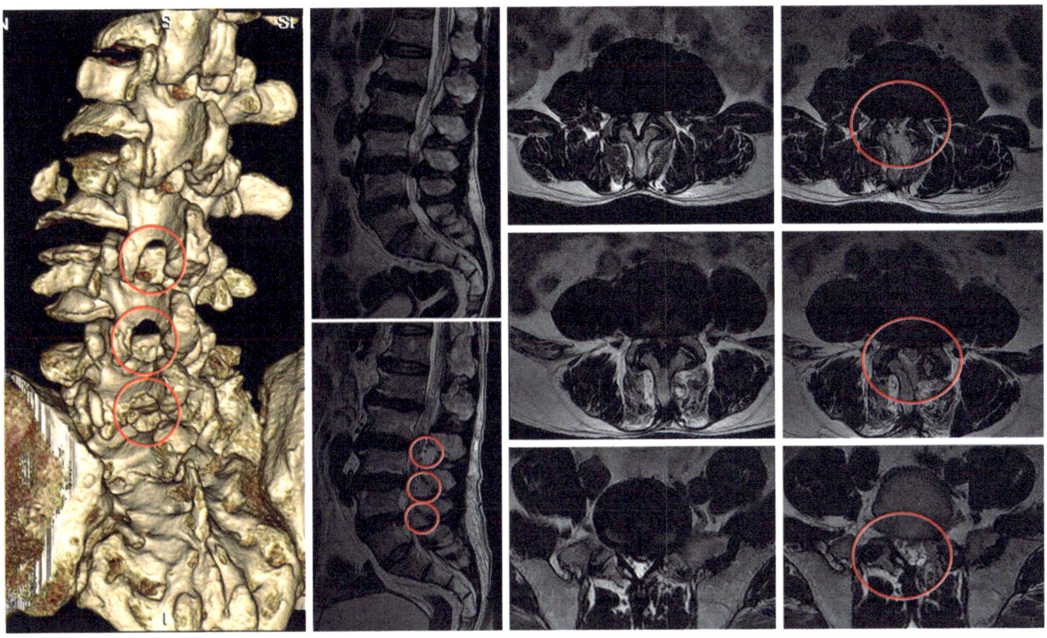

Fig. 8 Lumbar (segment) endoscopic unilateral laminotomy for bilateral decompression (procedure) (LE-ULBD)

tional open surgery, endoscopic surgery has similar treatment outcomes [32, 33]. The visualized field during an endoscopic procedure is wider than open surgery with the help of the variable angle of the scope lens.

In the future, this factor may lead to less injury of the facet joint complex compared to conventional surgery. Acute postoperative back pain after endoscopic surgery may be less than that in open surgery. Additionally, the duration of hospital stay may be reduced.

The goal of this procedure is complete central and lateral recess decompression of the neural elements spanning from the tip of the SAP to the midportion of the caudal pedicle. They suggested the term "lumbar endoscopic unilateral laminotomy for bilateral decompression" (LE-ULBD).

In the literature, the terms such as full-endoscopic bilateral interlaminar technique [33], full-endoscopic lumbar laminectomy [34], and percutaneous endoscopic laminotomy with flavectomy by a uniportal and unilateral approach [35] have been used (Fig. 8).

Endoscopic-Assisted Surgery

Unilateral Biportal Endoscopic (UBE) Surgery

In the field of endoscopic spine surgery (Fig. 1), Unilateral biportal endoscopic surgery (UBE) has been described as one of the endoscopy-assisted surgeries with MED, MEL, and Destandau. UBE or biportal endoscopic spine surgery (BESS), which has two portals (one for the lens and the other for the operative instrument), is growing in number. UBE is familiar for surgeons who can perform open microscopic spine surgery. Hence, various names have been used for these procedures. Historically, UBE was conceived as a translaminar lumbar epidural endoscopy procedure in 1996 and 1998 in the Arthroscopy journal by Dr. De Antoni [36, 37]. In 2013, the Egyptian surgeon Heshan Magdi Soliman performed and defined irrigation endoscopic discectomy [38]. Three years later, a team of Korean spine surgeons, including JH Eum, DW Heo, and SK Son, who have been pioneers of this surgery, suggested endoscopy for lumbar stenosis, which was described by the name of UBE, in an article [39]. Almost simultaneously, DJ Choi introduced the term, BESS, in 2016 [40]. At present, in October 2019, 12 papers, each containing either the term "BESS" or "UBE," can be searched in PubMed.

Conclusion

Endoscopic spine surgery will be performed more frequently with more robust methods owing to the advancement of evolving technology. Similar to the nomenclature system used in organic chemistry, the AOSpine nomenclature system has the advantage of introducing terms for newly developed surgical procedures. For example, the names for various lumbar fusion procedures can be added to the nomenclature system. Navigation-guided endoscopic spinal procedures will emerge as a new concept. Moreover, endoscopic surgical fields can be developed with a user-friendly learning curve for spine surgeons.

As of the writing of this chapter, many new techniques and endoscopic equipment are still being introduced, and related papers are increasing in number every year. Hence, it is time to establish a simple and expandable nomenclature system for endoscopic spinal procedures for the use of physicians, researchers, and students.

References

1. Roh SW, Kim DH, Cardoso AC, Fessler RG. Endoscopic foraminotomy using MED system in cadaveric specimens. Spine (Phila Pa 1976). 2000;25:260–4.
2. Burke TG, Caputy A. Microendoscopic posterior cervical foraminotomy: a cadaveric model and clinical application for cervical radiculopathy. J Neurosurg. 2000;93:126–9.
3. Fessler RG, Khoo LT. Minimally invasive cervical microendoscopic foraminotomy: an initial clinical experience. Neurosurgery. 2002;51:S37–45.
4. O'Toole JE, Sheikh H, Eichholz KM, Fessler RG, Perez-Cruet MJ. Endoscopic posterior cervical foraminotomy and discectomy. Neurosurg Clin N Am. 2006;17:411–22.
5. Ruetten S, Komp M, Merk H, Godolias G. A new full-endoscopic technique for cervical posterior foraminotomy in the treatment of lateral disc herniations using 6.9-mm endoscopes: prospective 2-year results of 87 patients. Minim Invas Neurosurg. 2007;50:219–26.
6. Ruetten S, Komp M, Merk H, Godolias G. Full-endoscopic cervical posterior foraminotomy for the operation of lateral disc herniations using 5.9-mm endoscopes: a prospective, randomized, controlled study. Spine (Phila Pa 1976). 2008;33:940–8.
7. Kim CH, Chung CK, Kim HJ, Jahng TA, Kim DG. Early outcome of posterior cervical endoscopic discectomy: an alternative treatment choice for physically/socially active patients. J Korean Med Sci. 2009;24:302–6.
8. Yang JS, Chu L, Chen L, Chen F, Ke ZY, Deng ZL. Anterior or posterior approach of full-endoscopic cervical discectomy for cervical intervertebral disc herniation? A comparative cohort study. Spine (Phila Pa 1976). 2014;39:1743–50.
9. Kim CH, Kim KT, Chung CK, et al. Minimally invasive cervical foraminotomy and diskectomy for laterally located soft disk herniation. Eur Spine J. 2015;24:3005–12.
10. Ahn Y. Percutaneous endoscopic cervical discectomy using working channel endoscopes. Expert Rev Med Devices. 2016;13:601–10.
11. Quillo-Olvera J, Lin GX, Kim JS. Percutaneous endoscopic cervical discectomy: a technical review. Ann Transl Med. 2018;6:100.
12. Youn MS, Shon MH, Seong YJ, Shin JK, Goh TS, Lee JS. Clinical and radiological outcomes of two-level endoscopic posterior cervical foraminotomy. Eur Spine J. 2017;26:2450–8.
13. Kambin P, Brager MD. Percutaneous posterolateral discectomy. Anatomy and mechanism. Clin Orthop Relat Res. 1987:145–54.
14. Yeung AT. Minimally invasive disc surgery with the Yeung endoscopic spine system (YESS). Surg Technol Int. 1999;8:267–77.
15. Yeung AT, Tsou PM. Posterolateral endoscopic excision for lumbar disc herniation: surgical technique, outcome, and complications in 307 consecutive cases. Spine (Phila Pa 1976). 2002;27:722–31.
16. Hoogland T, Schubert M, Miklitz B, Ramirez A. Transforaminal posterolateral endoscopic discectomy with or without the combination of a low-dose chymopapain: a prospective randomized study in 280 consecutive cases. Spine (Phila Pa 1976). 2006;31:E890–7.
17. Ruetten S, Komp M, Merk H, Godolias G. Full-endoscopic interlaminar and transforaminal lumbar discectomy versus conventional microsurgical technique: a prospective, randomized, controlled study. Spine (Phila Pa 1976). 2008;33:931–9.
18. Gibson JNA, Subramanian AS, Scott CEH. A randomised controlled trial of transforaminal endoscopic discectomy vs microdiscectomy. Eur Spine J. 2017;26:847–56.

19. Chen Z, Zhang L, Dong J, et al. Percutaneous transforaminal endoscopic discectomy compared with microendoscopic discectomy for lumbar disc herniation: 1-year results of an ongoing randomized controlled trial. J Neurosurg Spine. 2018;28:300–10.
20. Sinkemani A, Hong X, Gao ZX, et al. Outcomes of microendoscopic discectomy and percutaneous Transforaminal endoscopic discectomy for the treatment of lumbar disc herniation: a comparative retrospective study. Asian Spine J. 2015;9:833–40.
21. Wang B, Lu G, Liu W, Cheng I, Patel AA. Full-endoscopic interlaminar approach for the surgical treatment of lumbar disc herniation: the causes and prophylaxis of conversion to open. Arch Orthop Trauma Surg. 2012;132:1531–8.
22. Ruetten S, Komp M, Godolias G. A new full-endoscopic technique for the interlaminar operation of lumbar disc herniations using 6-mm endoscopes: prospective 2-year results of 331 patients. Minim Invas Neurosurg. 2006;49:80–7.
23. Casimiro M. Short-term outcome comparison between full-endoscopic interlaminar approach and open minimally invasive microsurgical technique for treatment of lumbar disc herniation. World Neurosurg. 2017;108:894–900.e1.
24. Shi C, Kong W, Liao W, et al. The early clinical outcomes of a percutaneous full-endoscopic Interlaminar approach via a surrounding nerve root discectomy operative route for the treatment of ventral-type lumbar disc herniation. Biomed Res Int. 2018;2018:9157089.
25. Choi G, Lee SH, Raiturker PP, Lee S, Chae YS. Percutaneous endoscopic interlaminar discectomy for intracanalicular disc herniations at L5-S1 using a rigid working channel endoscope. Neurosurgery. 2006;58:ONS59–68. discussion ONS59–68
26. Dabo X, Ziqiang C, Yinchuan Z, et al. The clinical results of percutaneous endoscopic Interlaminar discectomy (PEID) in the treatment of calcified lumbar disc herniation: a case-control study. Pain Physician. 2016;19:69–76.
27. Kim CH, Chung CK, Woo JW. Surgical outcome of percutaneous endoscopic Interlaminar lumbar discectomy for highly migrated disk herniation. Clin Spine Surg. 2016;29:E259–66.
28. Kim HS, Park JY. Comparative assessment of different percutaneous endoscopic interlaminar lumbar discectomy (PEID) techniques. Pain Physician. 2013;16:359–67.
29. Sasani M, Ozer AF, Oktenoglu T, Canbulat N, Sarioglu AC. Percutaneous endoscopic discectomy for far lateral lumbar disc herniations: prospective study and outcome of 66 patients. Minim Invas Neurosurg. 2007;50:91–7.
30. Koga S, Sairyo K, Shibuya I, et al. Minimally invasive removal of a recurrent lumbar herniated nucleus pulposus by the small incised microendoscopic discectomy interlaminar approach. Asian J Endosc Surg. 2012;5:34–7.
31. Ko S, Oh T. Comparison of bilateral decompression via unilateral laminotomy and conventional laminectomy for single-level degenerative lumbar spinal stenosis regarding low back pain, functional outcome, and quality of life - a randomized controlled, prospective trial. J Orthop Surg Res. 2019;14:252.
32. Huang YH, Lien FC, Chao LY, Lin CH, Chen SH. Full endoscopic uniportal unilateral laminotomy for bilateral decompression in degenerative lumbar spinal stenosis: highlight of ligamentum flavum detachment and survey of efficacy and safety in 2 years of follow-up. World Neurosurg. 2019;
33. Komp M, Hahn P, Oezdemir S, et al. Bilateral spinal decompression of lumbar central stenosis with the full-endoscopic interlaminar versus microsurgical laminotomy technique: a prospective, randomized, controlled study. Pain Physician. 2015;18:61–70.
34. Wagner R, Telfeian AE, Krzok G, Iprenburg M. Fully-endoscopic lumbar laminectomy for central and lateral recess stenosis: technical note. Interdisc Neurosurg. 2018;13:6–9.
35. Lee CW, Yoon KJ, Jun JH. Percutaneous endoscopic Laminotomy with Flavectomy by Uniportal, unilateral approach for the Lumbar Canal or lateral recess stenosis. World Neurosurg. 2018;113:e129–e37.
36. De Antoni DJ, Claro ML, Poehling GG, Hughes SS. Translaminar lumbar epidural endoscopy: anatomy, technique, and indications. Arthroscopy. 1996;12:330–4.
37. De Antoni DJ, Claro ML, Poehling GG, Hughes SS. Translaminar lumbar epidural endoscopy: technique and clinical results. J South Orthop Assoc. 1998;7:6–12.
38. Soliman HM. Irrigation endoscopic discectomy: a novel percutaneous approach for lumbar disc prolapse. Eur Spine J. 2013;22:1037–44.
39. Hwa Eum J, Hwa Heo D, Son SK, Park CK. Percutaneous biportal endoscopic decompression for lumbar spinal stenosis: a technical note and preliminary clinical results. J Neurosurg Spine. 2016;24:602–7.
40. Choi CM, Chung JT, Lee SJ, Choi DJ. How I do it? Biportal endoscopic spinal surgery (BESS) for treatment of lumbar spinal stenosis. Acta Neurochir. 2016;158:459–63.
41. Christoph P, Hofstetter M, Ahn Y, Gun Choi JNA, Gibson D, Ruetten S, Zhou Y, Zhen Zhou Li M, Siepe CJ, Wagner R, et al. A259: AO Consensus On Nomenclature for Working channel Endoscopic Spinal Procedures. Toronto: Global Spine Congress; 2019.

Part II

Lumbar Central Stenosis

Full Endoscopic Posterior Approach, In and Out

Han Ga Wi Nam, Kang Taek Lim, and Chun Kun Park

Introduction (Key Point and Purpose) of Approach

Many spine surgeons, who were familiar with conventional endoscopic transforaminal discectomy, have bestowed a consideration that a spine surgeon could do endoscopic spine surgery (ESS) in the other spine pathologies, but discectomy for once. Because the endoscope the spine surgeons could make use of was only the one for the transforaminal approach, it was not easy to carry out ESS, with a conventional endoscopic system (too small in diameter and too long in length), particularly in case approaching dorsally. In other words, the conventional endoscopic system should not be appropriate for pathology located in the posterior and epidural space. As a result, the spine surgeons designed a larger diameter and shorter length of endoscopy, compared to the conventional one, along with the development of surgical tools such as rongeurs, forceps, dissectors, and high-speed drills enough to remove ligamentous and bony tissues and bony fragments with the aid of industries. Thereafter, endoscopic surgeons tried to expand the surgical indications, representatively disc herniation regardless of its location, size, and the number of the lesion and degenerative canal stenosis. Nowadays, some spine surgeons succeeded a full endoscopic interbody fusion in the cervical (anterior approach) and lumbar (posterior approach) spines. The endoscopic fusion technology is on clinical trial. According to the title of this chapter, the editors recognized the authors' technique interestingly as an in-and-out procedure.

A representative surgical technology using the in-and-out procedure must be transforaminal endoscopic discectomy. At the early stage of the authors' procedure, a surgeon attempts to move an endoscopy to get close to the main pathology located in the back under the guidance of C-arm, followed by removal of the lesion and soon after endoscopy is taken out.

In this chapter, the authors tried to do their best for readers to understand how to handle this endoscopic system in central stenosis by demonstrating the figures of each surgical step and removal of the main pathology followed as well as presenting the overview of this surgical technique by briefly reviewing surgical indication, outcome, and other relevant issues.

Electronic Supplementary Material The online version of this chapter (https://doi.org/10.1007/978-981-15-8253-0_3) contains supplementary material, which is available to authorized users.

H. G. W. Nam · K. T. Lim (✉) · C. K. Park
Department of Neurosurgery, Good Doctor Teun Teun Hospital, Anyang, South Korea
e-mail: ckpmd@catholic.ac.kr

H. S. Kim et al. (eds.), *Advanced Techniques of Endoscopic Lumbar Spine Surgery*,
https://doi.org/10.1007/978-981-15-8253-0_3

Indication and Contraindication

Possible indications for the procedure include:

1. Unilateral or bilateral neurogenic claudication or lower limb radiculopathy with or without associated back pain not responding to conservative treatment.
2. Evidence of stenosis on magnetic resonance imaging and/or computed tomography correlating with clinical presentation.

Possible contraindications include:

1. Patients presenting with foraminal stenosis.
2. More than grade 1 degenerative spondylolisthesis.

Anesthesia and Position

Anesthesia

- Epidural anesthesia is performed on patients at a level 1 or 2 above the index level.
- Conscious sedation with sevoflurane (1–2 vol/%) was allowed. This method can be used for patients who cannot perform general anesthesia and reduces the side effects of general anesthesia, such as nausea, dysphagia, and memory loss.

Position

- The patient is positioned prone on a Wilson frame comfortably placed on a standard operating room table or a flat Jackson table to minimize abdominal pressure (Fig. 1).
- A waterproof surgical drape is applied due to continuous saline irrigation (Fig. 2.).
- The surgeon and a scrub nurse with the Mayo trolley stand on the side of the pathology (Fig. 3).
- Across from the surgeon stands the X-ray technician with a mobile or mounted C-arm.
- The anesthesia team stands at the head end of the patient with the anesthetic trolley.

Special Surgical Instruments

- All operative procedures were performed with a complete uniportal endoscopic instrument system: Techcord Endoscopic System (Techcord, Daejeon, Korea) (Fig. 4).
- Uniportal endoscopes are used in the different fashion as an operating microscope employed for open spinal surgery in aspects of 360° operating field rotation.
- The same instruments used for conventional surgery were used during endoscopic surgery by modifying the working length.
- Surgical instruments can be categorized into four groups (Fig. 5):
  - Mechanical instruments: long pituitary forceps (small/large), dissectors (small/large), up-angled curette, ball-tipped probe.
  - Special instruments: obturator, working sleeve, endoscopic customized root retractor.
  - Electrosurgical instruments: bipolar radiofrequency electro-coagulator (OK Medinet Korea, Seoul, Korea), DELPHI radiofre-

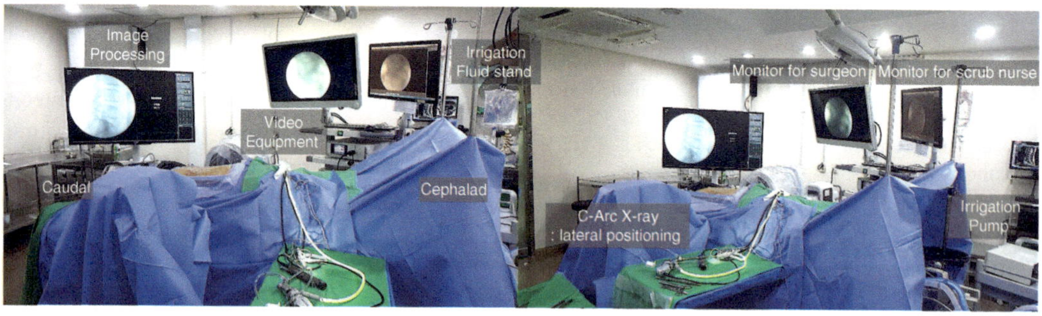

Fig. 1 Patient positioning and operating room setup

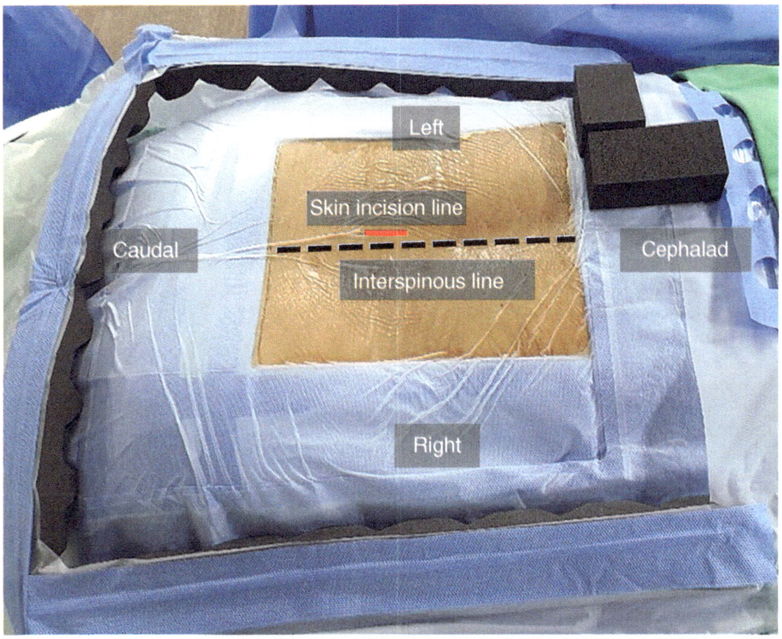

Fig. 2 Waterproof surgical drape for a left-sided L4–5 approach

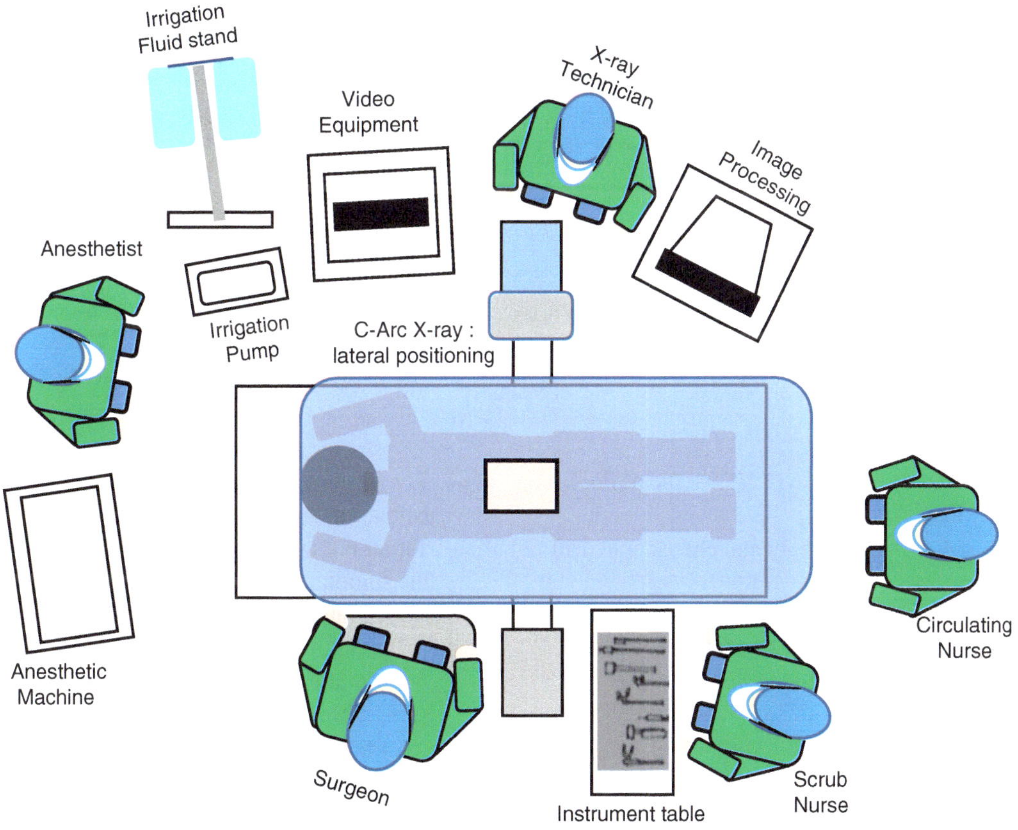

Fig. 3 Standard operating room setup

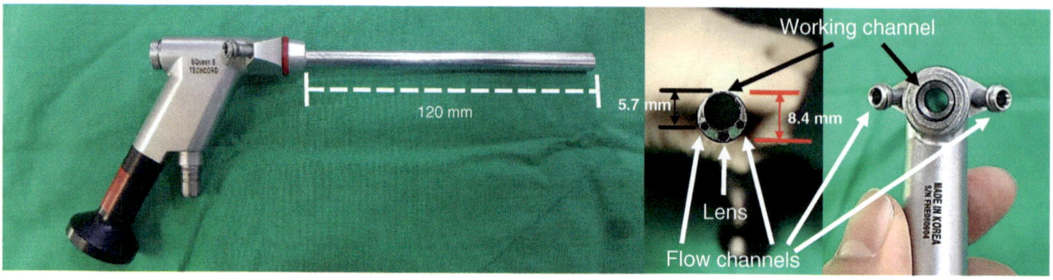

Fig. 4 Techcord Endoscopic System (8.4 mm outer diameter, 5.7 mm working channel and 12° direction of view, 80° field of view)

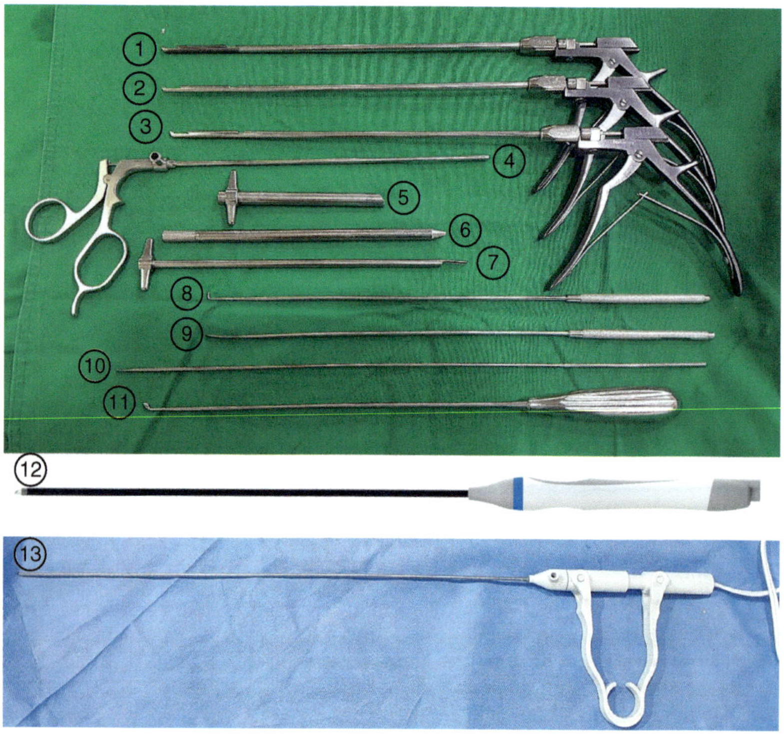

Fig. 5 Essential unit for uniportal endoscopic decompression: [1–3] Kerrison punches, [4] pituitary forceps (large), (5) working sleeve, (6) obturator, (7) endoscopic customized root retractor, (8) ball-tipped probe, (9–10) dissectors (small/large), (11) up-angled curette, (12) DELPHI radiofrequency electrode, (13) bipolar radiofrequency electro-coagulator

quency electrode (C&S Medical, Pocheon, Korea).
  - Motorized instruments: endoscopic drill.

Surgical Steps (Illustration, Photos, and Video)

- Step 1: Level marking (Fig. 6).
  - Target level end plates and interlaminar window are roughly marked with obturator under lateral fluoroscopic images.
- Step 2: Skin entry point (Fig. 7).
  - The skin incision is performed two fifth below the index lamina.
  - Target point—just below inferior border of the spinolaminar junction on the ipsilateral side in lateral view C-arm.
- Step 3: Dilation and endoscope insertion.
  - After making a 7–8 mm vertical skin incision, a blunt dilator that served as a guide for the 9.5 mm outer diameter working sleeve was advanced into the lamina on the ipsilateral side in a right-angle direction, just beside the spinous process (Fig. 8).

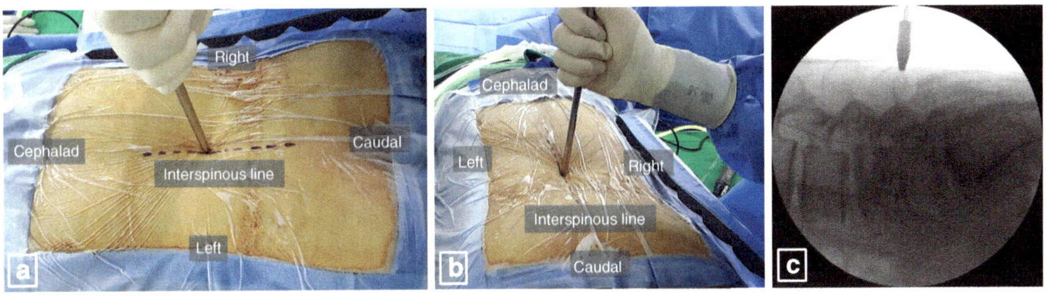

Fig. 6 Right-sided L4–5 uniportal endoscopic decompression. The inferior border of the L4 lamina, close to the base of the corresponding spinous process (**a**, **b**) are roughly marked with obturator under lateral fluoroscopic images (**c**) just beside the spinous process

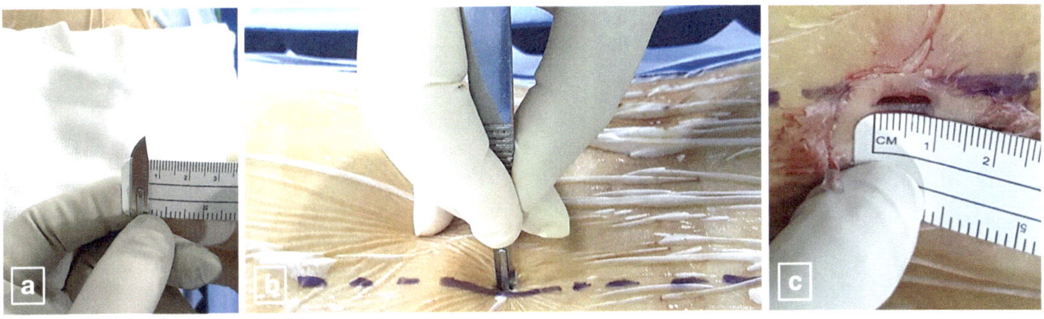

Fig. 7 Skin entry point and skin incision. The skin incision is performed at the previous level marking site with a scalpel blade #10 (**a**, **b**) less then 1cm sized (**c**)

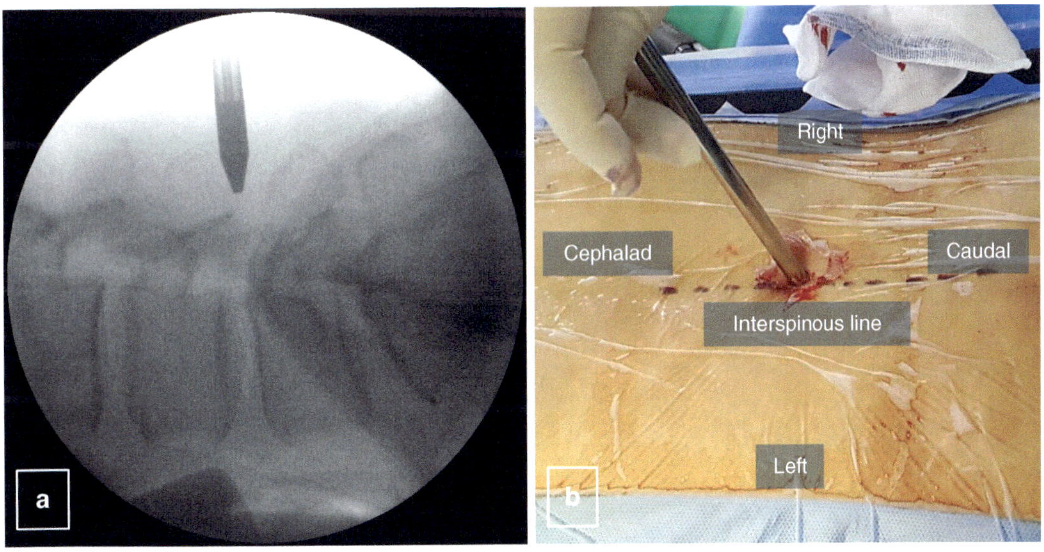

Fig. 8 Dilation for a right-sided L4–5 decompression. The surgeon advanced a blunt dilator with a 9.5 mm outer diameter as a guide for the working sleeve into inferior margin of the L4 lamina, close to the base of the corresponding spinous process under lateral fluoroscopic images (**a**), a photo in the surgical field (**b**)

- Subsequently, the working sleeve was inserted over the dilator and a rigid angle endoscope (8.4 mm outer diameter, 12° view) was introduced into the lesion from one side through the working sleeve (Fig. 9).
- The unique surgical approach through fatty atrophy between the spinous process and multifidus muscles helped decrease the postoperative muscle-origin back pain and is considered an advantage of this process.
- This full procedure is performed under continuous pressure irrigation using cold, antibiotic instilled normal saline. RF is used initially to clear the fat and paraspinal soft tissue and to enhance visibility.

• Step 4: Decompression, in-and-out technique.
  - The epidural space was opened via laminectomy, and the ligamentum flavum and superior articular process were removed to expose the traversing root sequentially

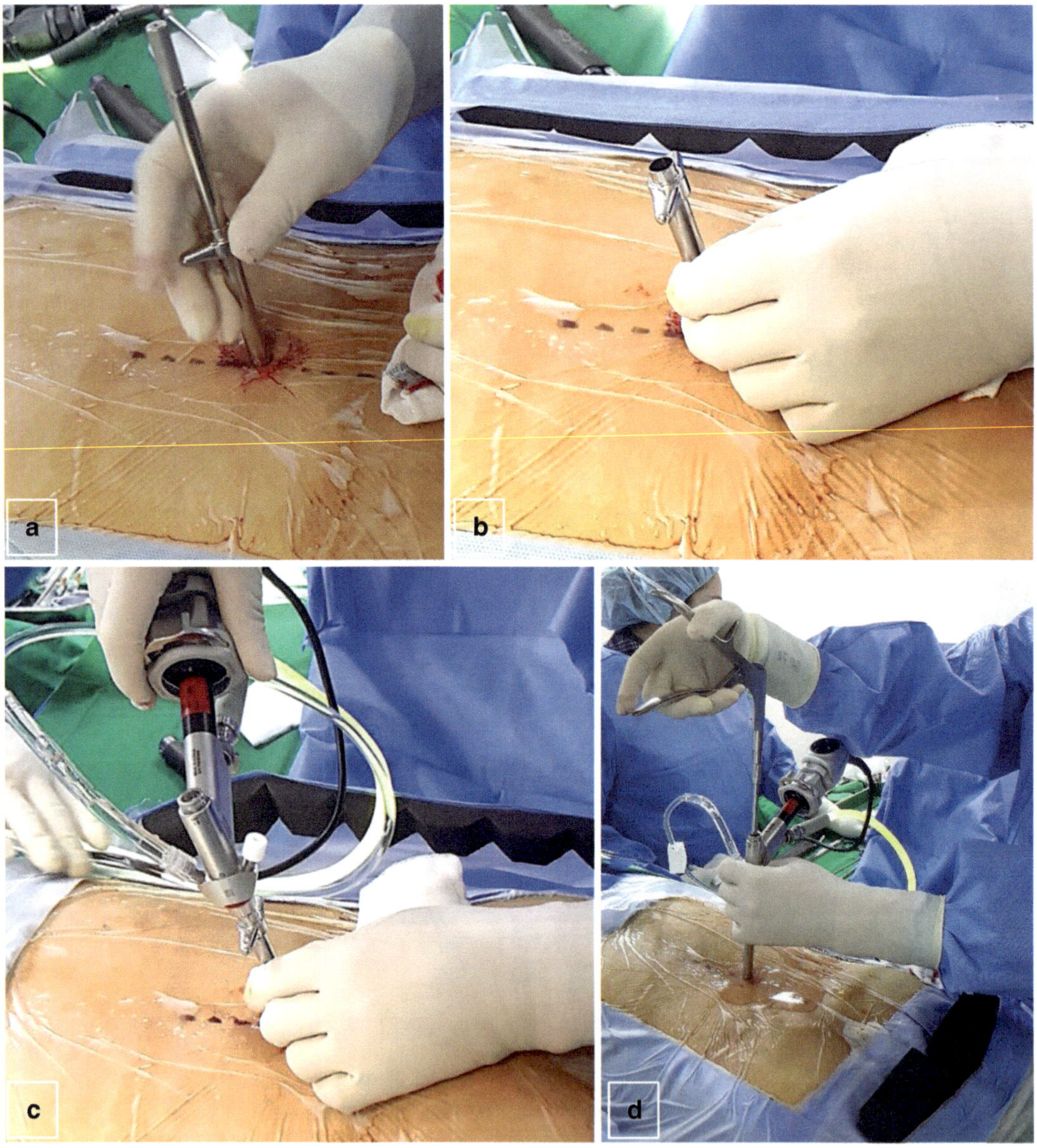

Fig. 9 Endoscope insertion for a right-sided L4–5 decompression. The surgeon inserted the working sleeve over the dilator (**a**, **b**) and introduced a rigid angle endoscope, with an 8.4 mm outer diameter and a 12° view (**c**, **d**)

using a 4 mm drill and 5 mm Kerrison punch through the 5.7 mm working channel of the endoscope.

- Laminotomy was performed to expose the uppermost portion of the ligamentum flavum, and as much of the ligamentum flavum was removed as possible (Video 1).
- Following ipsilateral decompression, the contralateral ligamentum flavum and superior articular process were removed to decompress the contralateral traversing nerve root. Minimal bone work, as much as required, was performed to preserve the facet joint, which was the first priority (Video 2).
- The contralateral approach with endoscope provides the angulation with which we can approach the facet joint, helping the surgeon to slide the cannula underneath it. This way, we can perform targeted decompression of the most pathological portion of the facet (ventral and medial portion of superior articular process) and preserve the rest of the facet.
- The operative field was irrigated continuously with normal saline using the irrigation pump to provide a clean view with good visualization of epidural anatomy for safety purposes.
- In case of multiple level stenoses, decompression through a single skin entry was achieved via a special technique called the jumping technique (Fig. 10).
- In this technique, after completion of one level, the working sleeve was completely removed and moved cranially or caudally to the other target within the subcutaneous space under image guidance, but still within the same skin incision. Skin has good elasticity and can be used to make another muscle layer tracts by subfascial dissection through a single incision (Fig. 11).
- Then, the same process as for the PSLD procedure was performed in a different direction, upper or lower, for decompression of the remaining lumbar stenosis. After the first muscle tract, the subsequent two muscle tracts have an inconvenient approach angle but do not interfere with decompression. After identification and confirmation of the interlaminar space and laminar space under the C-arm, the dilator was introduced into the created path by a small forceps, and the working sleeve was inserted over the dilator. Upward and downward retraction of the skin allowed the tubular working sleeve to be placed in the upper and lower interlaminar spaces, where the decompression will be performed.
- Every step of the procedure was done under image intensifier control to confirm the exact entry point. The stenoscope was introduced into the lesion and subsequent procedures were performed as described above. After the procedures, a drain was placed in the epidural space to prevent postoperative hematoma for 1 day.

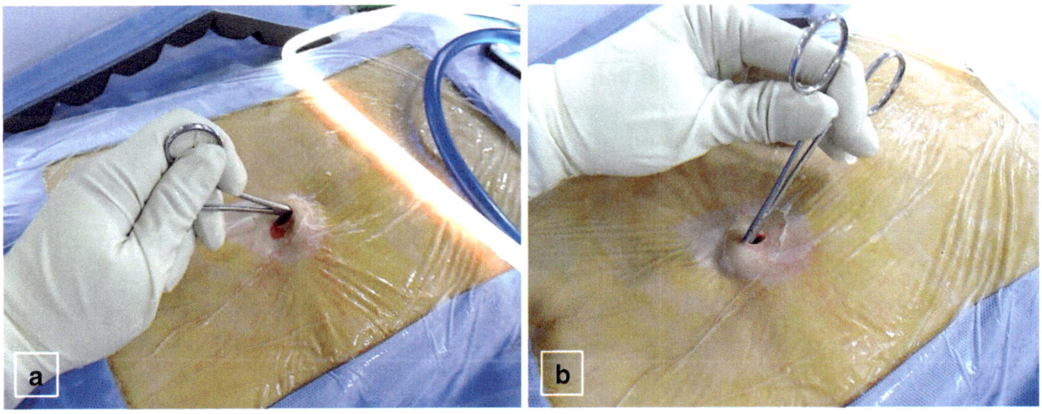

Fig. 10 The jumping technique. After one-level decompression, the upper (**a**) or lower (**b**) interlaminar space and laminar space confirmed with mosquito under the C-arm through the same skin incision site

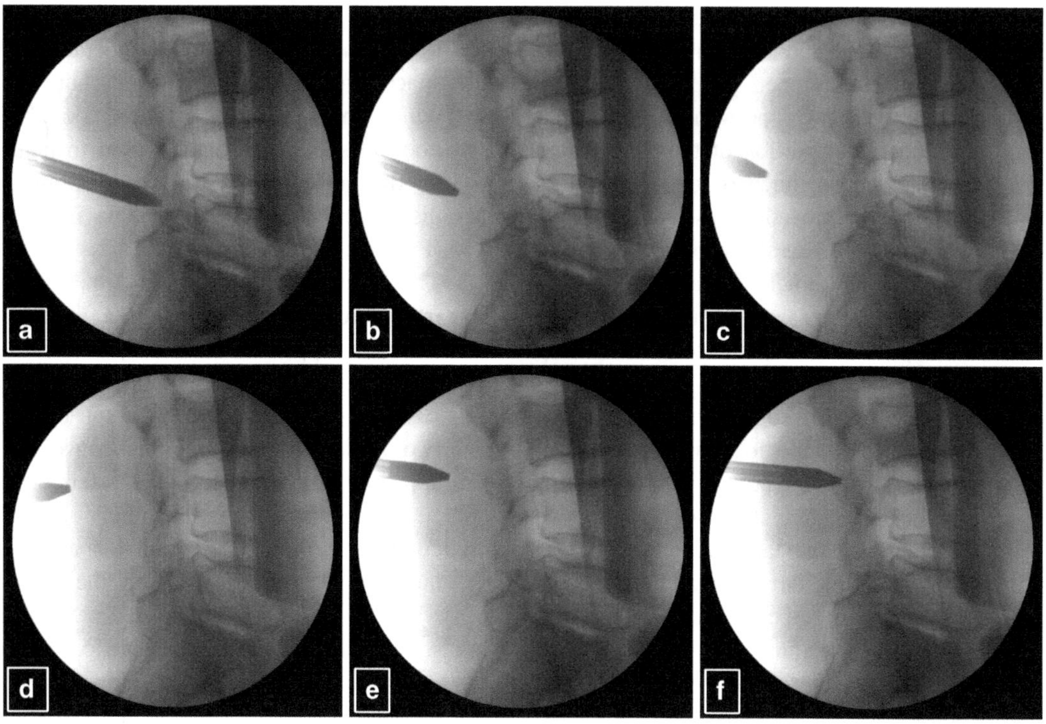

Fig. 11 Lateral fluoroscopic images of the jumping technique (A case of L3–4, L4–5 level decompression). After L4–5 level decompression (**a**), the obturator was moved cranially to the L3–4 interlaminar space within the subcutaneous space under image guidance (**b**–**f**), but still within the same skin incision

Illustrated Case or Cases

- Case 1: 1-level decompression (Fig. 12, Video 3).
  - A 76-year-old female complained of both buttock and radiating pain (L5 dermatome) refractory to conservative management. Preoperative MRI (magnetic resonance imaging) showed severe stenosis of L4–5 segment with protruded calcified disc. We performed uniportal endoscopic decompression (left-side unilateral laminotomy and bilateral decompression). Postoperative MRI shows complete bilateral decompression.
- Case 2: 2-level decompression (Fig. 13).
  - A 72-year-old female presented with both leg and buttock pain. Preoperative MRI showed severe multiple stenosis. We performed uniportal endoscopic multiple decompression with one skin incision. Postoperative MR images show enough decompression without paraspinal muscle damage.
- Case 3: 3-level decompression (Fig. 14).
  - A 76-year-old female presented with severe back pain, leg pain, and buttock pain. Preoperative MRI showed severe multiple stenosis at L2–3, L3–4, and L4–5. We performed uniportal endoscopic multiple decompression with one skin incision by the jumping technique. Postoperative MR images show enough bilateral decompression.

Complication and its Management

Surgery-related complications are incidental dural tears that include root herniation, epidural hematoma and infection, and facet damage. The incidence of dural tears appeared to be increased

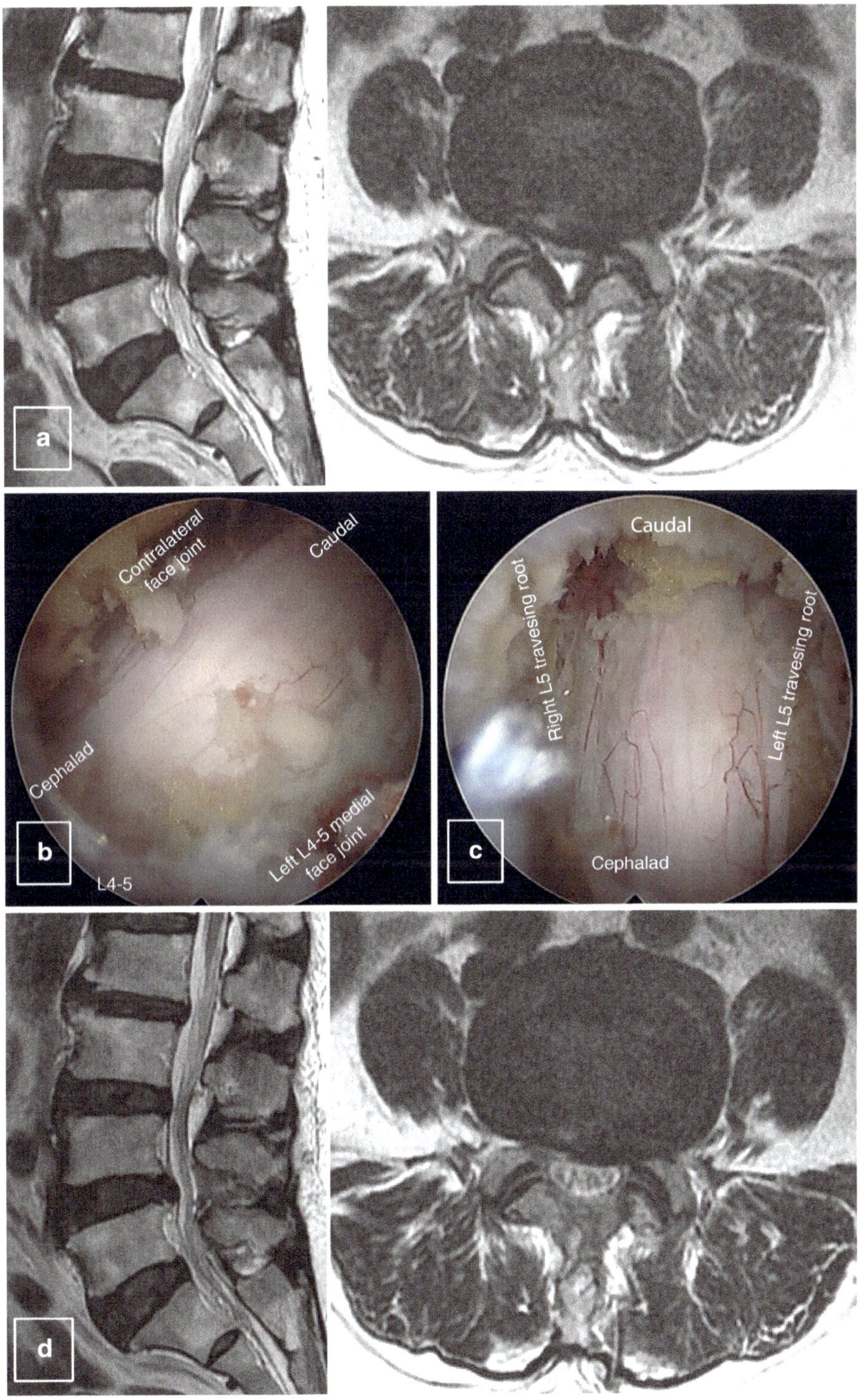

Fig. 12 Images of a 76-year-old woman with both buttock and radiating pain (L5 dermatome). Preoperative MR images show lumbar stenosis at L4–5 (**a**). Intraoperative endoscopic images show hypertrophic ligamentum flavum compressed left L5 nerve root (**b**) and the spinal canal was well decompressed (**c**). Postoperative MR images show enough decompression without paraspinal muscle damage (**d**)

when performing the resection of superior articular process of ipsilateral and contralateral side by Kerrison punch. Intraoperatively, a thin layer of TachoSil®, a hemostatic dural sealant, is provided locally at the site of the dural tear and defects [1]. The incidence of infection is very low in endoscopic surgery due to the use of a large amount of irrigation fluids resulting in an increased washout. C-reactive protein and ESR were the most sensitive clinical laboratory maker to assess the presence of infection and effectiveness of antibiotic treatment response. MRI is the imaging modality of choice in the diagnosis of postoperative infection. Infected patients were managed adequately with broad-spectrum antibiotics and immobilization. The incidence of facet damage is rare during decompression due to its steerability of endoscopy. It is easy to see ipsilateral anatomical structures in more detail compared to open microscopic decompression.

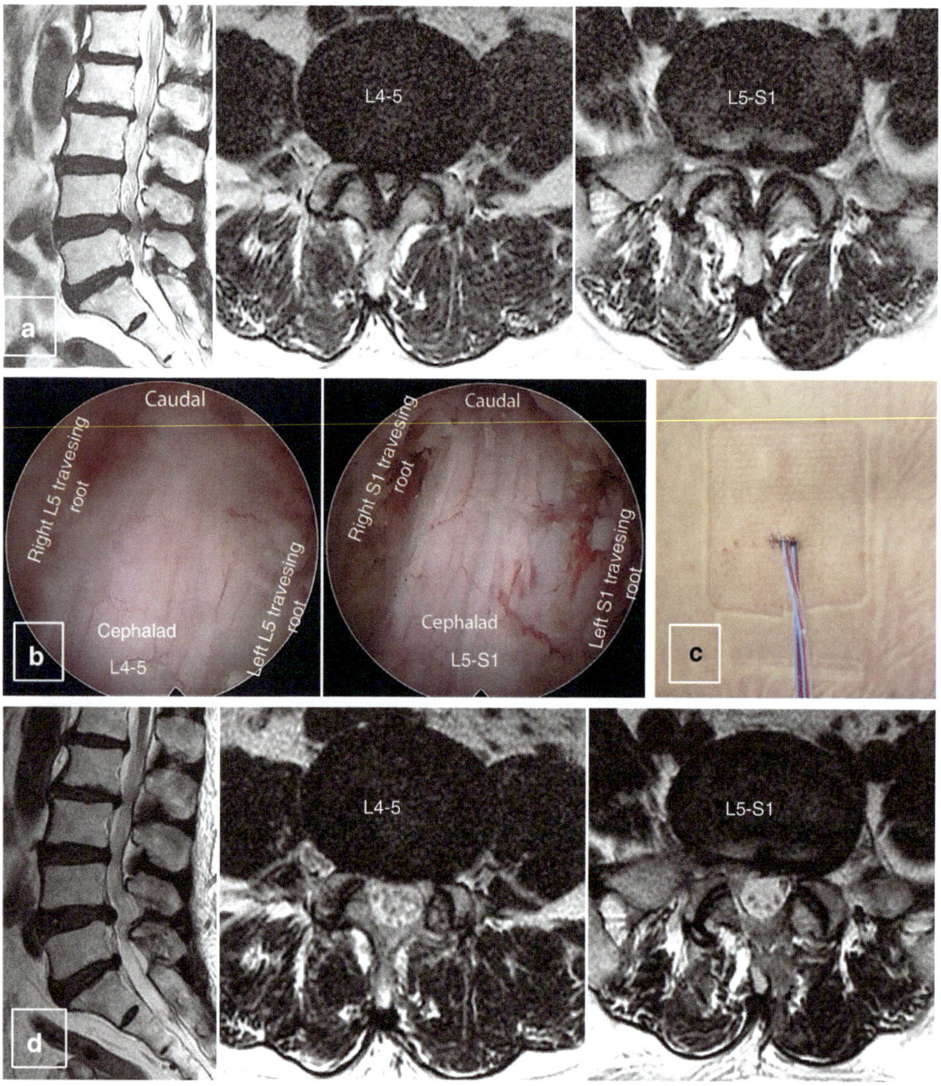

Fig. 13 Images of a 72-year-old woman with both buttock and leg pain. Preoperative MR images show severe lumbar stenosis at L4–5 and L5–S1 (**a**). Intraoperative endoscopic images show the spinal canal was well decompressed (**b**). Postoperative 1 day, two drainage were inserted on the skin incision site (**c**). Postoperative MR images show complete bilateral decompression (**d**)

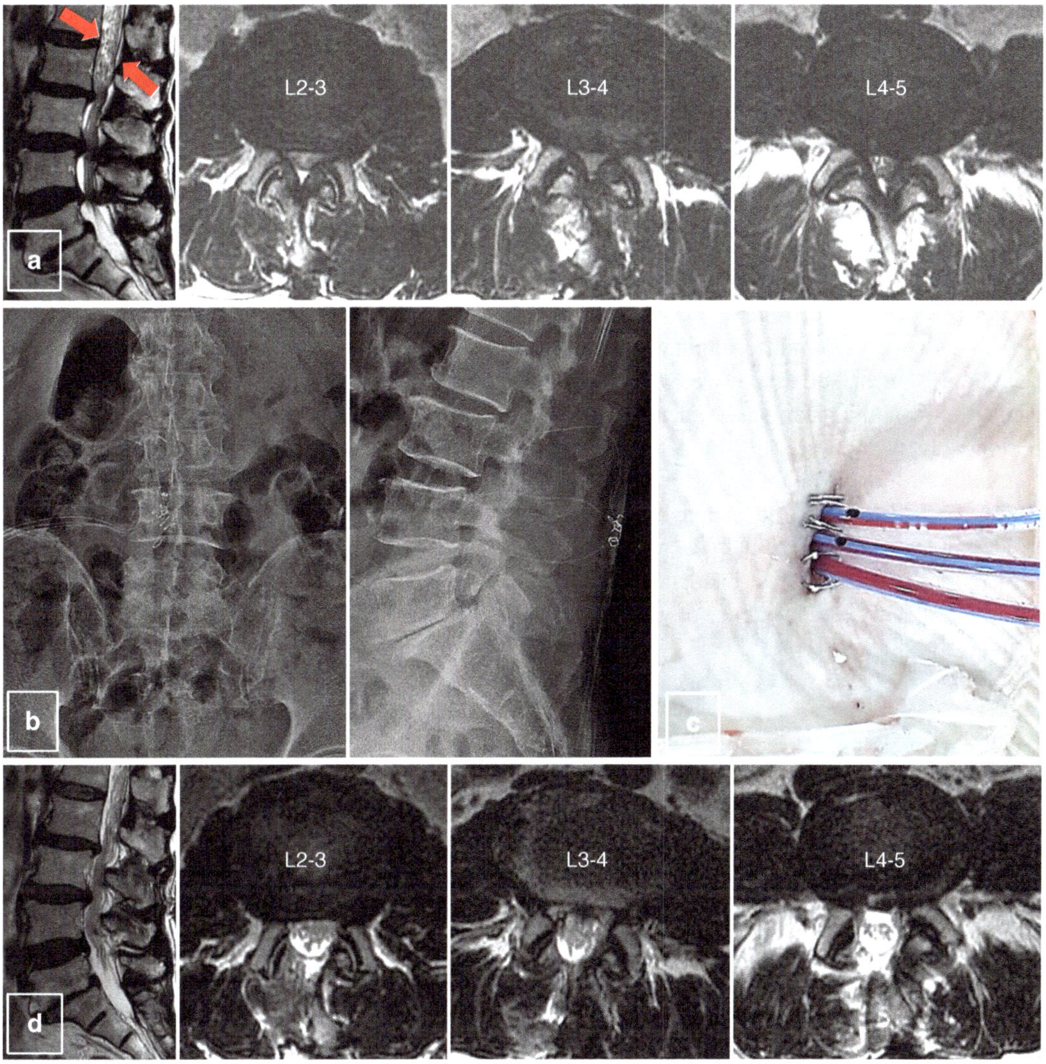

Fig. 14 Images of a 76-year-old woman with severe back pain, leg pain, and buttock pain. Preoperative MR images show severe lumbar stenosis at L2–3, L3–4, and L4–5 with hourglass appearance of lumbar spine. The tortuous nerve roots above the level of compression are depicted with red arrows (**a**). Postoperative X-ray after L3–4, L4–5, L5–S1, and 3-level decompression with one skin incision by the jumping technique (**b**). The jumping technique for multiple layer decompression with one skin incision. Three drainage were inserted on the skin incision site (**c**). Postoperative MRI shows enough bilateral decompression without paraspinal muscle damage (**d**)

Brief Discussion: Surgical Tip and Pitfall

Inside-out technique procedures for decompression of spinal canal include exposure of lateral margin of neural structures first, after removal of ipsilateral ligamentum flavum and superior articular process [2]. The main purpose of endoscopic surgery can be to save the bony structures that will act as a scaffold of body architecture. Bone work for decomperession should be calculated before removal of bone. Endoscopic approaches are feasible for central canal and lateral recess stenosis and are also found to be successful in huge herniated discs, or migrated disc, upward and downward, and for foraminal stenosis, extraforaminal disc herniation with paraspinal approach and cervical posterior decompression in foraminal cervical stenosis was a good option to relive cervical stenosis symptoms also. A 12° angle optic lens of endoscopy is helpful in watching ipsilateral facet during procedures after removal of ligamentum flavum (inside-out technique) so that surgeon can do minimum bone work to remove the hypertrophied superior articular process and can be beneficial in preventing root injury [1]. The patients who underwent inside-out technique had significant improvements in canal size without facet damages, radiating pain, and functional status postoperatively and were still statistically significant after 12 months of follow-up without iatrogenic spinal instability. Endoscopic surgery with inside-out technique would help decrease the use of narcotics and antibiotics, incidence of symptomatic CSF leaks, and incidence of wound infections [3, 4].

References

1. Nam HGW, Kim HS, Park JS, Lee DK, Park CK, Lim KT. Double-layer TachoSil packing for Management of Incidental Durotomy during Percutaneous Stenoscopic Lumbar Decompression. World Neurosurg. 2018;120:448–56.
2. Lim KT, Nam HGW, Kim SB, Kim HS, Park JS, Park CK. Therapeutic feasibility of full endoscopic decompression in one- to three-level Lumbar Canal stenosis via a single skin port using a new endoscopic system, percutaneous Stenoscopic lumbar decompression. Asian Spine J. 2019;13(2):272–82.
3. Nam HGW, Kim HS, Lee DK, Park CK, Lim KT. Percutaneous Stenoscopic lumbar decompression with Paramedian approach for Foraminal/Extraforaminal lesions. Asian Spine J. 2019;13(4):672–81.
4. Wi Nam HG, Lim KT, Park JS, Park CK, Kim HS. Endoscopic rescue technique for iatrogenic sacroiliac joint syndrome caused by sextant percutaneous pedicle screw fixation system: a case report. World Neurosurg. 2019;

Full Endoscopic Posterior Approach 'Out and In' Technique

Chul Woo Lee, Hyeun Sung Kim,
Harshavardhan Dilip Raorane, and Pang Hung Wu

Introduction

The Posterior microscopic decompression is an established gold standard treatment for spinal canal stenosis (SCS). However, it is associated with significant paraspinal muscle damage, atrophy, iatrogenic instability and chronic low-back pain in long-term follow-up. The posterior decompression can be combined with the fusion procedure with added stability. However, it is also associated with complications such as adjacent segment disease. At present, endoscopic spine surgery (ESS) is considered as the least invasive form of spine surgery surgery [1]. With the development of interlaminar approach, along with the improved endoscopic optics and instrumentations, endoscopic spine surgery (ESS) is applied for a wide spectrum of degenerative lumbar diseases [2].

Electronic Supplementary Material The online version of this chapter (https://doi.org/10.1007/978-981-15-8253-0_4) contains supplementary material, which is available to authorized users.

C. W. Lee
St. Peter's Hospital, Seoul, South Korea

H. S. Kim (✉)
Department of Neurosurgery, Gangnam Nanoori Hospital, Seoul, South Korea

H. D. Raorane · P. H. Wu
Nanoori Hospital Gangnam,
Seoul, South Korea

Advantages

- It minimizes trauma to the paraspinal muscles on the ipsilateral side and completely preserves paraspinal muscles of the contralateral side.
- It is associated with faster postoperative recovery and rehabilitation and minimal low-back pain in long-term follow-up, particularly in an older population of >70 years where rehabilitation is a major concern in postoperative period.
- It prevents the damage to the posterior ligamentous complex (supraspinous ligament, interspinous ligament and facet capsule) which acts as the posterior tension band to maintain spinal integrity.
- It is advantageous to preserve a facet joint to avoid iatrogenic instability [3, 7].

Indications

1. Spinal central canal and lateral recess stenosis.
   - Combined central and paracentral disc herniation.
   - Facet hypertrophy.
   - Ligamentum flavum hypertrophy.
2. Other pathologies.
   - Facet joint cyst.
   - Ligamentum flavum cyst.
   - Ossification of the Ligamentum flavum.

H. S. Kim et al. (eds.), *Advanced Techniques of Endoscopic Lumbar Spine Surgery*,
https://doi.org/10.1007/978-981-15-8253-0_4

Contraindications

- Gross segmental instability evident on dynamic radiographs (>4 mm of translation or >10° angular opening).
- Grade 2 or more spondylolisthesis according to Meyerding's criteria.
- Severe degenerative scoliosis.
- Infection.
- Malignancy.

Anatomical Consideration

It is important to understand the layered anatomy of the ligamentum flavum as it forms the basic principle of 'out and in' technique of endoscopic stenosis lumbar decompression (ESLD). The Ligamentum flavum consists of two layers: the superficial layer which consists of loose fibres arranged obliquely and can be easily removed with endoscopic forceps and the deep layer of the ligament flavum which stretches far beyond the upper margin of the superficial layer and consists of two parts—interlaminar part which is firm quadrangular sheets of fibres arranged cranio-caudally attached to the ventral surface of lamina and separated by the midline defect and foraminal part which extends deep into the foramen and merges with the facet capsule (Fig. 1).

Surgical Technique

Preoperative Planning

Plain Radiograph

We routinely perform plain radiograph AP, lateral, oblique and dynamic view of lumbar spine. Plain radiograph is evaluated for the curvature of spine (presence of degenerative scoliosis); dynamic view is assessed for the segmental instability. For surgical planning, AP view is evaluated for the extent of interlaminar window which is reduced in most of the cases of spinal canal stenosis. The width of cranial and caudal laminae and isthmus is evaluated for the safe bony decompression.

Magnetic Resonance Imaging (MRI) and CT Scan

Ligamentum flavum's sublaminar and subarticular extent along with thickness is evaluated in MRI. The axial cut of CT scan is evaluated for the size, shape and orientation of facets (facet tropism). It gives an idea about safe range of the medial facet resection without causing iatrogenic instability. 3D reconstructed CT scan image gives an exact 3D view of interlaminar window narrowed by deviated spinous process and hypertrophied bony spurs. The cross-sectional area of dural sac is measured preoperatively for the severity of stenosis and postoperatively for the adequacy of decompression.

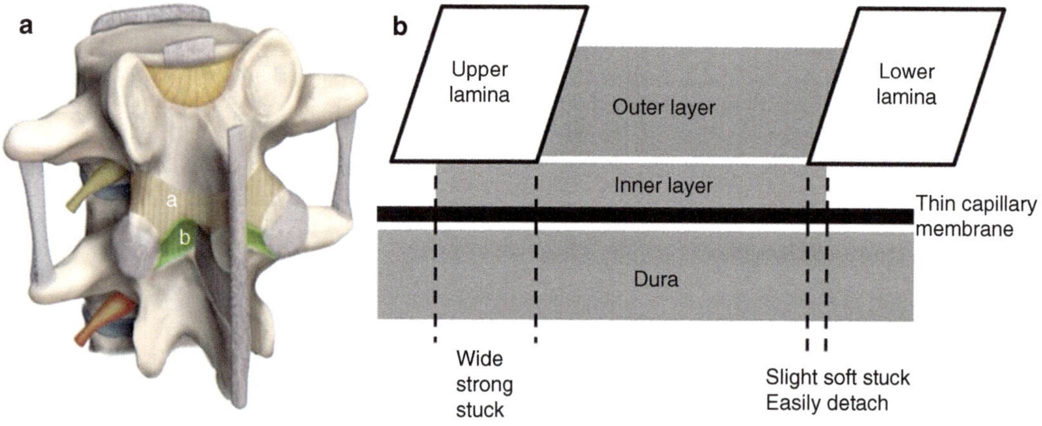

Fig. 1 Layered anatomy of the ligamentum flavum with its attachments. (**a**) 3D view (a. inner layer, b. outer layer). (**b**) Cross-sectional view

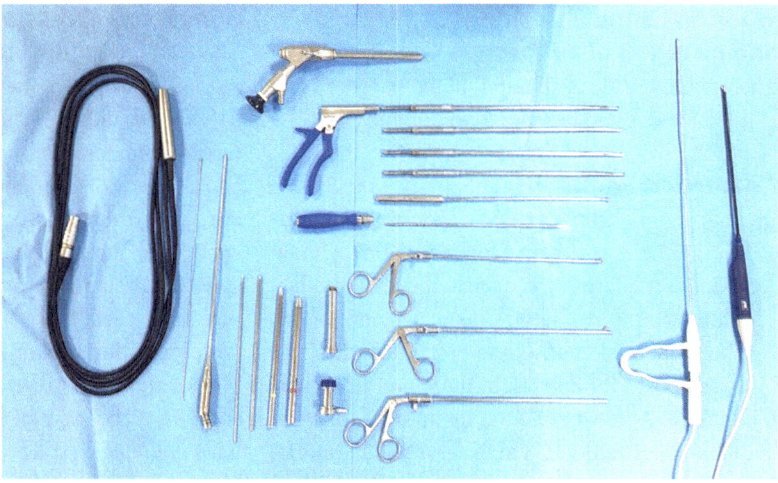

Fig. 2 Instruments for endoscopic posterior lumbar canal decompression

Anaesthesia and Position

The procedure is performed under epidural anaesthesia with sedation or general anaesthesia for ease of patient positioning and immobilization. Local anaesthesia is not preferred as interlaminar approach is associated with significant neural retraction which is a painful procedure for the patient.

The patient is placed in prone position on a radiolucent table with Wilson's frame. It obliterates the lumbar lordosis and widens the interlaminar window for the safe passage of the working cannula with minimal bony resection. A single dose of antibiotics is administered in preoperative period. The entire procedure is performed under constant saline irrigation. We prefer to use an arthro-pump with pressure set at 30–40 mm Hg. Irrigation fluid pressure should be adjusted according to the clarity of surgical fluid.

Special Surgical Instruments

1. Guide wire.
2. Obturator, serial dilators and working cannula 13.7 mm with bevel tip.
3. Endoscope with 15° viewing angle, outer diameter 10 mm, working channel diameter of 6 mm and working length 125 mm: for central decompression.
4. Endoscope with 30° viewing angle, outer diameter 6.5 mm, working channel diameter 3.7 mm and working length 208 mm (used in traditional transforaminal approach): for discectomy or contralateral foraminotomy by 'channel switching technique'.
5. High-speed endoscopic drill with 3.5 mm diamond tip.
6. Radiofrequency ablator with probe.
7. Endoscopic Kerrison's rongeurs.
8. Endoscopic disc forceps.
9. Endoscopic bone cutter.
10. Endoscopic blunt bent tip probe (Fig. 2).

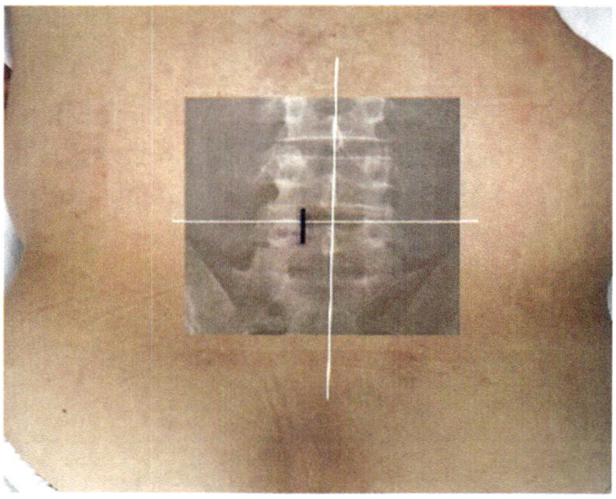

Fig. 3 Skin incision point: medial border of facet

Surgical Steps

Skin Incision

Longitudinal incision of size 1 cm taken over target point located about 1–1.5 cm from midline on the ipsilateral side at desired level (Fig. 3).

Working Cannula Docking and Insertion of Endoscope

The operative side is decided on the basis of clinical symptoms and preoperative planning.

Anatomical Points

In endoscopic spine surgery (ESS), the endoscopic image is different from the field of view seen under a microscope or naked eye, so understanding anatomical landmarks is very important for the sequential endoscopic procedures.

In the posterior approach, there are three anatomical points created by the ligamentum flavum and bone intersections, which serve as landmarks to facilitate the endoscopic procedure.

There are three target points which can be approached under fluoroscopy guidance in AP (Fig. 4).

Serial dilators, obturator and working cannula are inserted in order through the space between multifidus muscles adjacent to the spinous process, and finally endoscope is introduced along the working cannula. The bevel tip is docked over lateral bony structures with the working cannula facing medially towards the ligamentum flavum in order to avoid neural injury.

Bony Decompression

The soft tissue dissection and haemostasis are carried out with a radiofrequency ablator. The soft tissue and superficial layer of the ligamentum flavum are removed with endoscopic forceps. The bone drilling started at the medial border of the ipsilateral facet joint (point A) in caudal to cranial direction and from deeper to superficial plane up to the spino-laminar junction of cranial vertebra (point B) (Fig. 5a) and caudal vertebra (point C) until we observe the free margins of the deep layer of the ligamentum flavum (Fig. 5b). The base of the spinous process along with the undersurface of the contralateral lamina and lateral recess is decompressed according to the requirement (contralateral approach) (Fig. 5c, d). Hence during ESLD, it requires significant bone drilling of cranial lamina compared to caudal lamina. Interlaminar window is further narrowed with degenerative process; hence, it requires significant bony decompression apart from soft tissue decompression, which should be carried out before resection of the LF. It forms the basic principle of 'out and in' technique of ESLD where the deep layer of the ligamentum flavum acts as a protective barrier between the

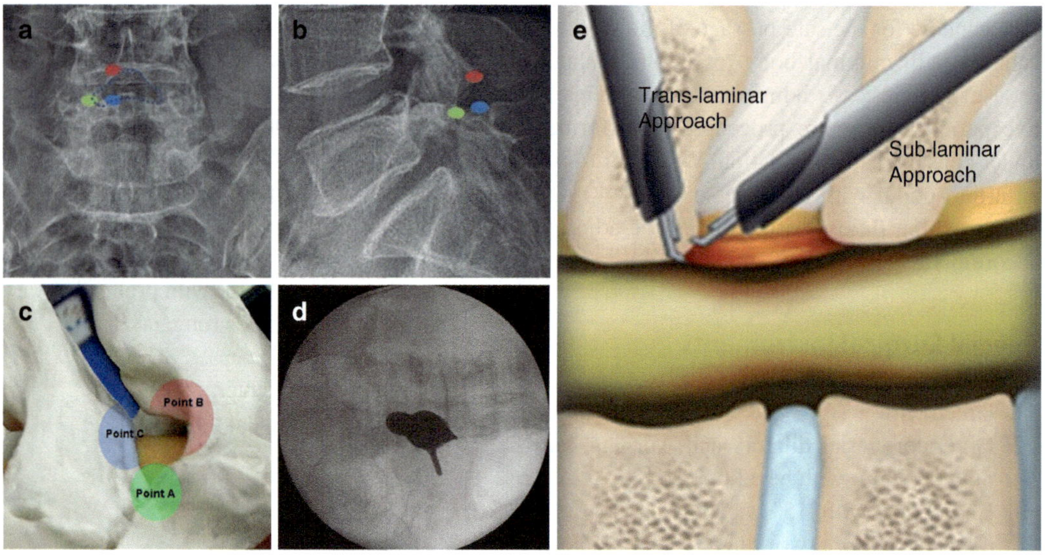

Fig. 4 Three anatomical landmarks: green circle (point A), junction of medial border of ipsilateral facet and caudal lamina (initial landmark of sublaminar approach); red circle (point B), spino-laminar junction of cranial vertebra (initial landmark of cranial outside in (over the top) approach); blue circle (point C), spino-laminar junction of caudal vertebra (landmark of caudal outside in (over the top) approach) in X-ray. (**a**) AP view. (**b**) Lateral view. (**c**) 3D model view. (**d**) Intraoperative fluoroscopic view. (**e**) Schematic illustration of posterior two approaches (translaminar and sublaminar)

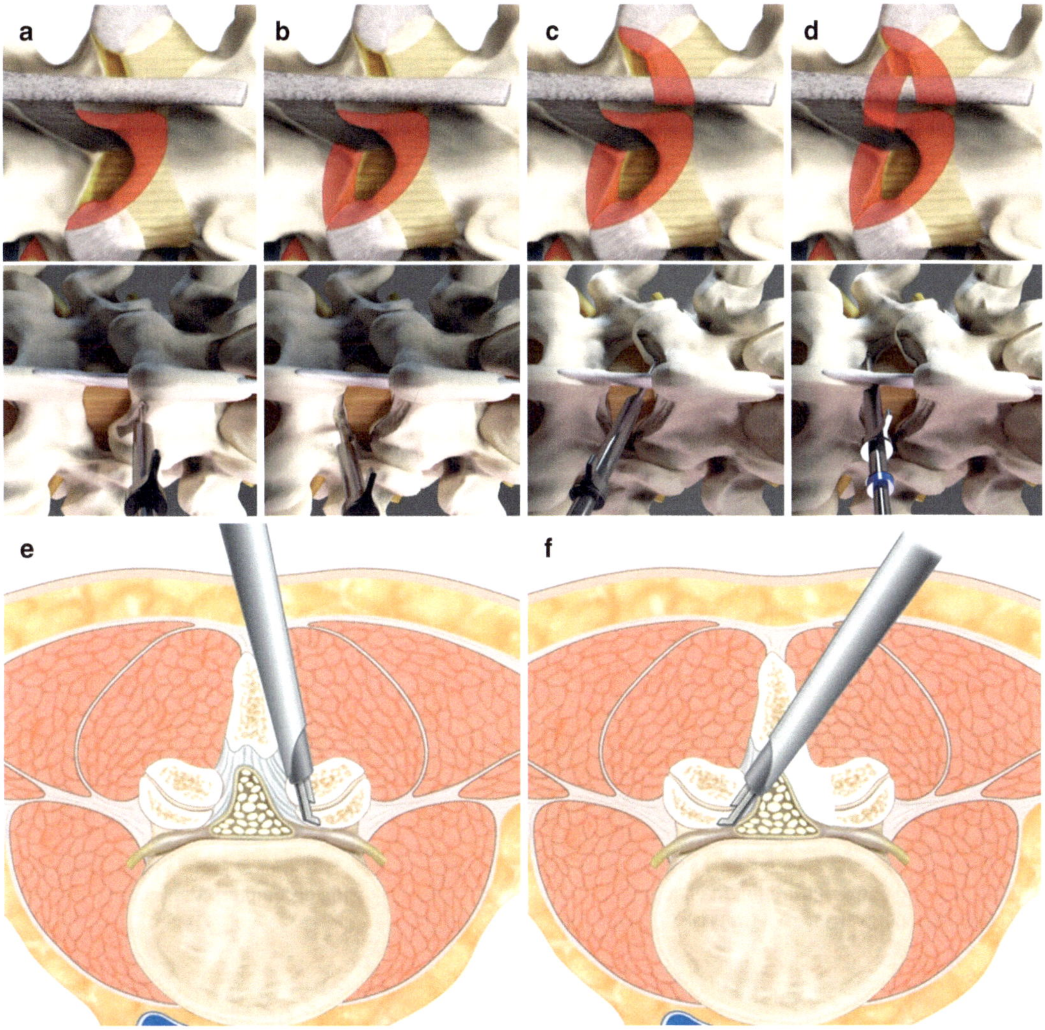

Fig. 5 Illustrative image of sequence of bony drilling for the bilateral decompression during endoscopic lumbar canal and lateral recess decompression. (**a**) Drilling of ipsilateral cranial lamina. (**b**) Drilling of ipsilateral caudal lamina. (**c**) Drilling of spinous process base and contralateral sublaminar area. (**d**) Drilling of medial border of contralateral caudal lamina and facet. (**e**, **f**) Illustrative concept of 'outside in' approach

working zone and vital structures inside the spinal canal.

Removal of the Ligamentum flavum and Confirmation of Decompressed Neural Structures

The bony procedures is performed outside the deep layer of the ligamentum flavum so that neural structures are protected by it throughout the procedure. Finally, the deep layer of the ligamentum flavum is elevated from its sublaminar attachment with endoscopic dissector and ligamentum is resected in 'en bloc' fashion with the help of Kerrison's punch and forceps (Video 1). The switch to smaller endoscope with an OD of 6.5 mm is preferred to perform ventral decompression or contralateral decompression with minimal neural retraction. Haemostasis is achieved with the help of a radiofrequency ablator. Finally, adequacy of a decompression is

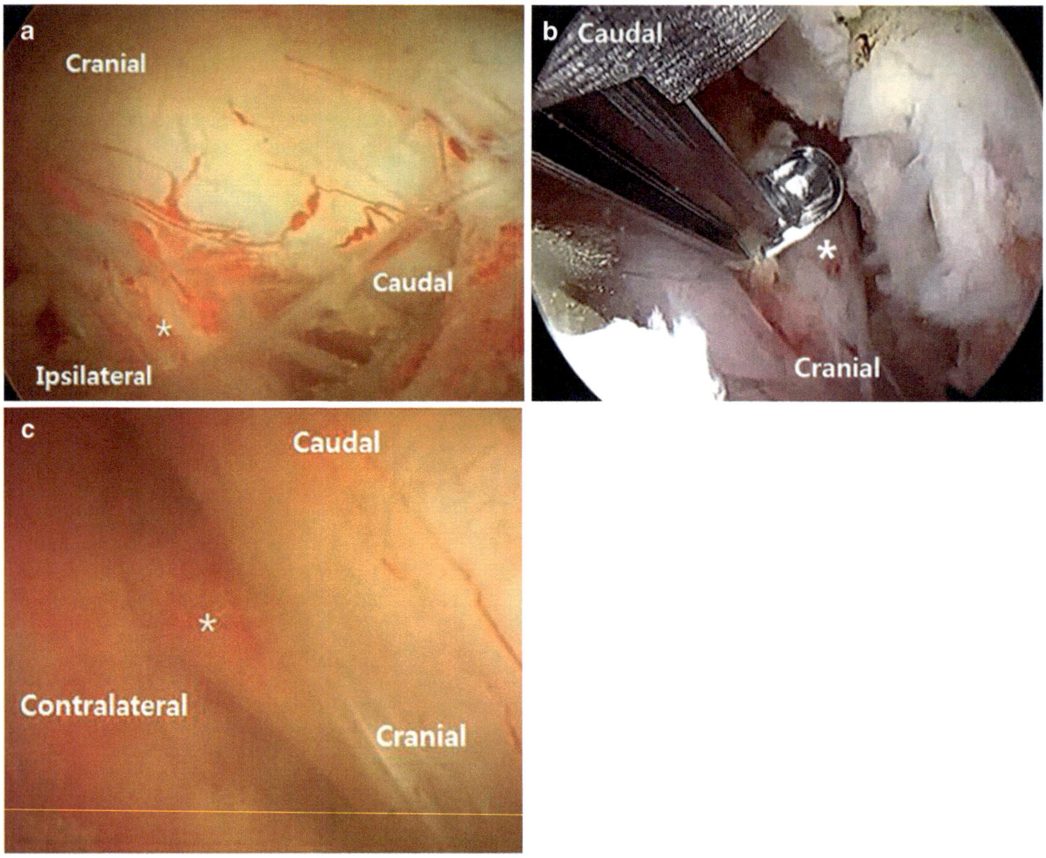

Fig. 6 (**a–c**) Operative illustration of endoscopic intraoperative findings showing decompressed thecal sac, ipsilateral and contralateral traversing root (asterisk)

checked by observing the free lateral recess, free floating dural sac and traversing nerve root in the epidural space (Fig. 6). Drain is inserted to avoid epidural haematoma collection in postoperative period. Fascia and skin are sutured with the absorbable sutures.

Postoperative Care

The patient is mobilized as soon as he/she recovered from anaesthesia with lumbosacral corset brace. Usually, the use of brace for 2–4 weeks in postoperative period is recommended. There is no specific rehabilitation protocol after the surgery. In endoscopic spine surgery The patient is allowed his/her daily routine activity as per patient's pain tolerance.

Complications and Management

Intraoperative

- Intraoperative bleeding.
  - Beforehand bleeding control is a solution to prevent troublesome intraoperative bleeding. Areas where frequently major bleeding is encountered are venous plexus at the cranial portion beyond the upper margin of the Ligamentum flavum and lateral recess.
  - It can be managed by temporary elevation of irrigation fluid pressure (40–50 mm Hg). When you meet the unknown origin bleeding, check the bleeding focus from outside of the working cannula. It can be muscles, bony damage by the tip of the

working cannula around bony resection margin or epidural capillary membrane. It can be coagulated with a radiofrequency ablator.
  - Haemostatic agents such as Floseal® and Gelfoam are useful to manage uncontrollable intraoperative bleeding from unknown origin.
  - Postoperative drain is recommended after operation to prevent postoperative haematoma.
- Incidental durotomy.
  - It is most common intraoperative complication. It is frequently associated with facet/ligamentum cyst and revision surgeries due to adhesion of the dura to the ligamentum flavum.
  - Small and late dural tear: endoscopic dural repair with TachoSil® fibrin patch (Nycomed, Linz, Austria) is recommended.
  - Large or early dural tear: conversion to open surgery and repair is needed.
- Injury to neural structures/transient dysesthesia.
  - Prevention is the best way of managing neural injury. Endoscopic vision should be always clear, which can be achieved by increasing the fluid pressure momentarily and adequate haemostasis.
  - Safe plane of dissection should be acquired between the neural structures and near structures. It can be achieved by rotating the bevel tip of the working cannula against the neural structures.
  - Blind closing of endoscopic forceps and punches should be avoided. Sharp instruments like Kerrison's punch should be used facing away from the neural structures. It is better to use endoscopic drills with protection sleeve.
  - 'Decompression first (by bony unroofing or discectomy) and manipulation second' is a strategic principle to minimize neural injury.
  - The radiofrequency ablator should be used with much caution. The surgeon should adhere to adequate power (soft tissue ablation and bone bleeding control, 250 Watts, but around the neural structures, below 90 Watts) and direction against neural structure in usage of RF.
- Incomplete decompression.
  - Revision ESLD.
  - Open posterior decompression.

Postoperative

- Surgical site infection.
  - Superficial (can be managed with IV antibiotics).
  - Deep (open debridement or open debridement and fusion).
- Iatrogenic instability.
  - Endoscopic transforaminal lumbar interbody fusion (E-TLIF).
  - Open TLIF.
- Early/late recurrence.
  - Revision ESLD/open decompression—endoscopic TLIF/open TLIF.

Illustrative Cases

Single-Level ESLD

Case 1 (Fig. 7)

Case 2 (Video 2) (Fig. 8)

Case 3 (Video 3) (Fig. 9)

Multilevel ESLD

Case 4 (Video 4) (Fig. 10)

Discussion (Surgical Tips and Pitfalls)

According to three stories of anatomical segment concept, the major lesions of degenerative central spinal canal stenosis are confined to first story (i.e. hypertrophied/buckled ligamentum flavum, hypertrophied superior articular facet and disc bulge). Successful endoscopic decompression of central spinal canal stenosis (ESLD) depends

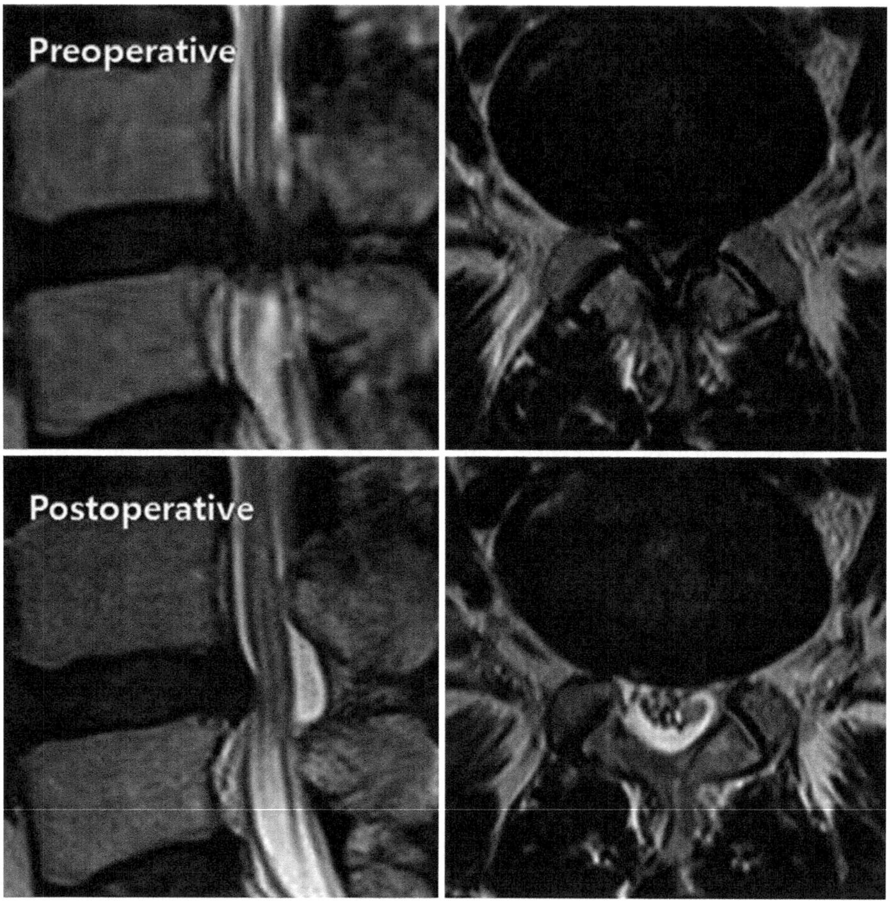

Fig. 7 Preoperative and postoperative T2 MR images of a 57-year-old female patient with L3–4 severe spinal canal stenosis (Schiza's grade D) treated with ESLD

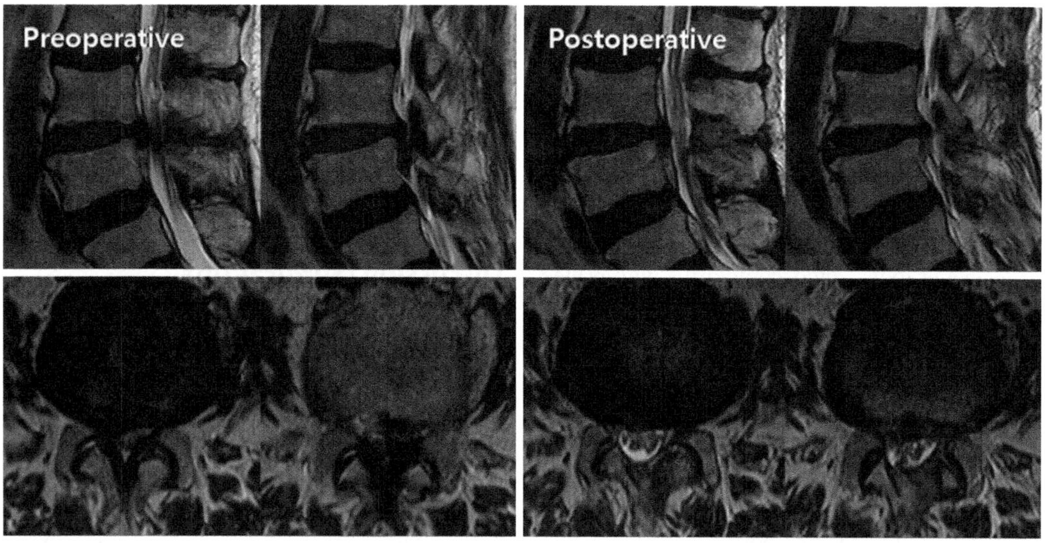

Fig. 8 Preoperative and postoperative T2 MRI images of a 76-year-old female patient with L3–4 severe spinal canal stenosis (Schiza's grade D) treated with ESLD

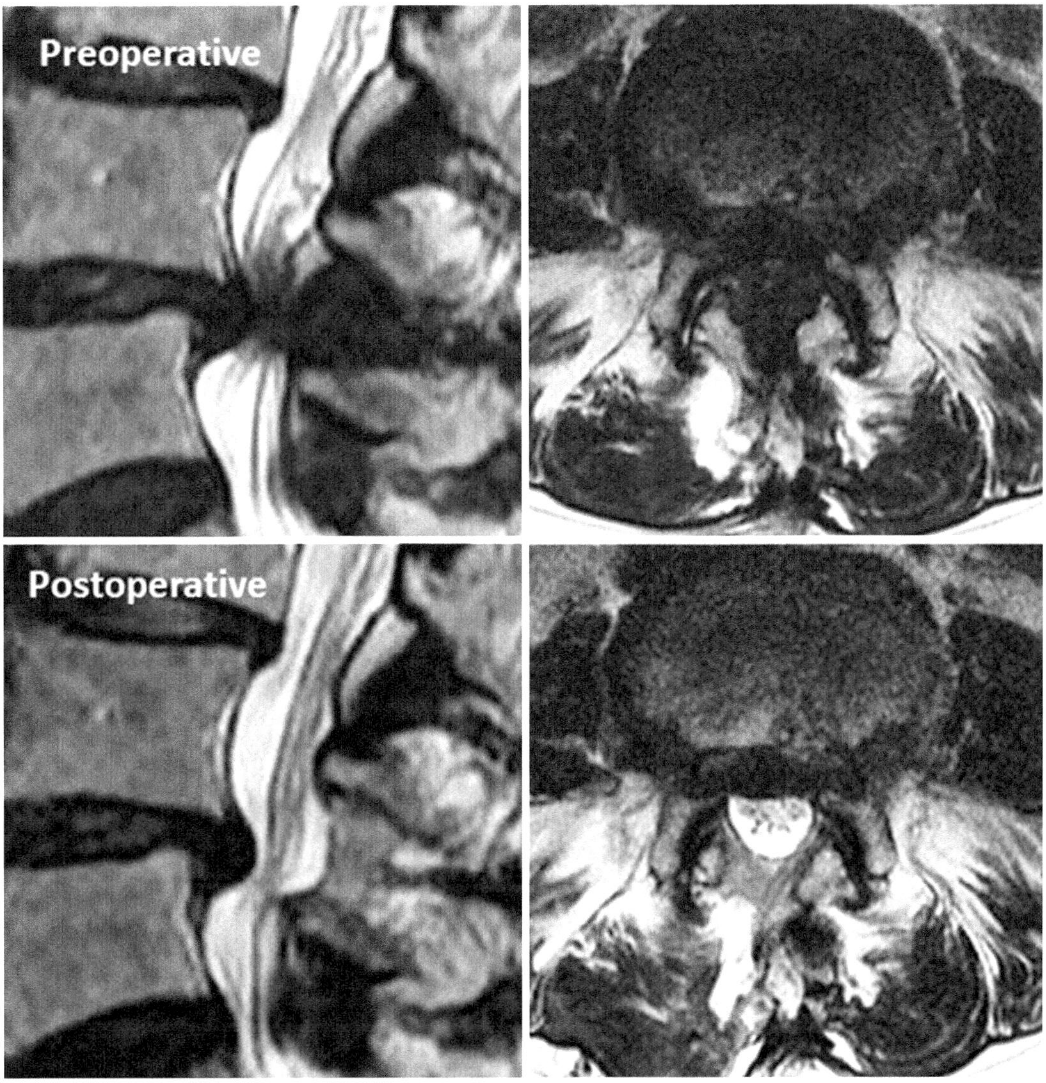

Fig. 9 Preoperative and postoperative T2 MR images of an 80-year-old female patient with L4–5 severe spinal canal stenosis (Schiza's grade D) treated with ESLD

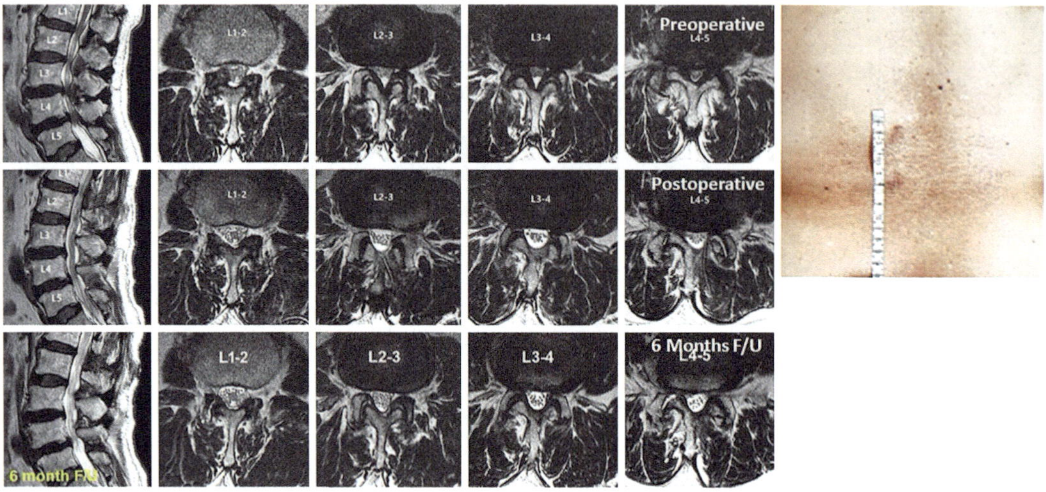

Fig. 10 Preoperative and postoperative T2 MR images of a 76-year-old male patient with multilevel spinal canal stenosis treated with ESLD with surgical scar

upon the resection of these lesions in first story of anatomical segment.

As compared to the tubular decompression, endoscopic decompression not only provides smaller size of access to the pathology but it also provides a flexible channel to reach the difficult part of spinal canal under direct vision. Docking of endoscope at point A ('V' point) provides the advantage point from where the surgeon can access the spinal canal by simply tilting and rotating the endoscope (Fig. 12). As the endoscope is docked at the deepest point of interlaminar window, it gives an idea about the depth of stenotic spinal canal to the surgeon. Bony decompression can be safely carried out from deep to superficial plane without further advancement of drill into the spinal canal.

The operative view in endoscopic spinal surgery is very narrow and magnified during the procedure. Additionally, the unique optical angle (20°–25°) of endoscope can induce the operator to have confusion in understanding the related anatomical structures. Accordingly, the knowledge of endoscopic landmarks is important for the successful decompression. The principal midline landmarks for the endoscopic ipsilateral decompression are the cranio-caudal orientation of fibres of the ligamentum flavum, the base of the spinous process with interspinous ligament and the midline defect in the deep layer of the LF. Laterally, the medial margin of SAP forms the lateral extent of endoscopic decompression [9] (Fig. 11).

One of the common causes of lateral recess stenosis is pinching of neural structures between hypertrophied facet/facet cyst and paracentral disc herniation. Hence, the adequate lateral recess decompression is an important step while performing the ESLD. However, excessive violation of the facet joint for complete decompression of the traversing root can cause postoperative instability. So, the operator always should be careful to preserve the facet joint. It can be achieved by rotating or tilting the endoscope towards the ipsilateral facet. Bone drilling should be followed in medial to lateral direction, at least, caudal to cranial or cranial to caudal direction along the medial margin of SAP (Fig. 12). Free traversing root in the lateral recess is the end point of decompression [5, 6].

The ligamentum flavum is preserved until the final step of the procedure, which protects the dura and neural structures from the sharp instruments. Sublaminar attachment is carefully elevated by curved blunt tip probe to observe epidural space. Pressure of irrigation fluid pushes the dura away from the LF and develops the plane between the LF and the dura. However, in certain

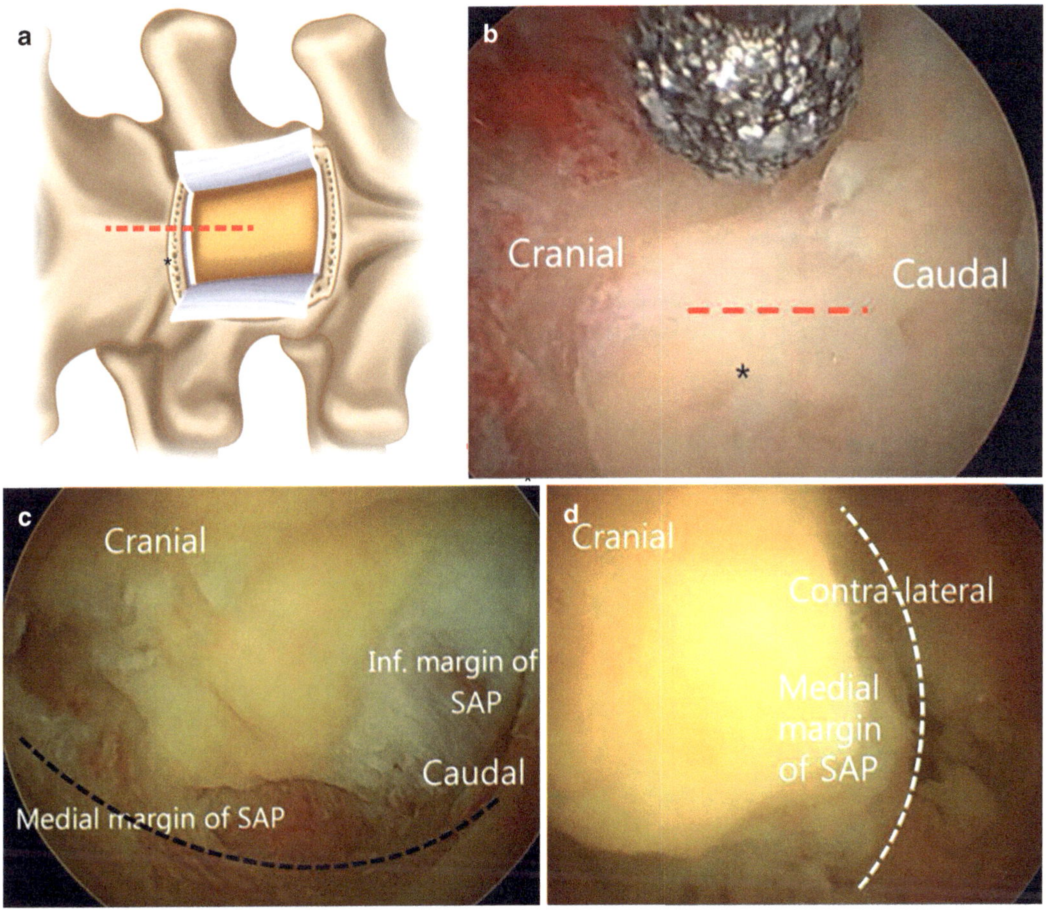

Fig. 11 (**a–d**) Anatomical landmarks in percutaneous endoscopic lumbar canal decompression showing the ligament flavum (asterisk), midline (red dotted line), medial margin of the ipsilateral superior articular process (SAP) (black dotted curved line) and medial margin of the contralateral SAP (white dotted curved line)

conditions such as facet cyst or ligamentum flavum cyst and revision surgeries, the dura is severely adhered to the LF. It needs careful manipulation of neural structures away from the LF. 'En bloc' resection of the ligamentum flavum avoids the possibility of incomplete decompression.

Dural tear is one of the serious complications in ESLD. It can lead to adverse consequences such as intraoperative increased intracranial pressure, postoperative rootlet expulsion and persistent CSF leakage from operative wound and pseudomeningocele, which need secondary revision surgery. Beforehand careful dissection and coagulation of peridural vessel and soft tissue are mandatory to prevent intraoperative dural tear. Avoid blind procedure and acquire the safe operative view between the dura and near structures by rotating the endoscope. Double-checking before the removal of peridural soft tissues and LF by punch also should be kept in mind. Most dural tears during operation can be figured out. Failure to detect it intraoperatively may cause further problems later.

Limitations

- Operative time for ESLD is slightly longer compared to an open decompression for single level. However, multilevel ESLD is associated with significantly longer operative time.

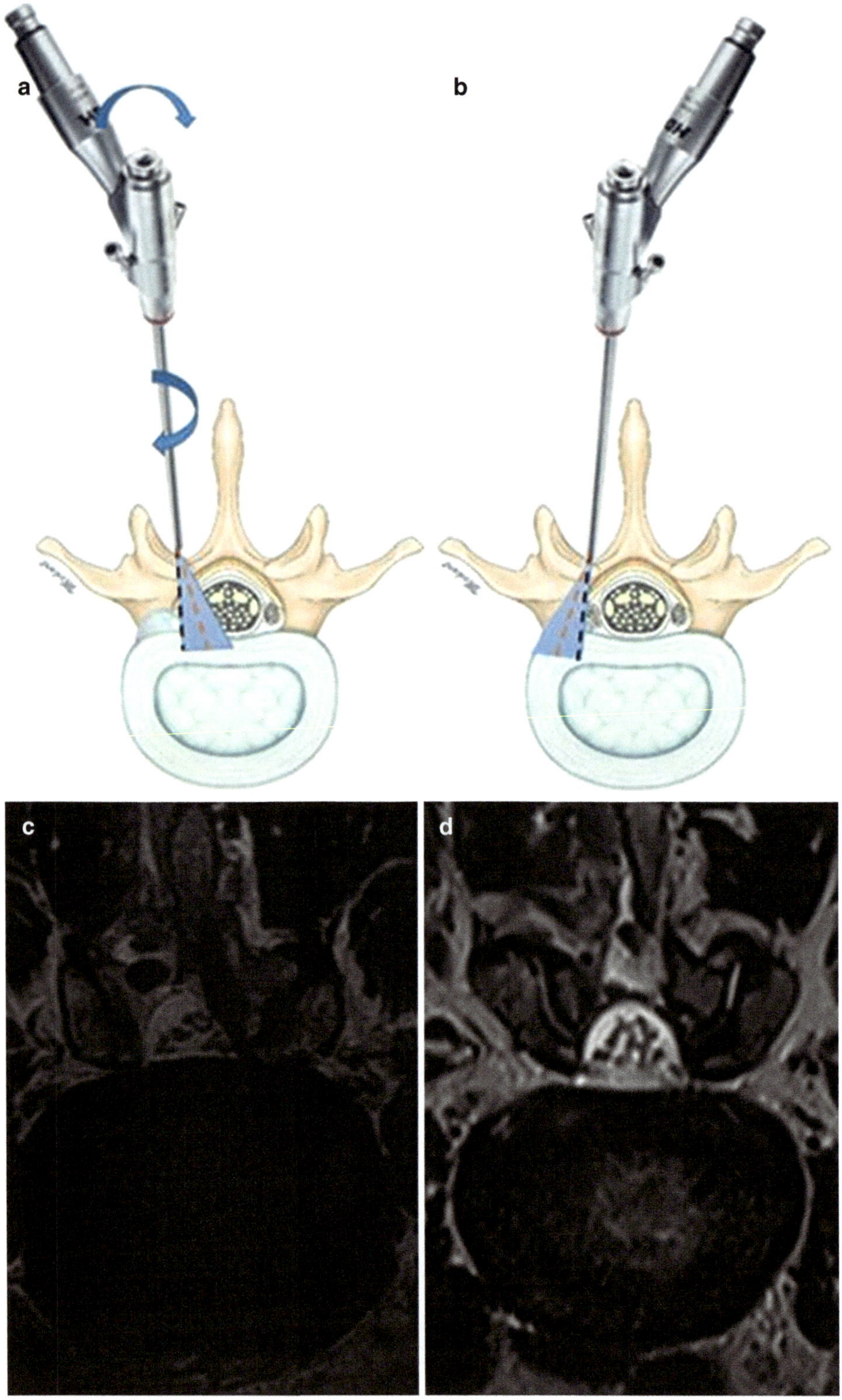

Fig. 12 Rotation and tilting manoeuvre of endoscope for facet joint preservation. (**a**) Operative angle in lateral to medial direction. (**b**) Operative angle in medial to lateral direction. (**c**) Postoperative axial MR image showing violated facet joint by bone drilling in lateral to medial direction. (**d**) Postoperative axial MR image showing preserved facet joint by bone drilling in medial to lateral direction. Blue triangle, endoscopic field of view; red dotted line, endoscopic optical angle for exploration of lateral recess; and black dotted line, operative surgical angle for drilling of bony structure

- The procedure is technically demanding and it has steep learning curve [4].

Summary

'Out and in' technique of ESLD provides safe and effective method for decompression of spinal canal stenosis in central canal and lateral recess. The advantages of techniques are considered in terms of less intraoperative blood loss, minimal damage to soft tissue, and early postoperative recovery with preservation of the spinal stability in long-term follow-up. The technique has long operative time and steep learning curve. However, it can be negotiated with development of surgical skills.

References

1. Kim M, Kim HS, Oh SW, Adsul NM, Singh R, Kashlan ON, Noh JH, Jang IT, Oh SH. Evolution of spinal endoscopic surgery. Neurospine. 16(1):6–14.
2. Ruetten S, Komp M, Merk H, Godolias G. Full-endoscopic interlaminar and transforaminal lumbar discectomy versus conventional microsurgical technique: A prospective, randomized, controlled study. Spine. 33:931–9.
3. Kim M, Lee S, Kim HS, Park S, Shim SY, Lim DJ. A comparison of percutaneous endoscopic lumbar discectomy and open lumbar microdiscectomy for lumbar disc herniation in the Korean: a meta-analysis. Biomed Res Int. 2018;2018:9073460.
4. Lee CW, Yoon KJ, Kim SW. Percutaneous endoscopic decompression in Lumbar Canal and lateral recess stenosis - the surgical learning curve. Neurospine. 2019;16(1):63–71.
5. Lee CW, Yoon KJ, Jun JH. Percutaneous endoscopic laminotomy with flavectomy by uniportal, unilateral approach for the lumbar canal or lateral recess stenosis. World Neurosurg. 2018;113:e129–37.
6. Ito F, Ito Z, Shibayama M, et al. Step-by-step sublaminar approach with a newly-designed spinal endoscope for unilateral-approach bilateral decompression in spinal stenosis. Neurospine. 2019;16(1):41–51.
7. Wang JC, Kim HS. Endoscopic spinal surgery (ESS): prepare for a happy 100-year-old! Neurospine. 2019;16(1):4–5.
8. Lim KT, Nam HGW, Kim SB, Kim HS, Park JS, Park CK. Therapeutic feasibility of full endoscopic decompression in one- to three-level Lumbar Canal stenosis via a single skin port using a new endoscopic system, percutaneous Stenoscopic lumbar decompression. Asian Spine J. 2019;13(2):272–82.
9. Siepe CJ, Sauer D, Michael MH. Full endoscopic, bilateral over-the-top decompression for lumbar spinal stenosis. Eur Spine J. 2018;27(Suppl 4):563–5.

Biportal Endoscopic Approach for Lumbar Central Stenosis

Hee-Seok Yang, Dong Hwa Heo, and Jeong-Yoon Park

Introduction

Lumbar central stenosis is a degenerative process that is frequent in the aging population. Lumbar spinal stenosis is a pathologic process where vertebral bodies, ligaments, and facet joints of the lumbar spine degenerate and overgrow, progressively compressing the neural and vascular elements in the spinal canal [1].

Recently, endoscopic techniques also have shown encouraging clinical results in the treatment of lumbar spinal stenosis [2]. Based on many studies and reports of successful decompression of the stenosis through uniportal and biprotal endoscopic approach, endoscopic spine surgery have evolved with less damage on normal structures and have demonstrated effective stenosis decompressions under direct visualization [2–5]. Recently, biportal endoscopic decompression is introduced. Uniportal endoscope uses single and same axis for endoscope and working channel, and it should have a close view. In addition, the instrument must be seen under close view and visual field during uniportal endoscopic surgery is narrow. On the other hand, biportal endoscopic spine surgery has a long and wide field of view, and the axes of the endoscope and working channel are separated. Therefore, the instrument can be used under a relatively long distance and wide field of view, and this unique feature of biportal endoscope made it easy to understand the anatomical orientation and to handle the surgical instruments. In biportal endoscopic spine surgery, endoscope and instrument approach angles are independent, and there is the freedom of vision and instrument angle during endoscopic spine surgery.

During biportal endoscopic spine surgery, we can use conventional retractor and instrument (drill, punch et al.) through a working portal and also can use the endoscopic cannula through endoscopic portal like uniportal endoscopic spine surgery. One of the main differences between biportal and uniportal endoscopic spine surgeries is that various general surgical instruments can be used during biportal endoscopic spine surgery because of independent working portal. In addition, we have to understand fluid dynamics during biportal endoscopic spine surgery and make cavitary water space, and there

Electronic Supplementary Material The online version of this chapter (https://doi.org/10.1007/978-981-15-8253-0_5) contains supplementary material, which is available to authorized users.

H.-S. Yang
Department of Neurosurgery, Seoul Barunsesang Hospital, Seoul, South Korea

D. H. Heo
Department of Neurosurgery, Seoul Bumin Hospital, Seoul, South Korea

J.-Y. Park (✉)
Department of Neurosurgery, Spine and Spinal Cord Institute, Gangnam Severance Hospital, Yonsei University College of Medicine, Seoul, South Korea
e-mail: spinepjy@yuhs.ac

H. S. Kim et al. (eds.), *Advanced Techniques of Endoscopic Lumbar Spine Surgery*,
https://doi.org/10.1007/978-981-15-8253-0_5

could be continuous flow between input and output channels. There were several papers about the behaviors of arthroscopic irrigation, and the authors recommend using an output cannula for biportal endoscopic spine surgery [6, 7]. In the text below, the surgical procedure for lumbar central stenosis using biportal endoscopic spine surgery will be described in detail.

Anesthesia and Position

The procedure is performed under general or epidural anesthesia. The patient is placed in the prone position with the abdomen free over the radiolucent frame in a flexed position to open the interlaminar space and foramen. A surgical drape designed to drain water well from the output channel can prevent the water leak from surgical field (Fig. 1).

Special Surgical Instruments

During the procedures, we used 3.5-mm spherical bur and diamond drill, 0° 4-mm-diameter arthroscope, 3.5-mm radiofrequency (RF) device, serial dilators, a specially designed dissector, and standard laminectomy instruments, such as hook dissectors, Kerrison punches, and pituitary for-

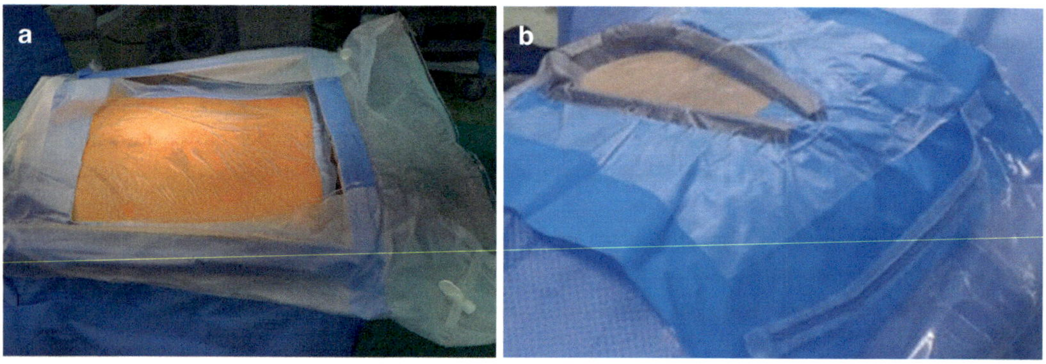

Fig. 1 Waterproof surgical drapes (A and B) for biportal endoscopic surgery

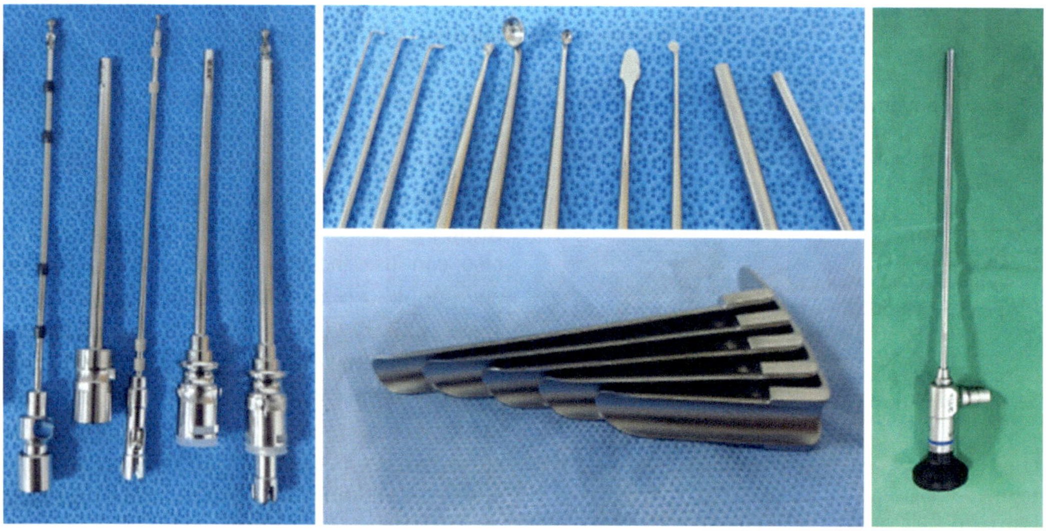

Fig. 2 Various kinds of surgical instruments of biportal endoscopic surgeries. 3.5-mm spherical bur and diamond drill (**a**), a specially designed dissector (**b**), 4-mm-diameter arthroscope (**c**), and semicircular cannula to keep proper outflow for working cannula (**d**). Clockwise from left. General spine surgical instruments were also available for biportal endoscopic surgeries

ceps (Fig. 2). The rest of the equipment uses the same endoscopy tower system. Instruments designed exclusively for biportal endoscopes are also available and could be more convenient. We use semicircular cannula to keep proper outflow through working cannula (Fig. 2d).

Surgical Steps (Illustration, Photos, and Video)

Skin Mark and Incision

Under image intensification, fluoroscopic confirmation of the level is made with a spinal needle inserted at the target area. Two portals are used: one portal was used for endoscope and the other working portal was used for instruments like drill, punch, and forceps. Skin entry points are determined according to the lesion site and the patient's anatomical variation. Because stenosis lesions differ from patient to patient and may combine central to lateral recess both side and foraminal lesions, portals should be created considering stenosis severity [8] and approach angles of instrument and scope to these combined lesions. Two standard entry points are made at 1 cm above and below the disc space for a posterior approach (Fig. 3). A 5-mm incision was given at the skin for the endoscope portal, and an 8-mm incision was given for the working portal along the skin crease. Docking point of two portals was over the lower portion of cranial laminae.

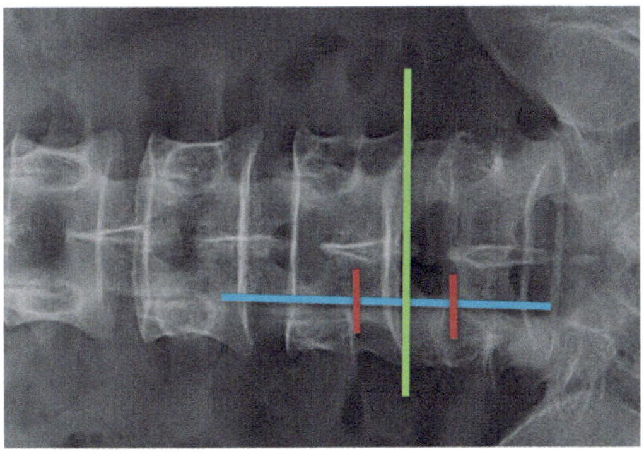

Fig. 3 Skin incision areas of biportal endoscopic lumbar surgery for L4–5 level. Anteroposterior X-ray view (**a**) and lateral X-ray view. From anteroposterior X-ray, draw line along the medical pedicle. From lateral X-ray, confirm the disc space. Two standard entry points are made at 1 cm above and below the disc space for a posterior approach. Upper portal was used for endoscope and the other working portal was used for instruments. Red lines are the skin incision

Two Portals (Biportal) Making

Serial dilators were then introduced to working portal and split the paraspinal muscles touching the spinous-laminar junction with minimal trauma. A 4-mm endoscope with trocar was then inserted into the endoscope portal, and a working sheath was inserted at the working portal (Fig. 4). RF device (for hemostasis and soft tissue dissection) was inserted into the working portal. A saline irrigation pump or just saline from 2 m height was connected to the endoscope and set to a pressure of 25–40 mm Hg during the procedure. Proper triangulation of the endoscope with the working instruments is vital for adequate visualization of the anatomical structures under keeping proper outflow with continuous irrigation of normal saline from endoscope to working portal. After exposing the lamina and the ligamentum flavum (LF), the levels are confirmed again with fluoroscopy.

Soft Tissue Dissection and Laminectomy

Muscle detachment using a dilator in the interlaminar space before inserting the endoscope helped secure sufficient visualization during the procedure. After triangulation with the endoscope and instrument, RF device and dissectors were used for bleeding control and detachment of the soft tissue remnants overlying the lamina and the ligamentum flavum.

Following complete exposure of the lamina and the ligamentum flavum in the targeted interlaminar space, an ipsilateral partial laminotomy was performed under magnified endoscopic vision. A laminotomy is performed using various burs initially to drill off the lower lamina of the cranial vertebra at the interlaminar space, similar to the decompression procedure with micro-

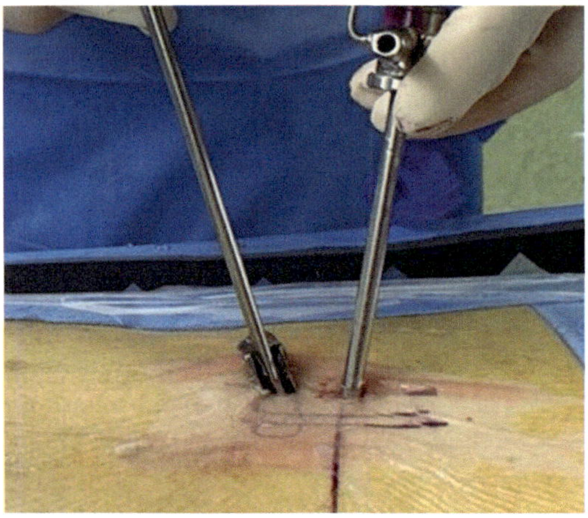

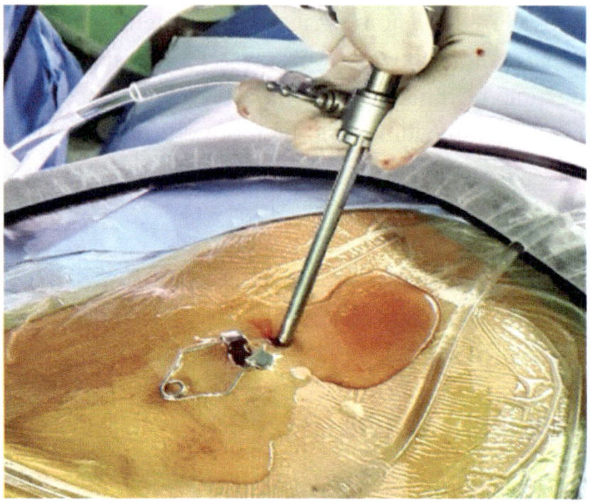

Fig. 4 Overview of biportal endoscopic surgeries. Endoscopic portal was used for only endoscopy and its trocar, and the other working portal was used for surgical instruments. Various kinds and sizes of working sheath were used for well drainage of irrigation fluid and smooth insertion of surgical instruments

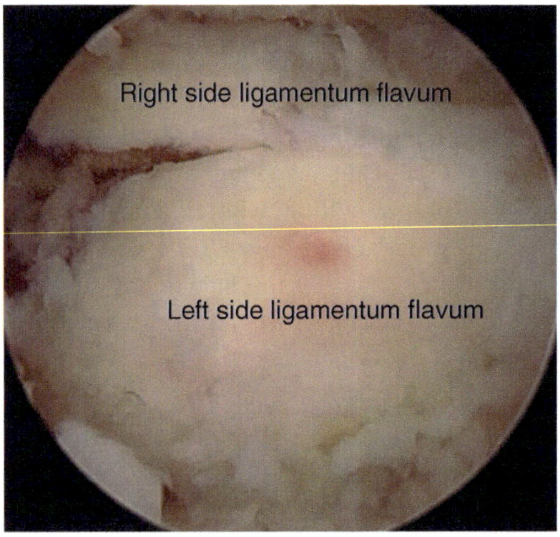

Fig. 5 Endoscopic view of unilateral laminectomy (left side approach). Ipsilateral ligamentum flavum as well as contralateral ligamentum flavum should be exposed after ipsilateral laminotomy

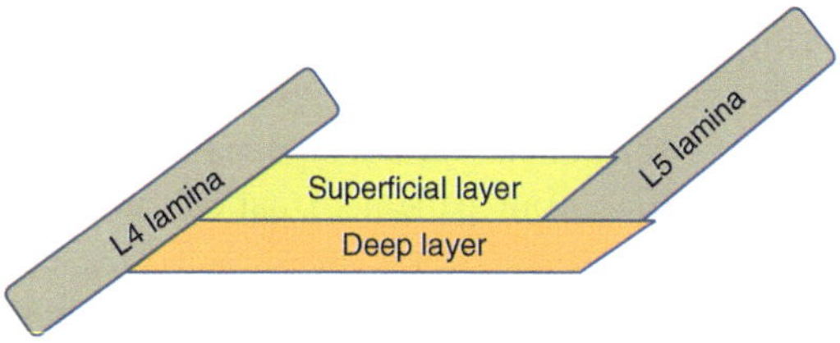

Fig. 6 Schematic illustration of the ligamentum flavum at lumbar area. Superficial layer was inserted over the caudal lamina. In contrast, deep layer was inserted below the caudal lamina

scopic approach with tubular retractor systems. Laminotomy of the upper laminar should be performed until exposure of proximal end of the ligamentum flavum. The upper lamina of the caudal vertebrae is partially removed using diamond drill and punches, continuing along the margins of the lateral recess and exposure of distal end of the ligamentum flavum. The thinned-off lateral recess and caudal laminar margin are then resected with the punch. In addition, midline spinous base area should be partially removed for exposure of contralateral ligamentum flavum (Fig. 5).

Ligamentum Flavum Removal and Decompression of Ipsilateral Traversing Nerve Root (Video 1)

Once adequate bony resection is achieved to the proximal and distal attachment of the ligamentum flavum, the superficial and deep layers of the ligamentum flavum are detached and removed. It may be removed with en bloc, but if adhesion is suspected due to severe stenosis, it may be necessary to separate and remove the superficial and deep layer (Fig. 6 and Video 1). In some cases, it is essential to check the lateral extent of the deep layer of the ligamentum flavum and remove to the lateral margin by using an angled curette [9]. A blunt hook dissector is used to identify the plane between the ligamentum flavum and the dura with saline irrigation, ensuring that it is free from adhesions. The ipsilateral ligamentum flavum was removed until full mobilization of the lateral border of the nerve root was achieved. The upper border of the lower lamina is removed for the ipsilateral foraminotomy as needed (Fig. 7).

Decompression of Contralateral Traversing Nerve Root (Video 2)

If bilateral decompression is required, the midline of the spinal canal must first be confirmed by resecting the base of the spinous process with a high-speed drill. The scope can then be adjusted medially. Usually, the base of the spinous process obstructs the placement of the scope; therefore, it may need to be partially resected to secure sufficient working space. Once exposed, the ligamen-

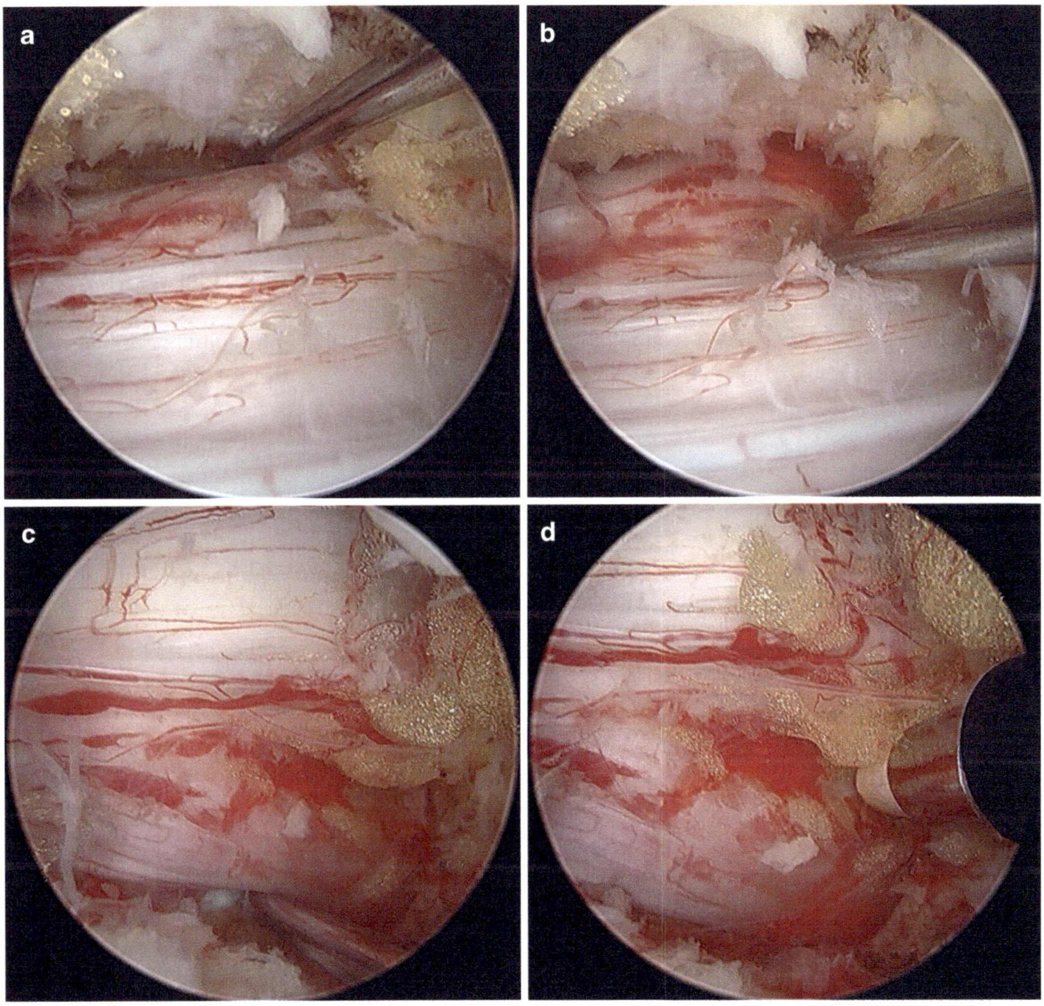

Fig. 7 Intraoperative endoscopic images showed complete decompression of bilateral traversing nerve roots. Medial margin of contralateral pedicle was checked for complete contralateral nerve root decompression of shoulder area (**a**). Also, axillar area of contralateral traversing nerve root was also checked (**b**). In addition, medical margin of ipsilateral pedicle (**c**) and ipsilateral axillar area (**d**) were carefully checked for complete decompression of ipsilateral nerve root

tum flavum can be detached from the contralateral lamina with angled curette and then undercut with a bur. After bony decompression, the thickened ligamentum flavum is resected with a curette and Kerrison punch to relieve the neural structures adequately. Contralateral decompression was performed until the contralateral traversing nerve root was identified and decompressed (Fig. 7).

Discectomy and Closure

If a patient is symptomatic and has ipsilateral disc herniation, it is possible to perform a discectomy under endoscopic view. The degree of neural decompression was assessed by normal respiratory-induced dural pulsation and confirmed with endoscopic viewing and use of a blunt probe. Bleeding is effectively controlled by the radiofrequency bipolar system under continuous irrigation. The skin incisions are closed after removal of the instruments and endoscope (Fig. 8). A surgical drain is inserted and kept for 24 h after surgery until spontaneous bleeding is controlled.

Illustrated Case or Cases

Case 1: A 79-year-old woman presented with a 1-year history of LBP and bilateral leg pain and numbness over the calf and dorsum of the foot. No benefit was obtained from the use of analgesic or nonsteroidal anti-inflammatory medications. She could not walk for over 5 min due to the pain and weakness. Neurologic examination revealed weakness of the right great toe dorsiflexion (Grade III). Magnetic resonance imaging (MRI) documented bilateral lateral recess stenosis at L3–4–5 level (Fig. 9a–c). The patient underwent biportal endoscopic decompression surgery with left side approach under general anesthesia. Postoperative back and leg pain VAS scores were decreased from 7 and 8 preoperatively to 3 and 2 after the operation, respectively. Weakness of the right great toe dorsiflexion was also recovered gradually to Grade IV in 3 weeks after operation, and neurogenic intermittent claudication also improved more 30 min. Postoperative MRI revealed satisfactory decompression of bilateral lateral recesses at L3–4–5 (Fig. 9d–f).

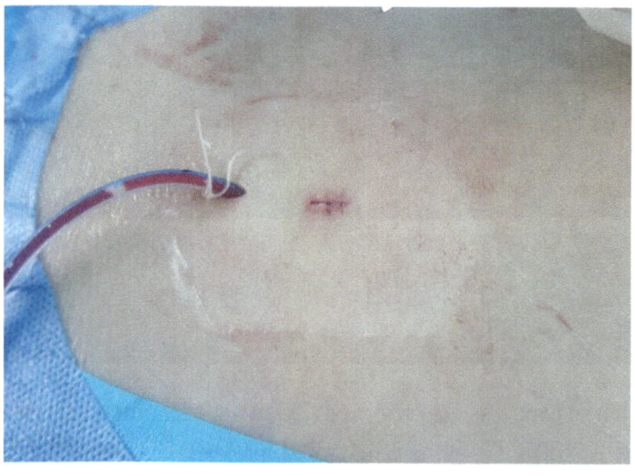

Fig. 8 Wound image of biportal endoscopic approach for lumbar stenosis. Hemovac drainage catheter was inserted for prevention of postoperative epidural hematoma

Case 2 (Video 2): A 71-year-old male patient presented with severe radicular pain of both legs and neurological intermittent claudication. Preoperative MR images reveal severe central and lateral recess stenosis of L4–5 (Fig. 10). This patient was received left sided unilateral laminotomy with bilateral decompression by biportal endoscopic approach (Video 2). Intraoperative endoscopic image and postoperative MR images demonstrated complete decompression of central canal and lateral recess of L4–5 (Fig. 10). Postoperatively, his symptoms were significantly improved.

Complications and its Management

Bleeding

To reduce the occurrence of the technical complications, the most important factor is to keep the surgical field clear by blocking epidural bleeding. Fluent water flow and bleeding control from edge bone or epidural small vessels were ensured before processing with flavectomy or laminectomy especially on the contralateral side. A bleeding from the laminectomy bone edge was compressed by squashing a piece of bone wax on

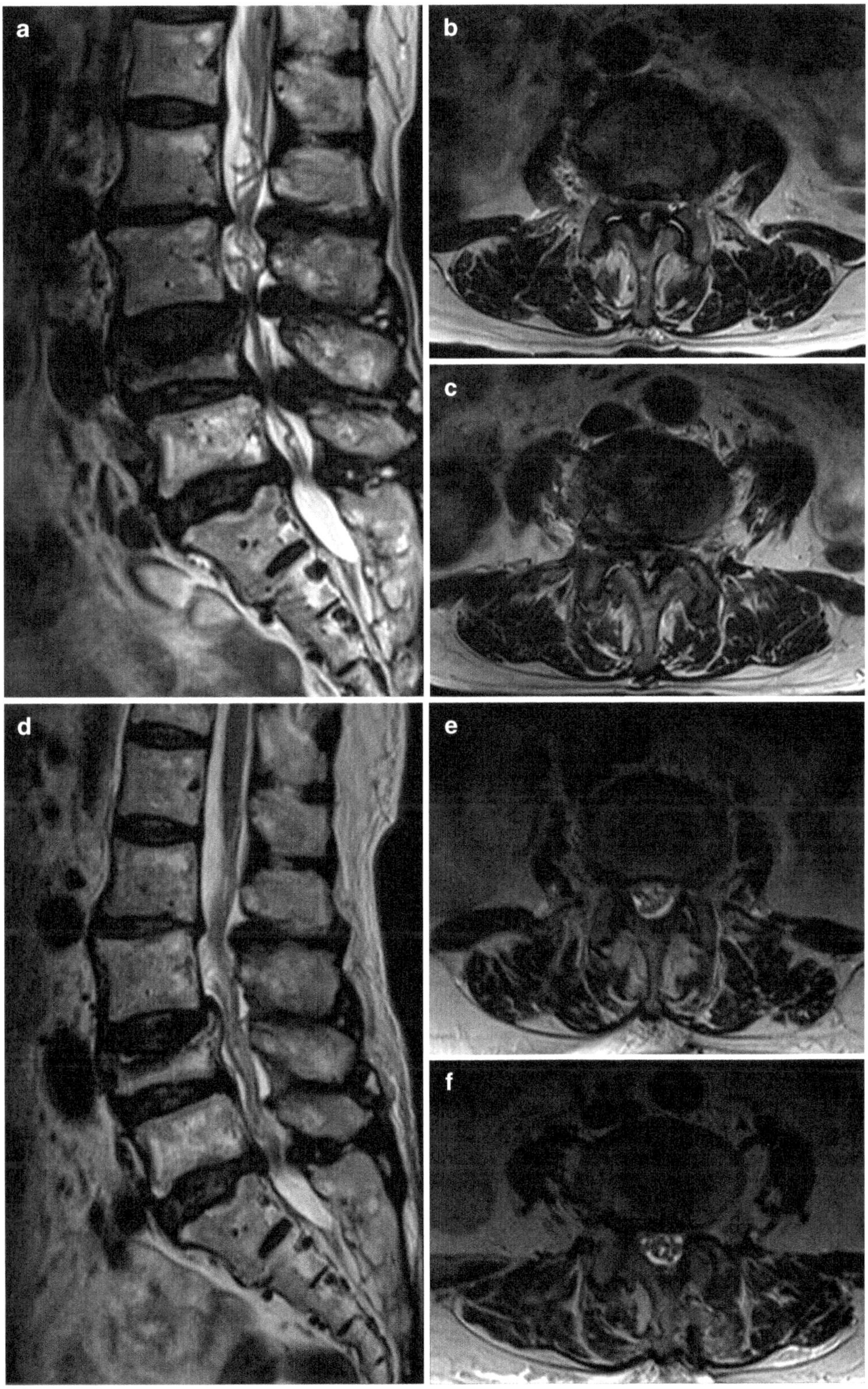

Fig. 9 Preoperative MRI showed severe central and lateral stenosis at L3–4–5 ((**a**) sagittal image; (**b**) axial image of L3–4; (**c**) axial image of L4–5). Postoperative MRI showed full decompression of lateral recess stenosis at L3–4–5 ((**d**) sagittal image; (**e**) axial image of L3–4; (**f**) axial image of L4-5). Clockwise from left

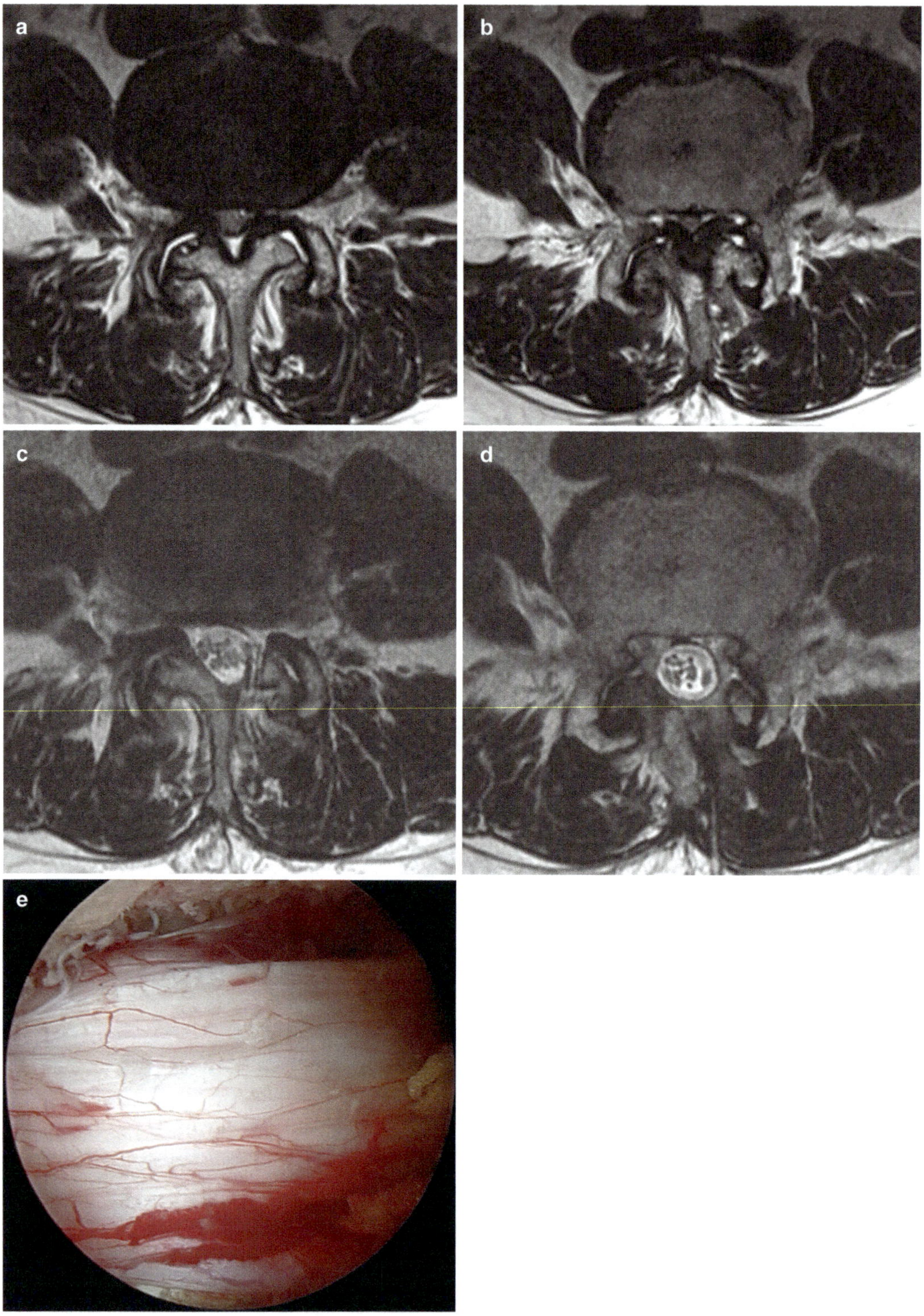

Fig. 10 Preoperative MR images show central and lateral recess stenosis of L4–5 (**a**, **b**). Postoperative MR images reveal complete decompression of central and lateral recess stenosis of L4–5 (**c**, **d**). Intraoperative endoscopic view image also demonstrated well decompression of central canal and bilateral traversing nerve roots (**e**)

the bleeding sites. A bleeding from the epidural edge just after flavectomy from the small epidural vessels could be coagulated using a small-sized RF device. If the bleeding cannot be controlled with these efforts, lowering the blood pressure to around 100 mm Hg can be helpful in some cases.

Dural tear

Several papers were reporting no differences in the incidence of complications between biportal endoscopic and microscopic groups [10]. The most common complication reported with a systematic review was a dural tear [11]. Biportal endoscopic spine surgery allows the surgical field to be viewed at high magnification, and the fluid from continuous pressure irrigation enables slight compression of the dura and widening of the contralateral epidural space during procedures. The risk of dural tear is reported to be increased in bilateral decompression procedures via a unilateral approach. Irrigation is continuous during biportal endoscopic surgery, which can make it difficult to confirm CSF leakage during the procedure. A significant dural defect should be repaired directly under the operative microscope, and small intraoperative durotomy can be resolved with the application of sealant materials and placing the patient on bed rest. The best treatment of dural tear is prevention with the exercise of several precautions. Aggressive surgical action to expose neural tissues through decompression may be harmful to the dural membrane. Instrumental manipulation of the narrow, invisible epidural space should be avoided. Keeping the cutting surface of the instruments (Kerrison punches and forceps) visible while removing structures identified by the endoscope also helps prevent dural tear.

Brief Discussion: Surgical Tip and Pitfall

For biportal endoscopic spine surgery, the axes of the endoscope and working channel are separated, making it easier for anatomical orientation and handling of instruments. The freedom of instrument angle is elevated and has made many technical advances, especially in the use of drills. Since biportal endoscopic spine surgery has a continuous water flow from the endoscopic portal to working portal, it is possible to maintain a clear view during bleeding.

From an anatomical perspective, the contralateral approach gives the most facile access to the lateral recess and intra-foraminal space. Using advantages of more freedom to manipulate instruments with biportal endoscopic spine sugery, endoscopic surgery for lumbar degenerative pathologies has been making rapid strides. Along with this, the efforts continue to find a useful and reliable classification system of lumbar spinal stenosis, which could be an index for preoperative evaluation and in determining the proper technique [12].

It was difficult to find the proper definition or criteria for the adequate decompression of spinal stenosis. The surgeon should perform surgery to keep the patient safe and to maximize the clinical results, and the spine surgeon must evaluate and take responsibility for the appropriate decompression, based on their experience and knowledge. The authors think the biportal endoscopic spine surgery has many advantages over the safety and stable outcome for the decompression of spinal stenosis.

The biportal endoscopic decompression method represents a viable option for lumbar spinal stenosis with good results. It was evolving with understanding other techniques and specialized in the benefits of the endoscopy. This biportal endoscopic technique is worth further developing and application.

References

1. Yong-Hing K, Kirkaldy-Willis WH. The pathophysiology of degenerative disease of the lumbar spine. Orthop Clin North Am. 1983;14(3):491–504.
2. Komp M, Hahn P, Oezdemir S, Giannakopoulos A, Heikenfeld R, Kasch R, et al. Bilateral spinal decompression of lumbar central stenosis with the full-endoscopic interlaminar versus microsurgical laminotomy technique: a prospective, randomized, controlled study. Pain Physician. 2015;18(1):61–70.
3. Hwa Eum J, Hwa Heo D, Son SK, Park CK. Percutaneous biportal endoscopic decompres-

sion for lumbar spinal stenosis: a technical note and preliminary clinical results. J Neurosurg Spine. 2016;24(4):602–7.
4. Kim HS, Paudel B, Jang JS, Oh SH, Lee S, Park JE, et al. Percutaneous full endoscopic bilateral lumbar decompression of spinal stenosis through Uniportal-contralateral approach: techniques and preliminary results. World Neurosurg. 2017;103:201–9.
5. Choi CM, Chung JT, Lee SJ, Choi DJ. How I do it? Biportal endoscopic spinal surgery (BESS) for treatment of lumbar spinal stenosis. Acta Neurochir. 2016;158(3):459–63.
6. Tuijthof GJ, Dusee L, Herder JL, van Dijk CN, Pistecky PV. Behavior of arthroscopic irrigation systems. Knee Surg Sports Traumatol Arthrosc. 2005;13(3):238–46.
7. Tuijthof GJ, de Vaal MM, Sierevelt IN, Blankevoort L, van der List MP. Performance of arthroscopic irrigation systems assessed with automatic blood detection. Knee Surg Sports Traumatol Arthrosc. 2011;19(11):1948–54.
8. Lee CK, Rauschning W, Glenn W. Lateral lumbar spinal canal stenosis: classification, pathologic anatomy and surgical decompression. Spine (Phila Pa 1976). 1988;13(3):313–20.
9. Chau AM, Pelzer NR, Hampton J, Smith A, Seex KA, Stewart F, et al. Lateral extent and ventral laminar attachments of the lumbar ligamentum flavum: cadaveric study. Spine J. 2014;14(10):2467–71.
10. Heo DH, Quillo-Olvera J, Park CK. Can percutaneous Biportal endoscopic surgery achieve Enough Canal decompression for degenerative lumbar stenosis? Prospective case-control study. World Neurosurg. 2018;120:e684–e9.
11. Lin GX, Huang P, Kotheeranurak V, Park CW, Heo DH, Park CK, et al. A systematic review of unilateral Biportal endoscopic spinal surgery: preliminary clinical results and complications. World Neurosurg. 2019;125:425–32.
12. Wang Y, Dou Q, Yang J, Zhang L, Yan Y, Peng Z, et al. Percutaneous endoscopic lumbar decompression for lumbar lateral Spinal Canal stenosis: classification of lateral region of lumbar Spinal Canal and surgical approaches. World Neurosurg. 2018;119:e276–e83.

Part III

Lumbar Foraminal Stenosis

Uniportal Full Endoscopic Contralateral Approach for Lumbar Foraminal Stenosis

Chang-il Ju, Hyeun Sung Kim, Pang Hung Wu, and Harshvardhan Raor

Introduction

In recent years, the incidence of spinal canal stenosis has increased steeply as the elderly population increases.

Incidence of Foraminal stenosis is proportional to increase in overall incidence of spinal canal stenosis.

Rationale of Endoscopic Contralateral Interlaminar Lumbar Foraminotomy

1. Reduce the lateral wedging instability violation (Fig. 1).
2. Triple crush decompression (Figs. 2 and 3).
3. Reduce the retraction of DRG.

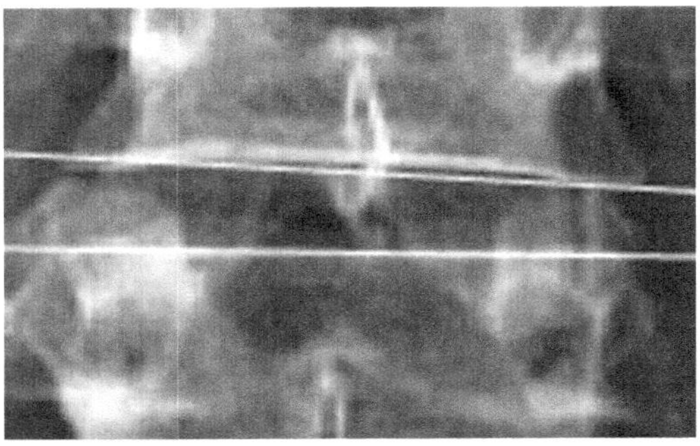

Fig. 1 Lateral wedging instability

Electronic Supplementary Material The online version of this chapter (https://doi.org/10.1007/978-981-15-8253-0_6) contains supplementary material, which is available to authorized users.

C.-i. Ju
Department of Neurosurgery, Chosun University Hospital, Gwangju, South Korea
e-mail: jchangil@chosun.ac.kr

H. S. Kim (✉) · H. Raor
Department of Neurosurgery, Nanoori Hospital Gangnam, Seoul, South Korea

P. H. Wu
Department of Neurosurgery, Nanoori Hospital Gangnam, Seoul, South Korea

National University Health Systems, JurongHealth Campus, Singapore, Singapore

H. S. Kim et al. (eds.), *Advanced Techniques of Endoscopic Lumbar Spine Surgery*,
https://doi.org/10.1007/978-981-15-8253-0_6

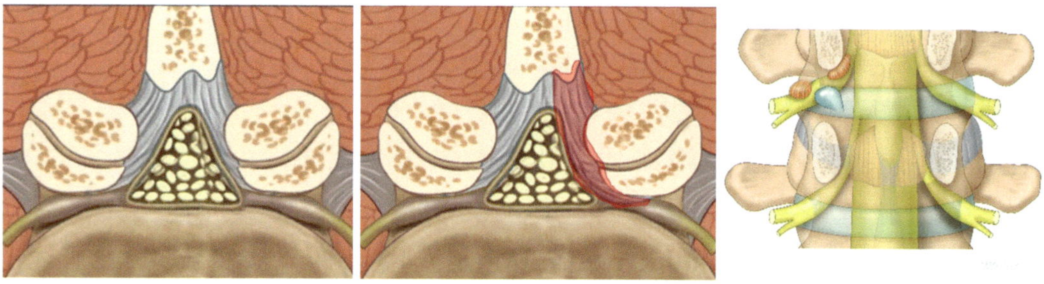

Fig. 2 Concept of triple crush compression of foraminal stenosis

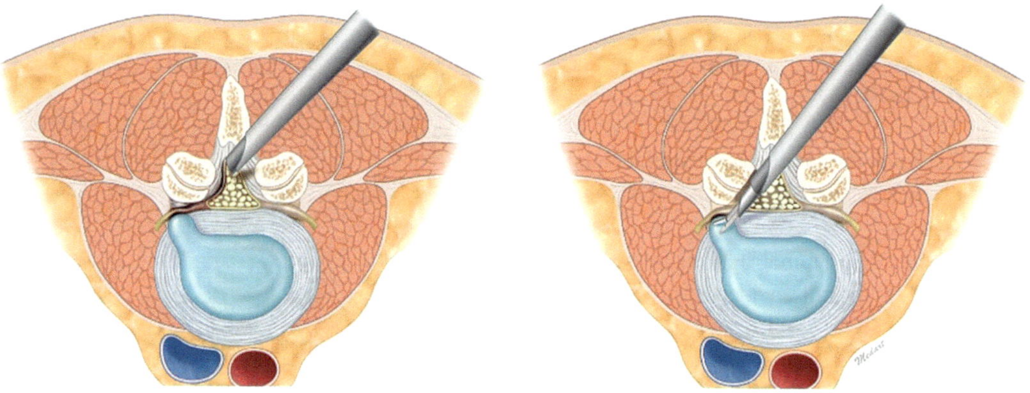

Fig. 3 Illustration of Endoscopic Contralateral Interlaminar Lumbar Foraminotomy

Three important principles to consider in endoscopic foraminal stenosis decompression are (1) successful decompression, (2) reduced neural retraction, and (3) anatomically less violation to preserve stability of facet joints.

The intervertebral foramen is bounded anteriorly by posterior wall of segmental vertebra 1 body and intervertebral disc, superiorly and inferiorly by the pedicles of cranial and caudal corresponding vertebra, and posteriorly by facet joint. Exiting nerve root and blood vessels are held in place by intervertebral foraminal ligaments (Fig. 4). Hypertrophy of any of these structures due to degenerative processes can lead to foraminal narrowing. Narrowing of foraminal dimensions can occur due to disc degeneration and overriding of superior articular facet on inferior articular facet, such loss in foraminal height traditionally are restored by interbody fusion device to jack up the foraminal height. Anterior-posterior foraminal narrowing can occur due to disc bulge, foraminal disc herniation, facet cyst or osteophyte, buckling of the ligamentum flavum, thickening of foraminal ligaments, or any combination of the above. Such narrowing is not easily corrected by restoration of foraminal height by interbody fusion. In both of the scenarios, uniportal full endoscopic contralateral approach for lumbar foraminal stenosis can provide direct decompression of the nerve with maximally preserving the patient's anatomical structures in comparison with the fusion procedure. It can also be done under epidural anesthesia with potentially wider indication to patients with multiple medical comorbidities.

The endoscopic uniportal contralateral endoscopic foraminotomy is a more advanced level of endoscopic decompression which required the

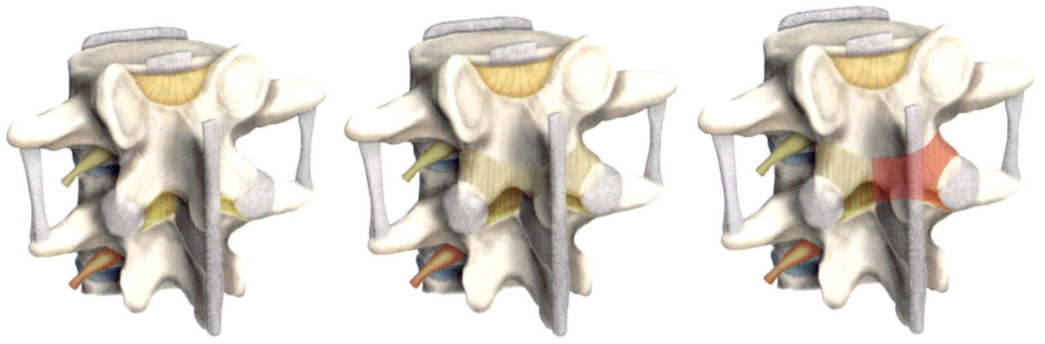

Fig. 4 Outer layer/inner layer/contralateral inner layer to foramen. Layered anatomy showing our target area of ligamentum flavum resection in red

surgeon to have background experience in endoscopic spine surgery.

We present to you the current application of uniportal full endoscopic contralateral approach for lumbar foraminal stenosis secondary to prolapsed foraminal disc (Video Reference).

Indication/Contraindication

Indication

1. Foraminal stenosis.
   (a) Presence of overriding superior articular process and narrowing of foraminal height.
   (b) Hypertrophy of the ligamentum flavum and foraminal ligament.
   (c) Disc protrusion.
   (d) Presence of osteophytes in facet joint and syndesmophytes in disc.
2. Contralateral foraminal HNP.
3. Combined foraminal and extraforaminal HNP.
4. Contralateral facetal cyst.
5. Contralateral pedicle fracture malunion.
6. Segmental instability with lateral wedging.

Contraindication

1. Infection.
2. Tumor.
3. Gross segmental instability.
4. Significant spinal deformity with poor sagittal and coronal balance.
5. Acute traumatic fracture complicated by foraminal stenosis.
6. Presence of central and/or bilateral lateral recess stenosis combined with foraminal stenosis (suitable for bilateral decompression of foraminal stenosis).

Anesthesia/Position

Anesthesia

- Epidural anesthesia with sedation
- In our institution, we use 0.75% ropivacaine mixed with equivalent amount of radiocontrast dye and 1:4,000,000 to make a concoction of epidural anesthetics. We use 10–15 mL of epidural anesthetics depending on spine levels to be done and dermatomes involved. For example, of 10 mL epidural anesthetics, we would add 5 mL 0.75% ropivacaine with 5 mL of radiocontrast dye and 1:400,000 epinephrine.
- General anesthesia
- We do not advocate doing local anesthesia with sedation in uniportal contralateral approach for contralateral foraminal decompression as direct contact of the nerve root with the dura of the neuropathic state causes severe pain in the patient. Therefore, local procedures have a high risk of surgery failure. If the patient moves, there is a high risk of nerve damage.

Position

- Prone position with Wilson frame.

Special Surgical Instrument

Basic Instrument

1. Irrigation pump.
2. C-arm image intensifier.
3. Guidewire.
4. Working channel and serial dilators with a gradual dilation of up to 10–16 mm.
5. Endoscope of a 30° viewing angle, 7.3 mm outer diameter or equivalent, and a working length of 171 mm.
6. The radiofrequency probe.
7. Endoscopic high-speed drill system typically 3.5 mm coarse diamond tip drill.
8. Endoscopic pituitary forceps.
9. Endoscopic Kerrison rongeurs.
10. Endoscopic probe.

Special Instrument

1. Flexible bend drill.
2. Side firing laser.

Both of these special equipment are seldom used by the authors of this chapter.

Surgical Steps

Anatomical Consideration

We are exploring the sublaminar space between contralateral ligamentum flavum and bony structures, namely, spinous process, lamina, inferior articular facet, and superior articular facet en route to the contralateral foramen. The 2 ligamentum flavum are separated at the midline which is filled with a slit of epidural fat which helps mark the margin of the ligamentum flavum. The other tell-tale sign of crossing into contralateral flavum is the presence of interspinous ligaments in the space at the midpoint. Our aim is to remove contralateral ligamentum flavum attachment on the ventral surface of the lower half of the cephalad vertebral lamina and attach to the dorsal surface and upper lip of caudal vertebral lamina, extending laterally to a variable distance on the ventral surface of the tip of superior articular process (Fig. 4).

Skin Marking/Skin Incision

Skin Marking

Skin Incision

(a) All aseptic precautions were maintained throughout the procedure. The image intensifier was brought into the surgical field and disc level and interlaminar space identified on posteroanterior view.
(b) Some variation of skin incision is calculated based on the midline to the extrapolated point of intersection which subtends the angle of contralateral lamina with the horizontal line on MRI. The skin incision was marked typically 1.5 cm lateral to the midline contralateral to the side of foramen to be decompressed and directed towards the side of stenosis. We check with intraoperative image intensifier with an oblique wire aiming towards the contralateral foramen. The skin incision should lie within this trajectory (Fig. 5).

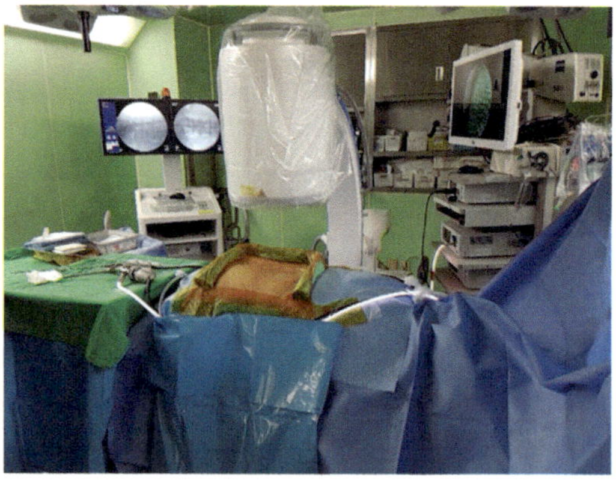

Fig. 5 Patient is in prone position for a right side approach to the left (contralateral side) foramen. Patient underwent epidural anesthesia and sedation placed on Wilson frame. C-arm, scope and video output screen are placed in position, head of the patient is on the right in this case

Approach and Docking

Docking can be done at either point A (the base of spinolaminar junction on the ipsilateral side cranial laminae) or point B (the deepest point of caudal laminae which would then move up to point A) (Figs. 6b and 7a). We start our docking with introduction of 18G spinal needle of 90 mm in length followed by blunt tip guidewire and serial dilation obturator. Once we are satisfied with docking on our AP and lateral intraoperative XR. We use endoscope for foraminal work with a 30° viewing angle, a 7.3 mm outer diameter, and a 4.7 mm working channel endoscope system of 171 mm length (Joimax GmbH) for better visualization of the foramen and lateral recess. The entire process is done under saline irrigation.

Sublaminar Approach Drilling

We typically use the sublaminar approach to contralateral foramen. Begin drilling on the ventral surface of distal spinous process and some part of interspinous ligament to get access of the working channel and drill to the contralateral sublaminar space (Figs. 6 and 9). We removed the superficial layer of the ligamentum flavum to create more working space to proficiently remove the inner layer of contralateral ligamentum flavum. Once we reached the contralateral sublaminar space, we proceed to drill inner lamina towards to contralateral ventral surface of the tip of superior articular process to detach the lateral margin of ligamentum flavum attachment (Fig. 10). Next, we drill cephalad towards the inner ventral lower half of the cephalad vertebra lamina to detach the cephalad ligamentum flavum attachment.

In patients with contralateral lateral recess stenosis, we can perform translaminar approach which would involve contralateral laminectomy (Fig. 7b).

Detachment of the Ligamentum Flavum

Follow the cranial margin of the inner layer of the ligamentum flavum and systematically detach the ligamentum flavum starting from middle to lateral attachments with endoscopic probe as shown in Fig. 10. Once the ligamentum flavum is detached.

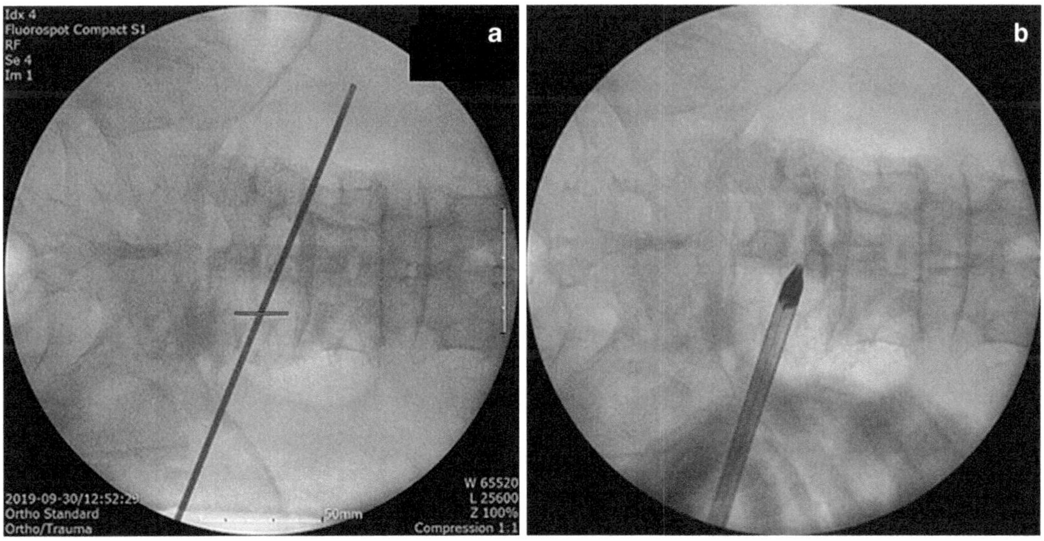

Fig. 6 (**a**) (in red) incision over the middle (for L1–4)/ medial pedicle line (for L5 and S1) and lateral edge of interlaminar window and perpendicular to end plate of caudal vertebra body. Intraoperative image of guidewire pointing towards contralateral foramen showing direction of approach to contralateral foramen. (**b**) Docking on the spinolaminar junction.

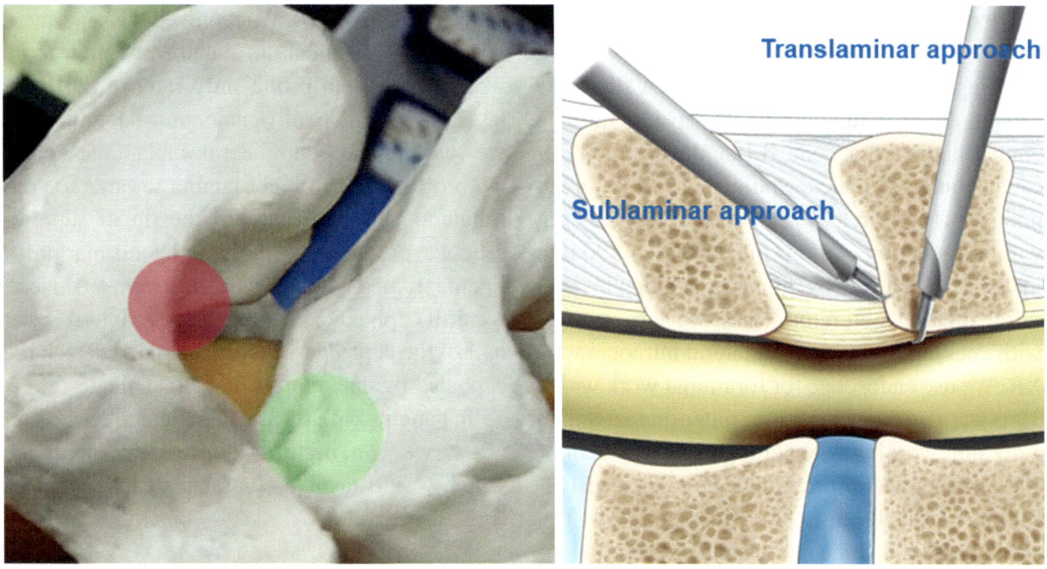

Fig. 7 (**a**) Docking sites. Point A in red: spinolaminar junction. Point B in green: deepest point of caudal lamina. (**b**) Sublaminar and translaminar approach

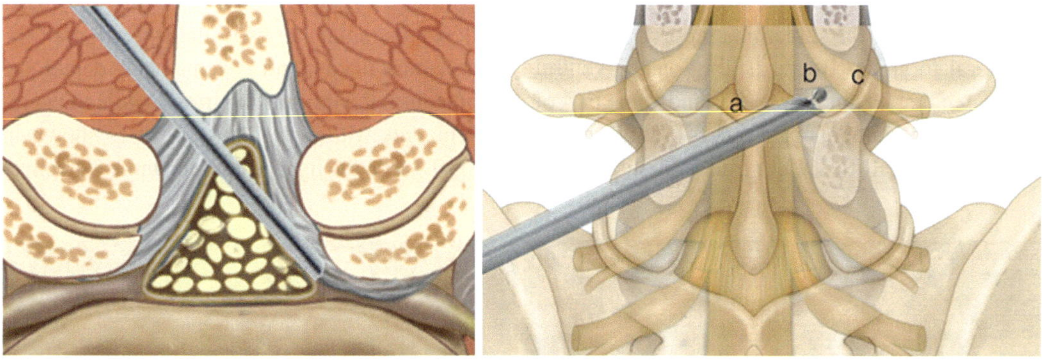

Fig. 8 Left diagram showing direction of scope to avoid inadvertent compression of neural element and detachment of the ligamentum flavum on superior articular process. Right diagram showing systematic drilling of point A, spinolaminar junction to reach the contralateral side and perform some central and lateral recess decompression; point B, ventral lower half of cephalad lamina attachment of the ligamentum flavum; and point C, ligamentum attachment on superior ventral edge of superior articular process

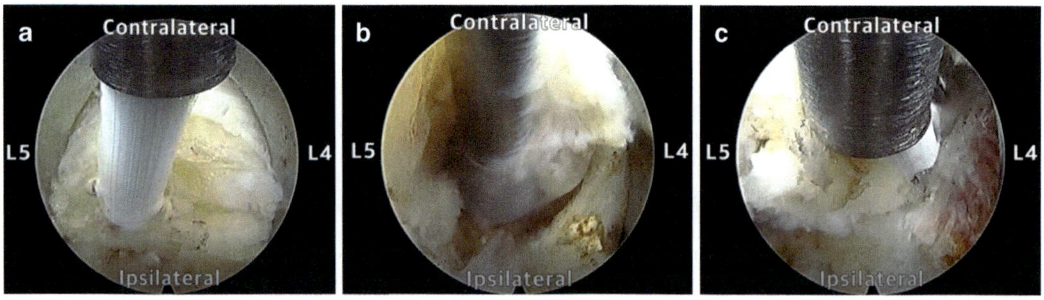

Fig. 9 Showing ipsilateral sublaminar approach with dissection of interspinous ligament (**a**), drilling of interspinous ligament and midline base of spinolaminar junction (**b**), and dissection of flavum off the midline spinolaminar junction (**c**) and Video 1

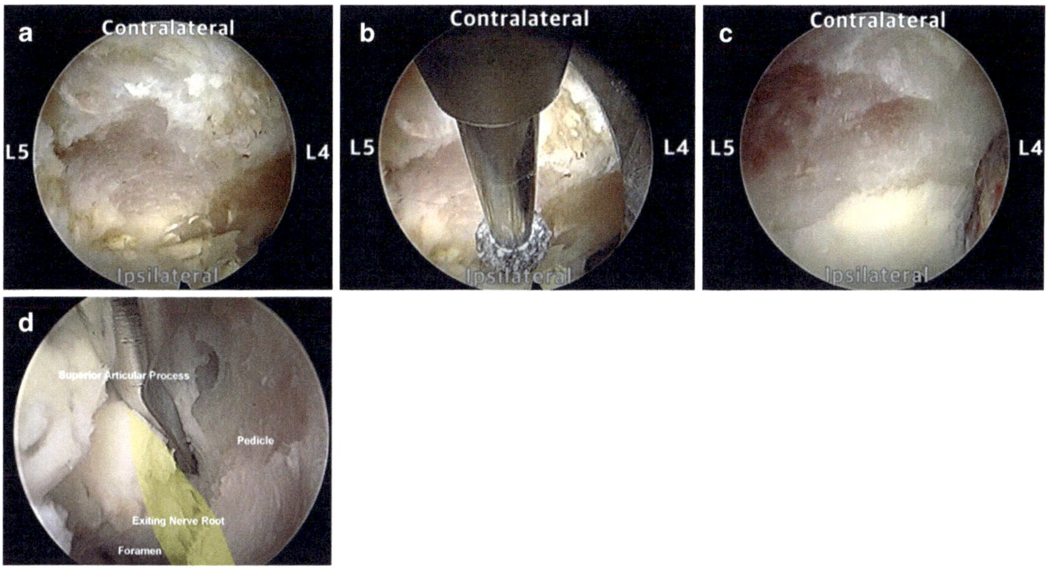

Fig. 10 Detachment of the ligamentum flavum with endoscopic probe off the superior articular process (SAP). Exposure of contralateral lamina, SAP (**a**, **b**). Using working channel to push in and stretch the ligamentum flavum attachment on SAP (**c**). Rotate and tilt the working channel and endoscope to expose the edge of superior articular process and lateral recess for decompression (**d**) (Video 2)

It is removed with endoscopic forceps. Bony and soft tissue lesions leading to foraminal stenosis is identified and decompressed systematically.

Foraminotomy

(a) Resection of foraminal ligament done with endoscopic Kerrison rongeur.
(b) Resection of inferior articular process and superior articular process done with drill (Fig. 10).
(c) Resection of foraminal disc first by coagulation with RF followed by drill and probe (Fig. 11a, b).
(d) Resection of osteophytic upper vertebrae and ventral vertebrae (Fig. 11c).

Final Confirmation Decompression of Foramen

(a) Free exiting nerve root (Fig. 11d).
(b) Checking the free lateral margin of the exiting nerve root: angle area in the lateral margin (Fig. 11e).

Illustrative Case Figures

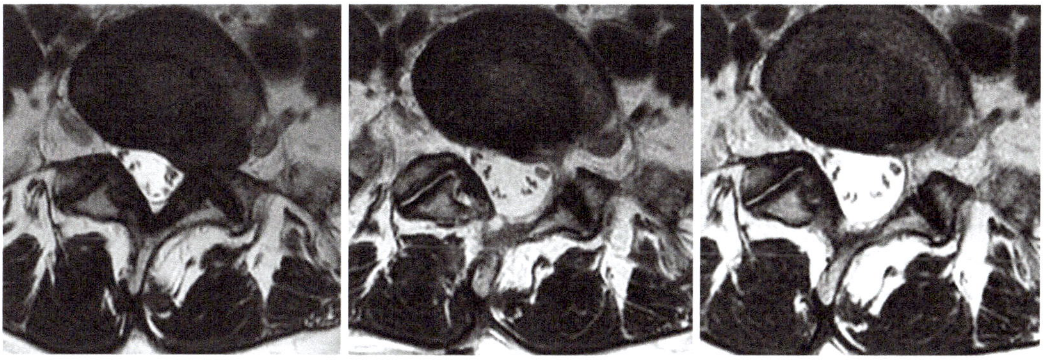

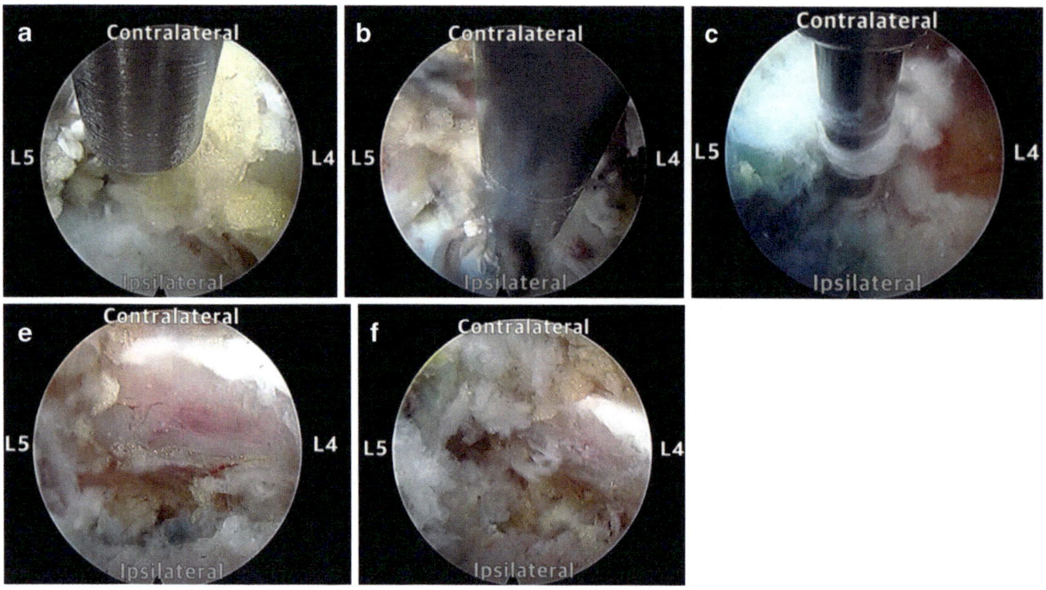

Fig. 11 Foraminal decompression. Exposure of lateral recess and disc (**a**). Discectomy (**b**). Foraminal syndesmophyte decompression (**c**). Tracing exiting nerve root out of foramen without need of retraction in ventral decompression (**d**, **e**) (Video 3)

- Preop/Postop/6 months FU.

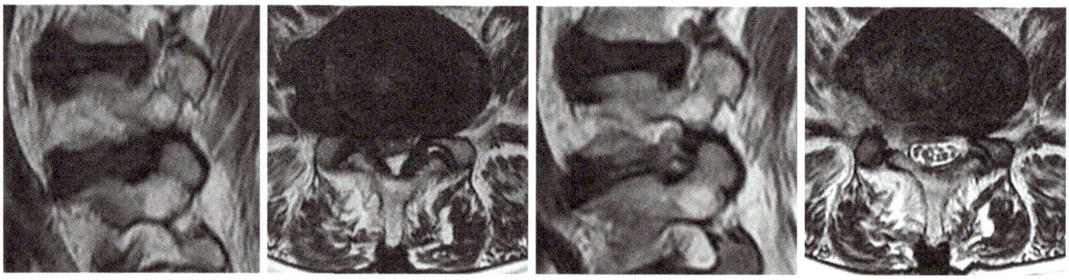

- Preop/Postop.

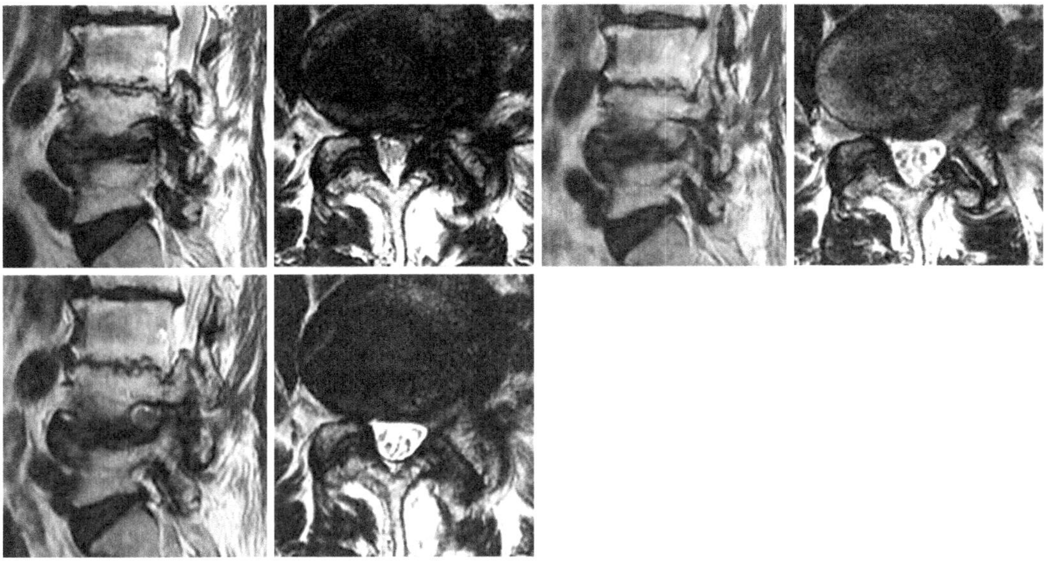

- Preop/Postop/6 months FU.

Complication/Management

1. Incomplete decompression.
   - Revision decompression.
   - Revision fusion with interbody cage.
2. Dural tear.
   - Patch blocking dural repair technique.
   - Open suture.
3. Infection.
   - Antibiotics.
   - Open decompression and drainage.
4. Recurrence.
   - Revision endoscopic decompression.
   - Fusion.
5. Instability.
   - Fusion.
6. Worsening of coronal imbalance.
   - Deformity correction.

Discussion

With the evolution of endoscopic spine surgery, foraminal stenosis treatment is very diverse at the moment. Endoscopic surgical options of foraminal stenosis are uniportal full endoscopic contralateral approach for lumbar foraminal stenosis, percutaneous full endoscopic bilateral lumbar decompression of spinal stenosis through uniportal-contralateral approach [1, 2], uniportal endoscopic transforaminal approach [3], biportal paraspinal approach, biportal contralateral approach [4], and endofusion with uniportal or biportal techniques [5]. Traditional techniques such as tubular microscopic contralateral decompression [6], open laminectomy and foraminotomy, Wiltse tubular approach and/or open posterolateral approach for decompression and/or fusion, and indirect decompression by anterior/lateral approach fusion techniques are other options for spine surgeons who are not practicing endoscopic technique [7]. A wide diversity of options suggest that there is no gold standard as many factors affect the outcome of surgery. For uniportal full endoscopic contralateral approach for lumbar foraminal stenosis, a certain level of endoscopic experience will be paramount to produce consistent good outcomes. In our opinion among these options, uniportal full endoscopic contralateral approach for lumbar foraminal stenosis is superior in conservation of the native anatomy with main focus on direct decompression of the elements which caused foraminal stenosis.

Some tips and pitfalls applied in this technique are:

1. Create sufficient sublaminar working space for the drill and working channel to allow contralateral ligamentum flavum resection without pressure of retraction and compression of the ligamentum flavum and underlying dura.
2. Contralateral lateral recess decompression with Kerrison punch on superior articular process can be challenging; we need to tilt and rotate the scope with full view of traversing nerve root and pointing punch away from the nerve root (Fig. 8).
3. When there is significant foraminal stenosis, drilling of the ventral syndesmophyte of the adjacent vertebra bodies and discectomy should be done to create space ventral to the exiting nerve root rather than excessive retraction of the nerve root.
4. Check intraoperative image when crossing the midline and when completion of foraminal stenosis. It can be confusing especially for beginners on the adequacy of contralateral decompression.
5. If lateral wedging and overriding superior articular facet is secondary to lateral listhesis and instability, fusion surgery should be considered instead of decompression.

Summary

The management of foraminal stenosis of the nerve root by uniportal full endoscopic contralateral approach for lumbar foraminal stenosis provides effective and safe decompression with facet joint preservation and other benefits of the minimally invasive spine procedure [2, 8].

References

1. Zygourakis CC, DiGiorgio AM, Crutcher CL, Safaee M, Nicholls FH, Dalle Ore C, et al. The safety and efficacy of CT-guided, fluoroscopy-free Vertebroplasty in adult spinal deformity surgery. World Neurosurg. 2018;116:e944–e50.
2. Kim H-SMDP, Paudel BMDMS, JSMDP J, SHMDP O, Lee SBE, Park JEBS, et al. Percutaneous full endoscopic bilateral lumbar decompression of spinal stenosis through Uniportal-contralateral approach: techniques and preliminary results. World Neurosurg. 2017;103:201–9.
3. Kim HS, Sharma SB, Raorane HD. How I do it? Transforaminal endoscopic decompression of intraspinal facet cyst. Acta Neurochir. 2019;161(9):1895–900.
4. Heo DH, Kim JS, Park CW, Park CK, Quillo-Olvera J. Contralateral sublaminar endoscopic approach for removal of lumbar Juxtafacet cysts using percutaneous Biportal endoscopic surgery: technical report and preliminary results. World Neurosurg. 2019;122:474–9.
5. Son SK, Park WW, Choi SH, Ahn Y, Youn MS, Heo DH. Endoscopic transforaminal lumbar interbody fusion: a comprehensive review. Neurosurg Rev. 2019;16(5):373–80.
6. Yamada K, Matsuda H, Cho H, Habunaga H, Kono H, Nakamura H. Clinical and radiological outcomes of microscopic partial pediculectomy for degenerative lumbar foraminal stenosis. Spine. 2013;38(12):E723–E31.
7. Orita S, Inage K, Eguchi Y, Kubota G, Aoki Y, Nakamura J, et al. Lumbar foraminal stenosis, the hidden stenosis including at L5/S1. Eur J Orthop Surg Traumatol. 2016;26(7):685–93.
8. Hwang JHMD, Park CWMDP. Contralateral interlaminar keyhole percutaneous endoscopic surgery in patients with unilateral radiculopathy: technical notes. World Neurosurg. 2017;

Lumbar Foraminal Stenosis: Full Endoscopic Transforaminal Approach

Sang-Ha Shin, Jun Seok Bae, and Jun Ho Lee

Introduction (Key Point and Purpose) of Approach

Open foraminal decompression with/without fusion has been performed as a standard surgical treatment for lumbar foraminal stenosis. Total facetectomy provides complete nerve decompression but often leads to spinal instability and usually requires additional fixation [1–3]. Wiltse et al. [4] reported a paraspinal approach as a method for decompression of foraminal stenosis. Because this technique preserves much of the facet joint, it is now widely used as a standard surgical treatment for decompression in patients with foraminal stenosis.

The full endoscopic transforaminal approach has less muscle trauma and less blood loss than open decompression. It can also be done under local anesthesia. Thus, reduced hospital stay, early functional recovery, and better cosmesis are shown [5, 6]. With the desire of patients and the development of endoscopic instruments, the transforaminal approach is gaining in popularity. To date, endoscopic transforaminal decompression has been predominantly performed in patients with disc herniation. For spinal stenosis, endoscopic working mobility is limited due to foraminal bony structure and exiting nerve root [7–10]. Recently reported endoscopic approach through extraforaminal landing enables working mobility after partial removal of superior articular process. After that, it was possible to approach the foraminal zone safely and to treat decompression for foraminal stenosis. We will describe this technique in this chapter.

Indication and Contraindication

Indication

This technique can be applied to patients with foraminal stenosis who do not respond to preservation therapy and whose symptoms persist. It is appropriate to perform in patients with unilateral radicular symptom.

Contraindication

This technique is not appropriate in patients with segmental instability or spondylolisthesis. In

Electronic Supplementary Material The online version of this chapter (https://doi.org/10.1007/978-981-15-8253-0_7) contains supplementary material, which is available to authorized users.

S.-H. Shin (✉) · J. S. Bae
Department of Neurosurgery, Wooridul Spine Hospital, Seoul, South Korea
e-mail: burrhoer@wooridul.co.kr

J. H. Lee
Department of Neurosurgery, Kyung Hee University Hospital, Seoul, South Korea
e-mail: moo9924@khu.ac.kr

H. S. Kim et al. (eds.), *Advanced Techniques of Endoscopic Lumbar Spine Surgery*,
https://doi.org/10.1007/978-981-15-8253-0_7

these cases, fusion surgery should be considered. It is also difficult to apply to patients with profound motor weakness or revision surgery. Approach is also difficult in patients with high iliac crest at L5/S1 level. Coexisting pathological conditions such as acute inflammation, infection, or tumor can also be difficult to apply.

Anesthesia and Position

Endoscopic foraminal decompression can be performed under local anesthesia. Midazolam or fentanyl may be given intravenously to relieve pain and sedation during procedure. The degree of sedation is controlled to respond to the physician's verbal command during the procedure. The patient is placed in the prone position after flexion of the knee and hip on the radiolucent table with fluoroscopic guidance. Knee and hip flexion postures provide foraminal widening to provide a wider working space during decompression.

Special Surgical Instruments

Unlike disc herniation, in patients with foraminal stenosis, the target of removal is not a soft cartilage but a bony structure or thickened foraminal ligament. Endoscopic drills, bone reamers, shavers, etc., can be used to remove bony structures (Fig. 1). And endoscopic punches or lasers are useful for the removal of thickened ligamentum flavum. Also, endoscopic scissor or endoscopic probe may be useful for dissection between the exiting nerve root and the surrounding tissue.

Surgical Steps

Preoperative MRI should be carefully checked to determine the appropriate skin entry point and approaching angle. The distance from the midline to the skin entry point can be calculated in the axial image of the MRI, usually 6–13 cm. The appropriate approach angle is determined by the location of the lesion. An angle of about 15° is recommended for the decompression of the subarticular zone and an angle of about 30–45° for the decompression of the foraminal or extraforaminal zone.

After determining the proper approach angle and skin entry point, insert an 18 gauge spinal needle under the superior articular process using a fluoroscope. Then insert the guide wire and place the obturator into the foramen. Along the obturator, the bevel-ended working cannula is introduced and placed on the undersurface of the

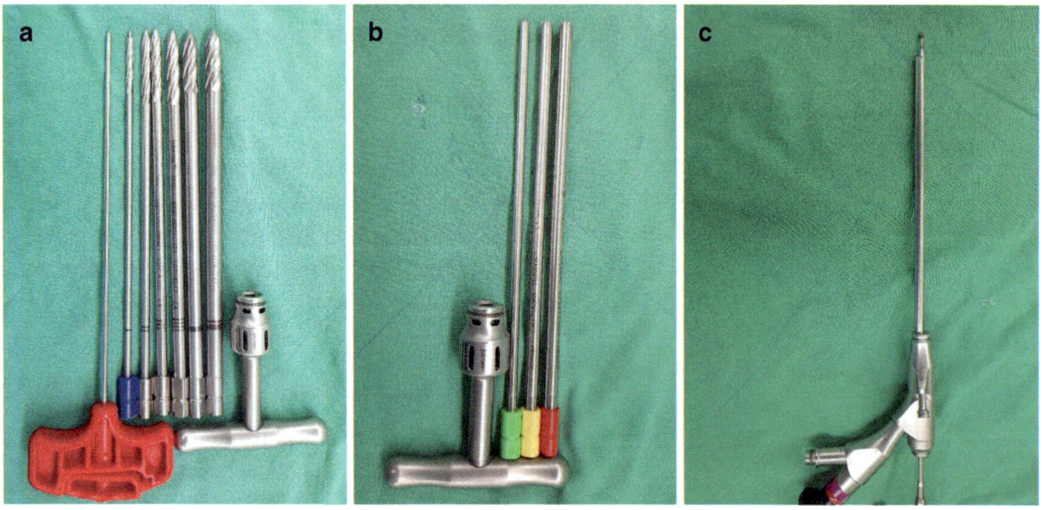

Fig. 1 special surgical instrument used for endoscopic foraminotomy. (**a**) Manual bone drill. (**b**) Manual bone reamer. (**c**) Electrical endoscopic drill

facet joint. The obturator is removed and the ellipsoidal working channel endoscope is inserted. The surgeon can see the superior facet through endoscopic visualization. Hypertrophied part of facet joints can be safely removed using an endoscopic burr or bone reamer with both endoscopic and fluoroscopic guidance. The direction of the bone removal should be from the outside to the inside and form the inferior pedicle to the superior pedicle. If resistance is lost during facet joint undercutting, bone work can be stopped and then foraminal ligament can be observed. When the foraminal ligament is removed, the perineural fat, exiting nerve root, traction spur, and disc surface can be observed. While moving the working cannula, decompression may be selectively carried out to the desired area. Hypertrophied foraminal ligaments can be removed using endoscopic punches, graspers, or scissors, and extruded discs or soft tissues can be coagulated or ablation using bipolar radiofrequency. Holmium:yttrium-aluminum-garnet (HO: YAG) lasers can provide clear vision by removing tissue debris. After decompression, the surgeon can fully observe the course of the exiting nerve root from the pedicle medial margin to the extraforaminal area through endoscopic vision. The endpoint of this procedure is when the exiting nerve root is observed free of the surrounding structure (Fig. 2). After complete decompression, the endoscope is

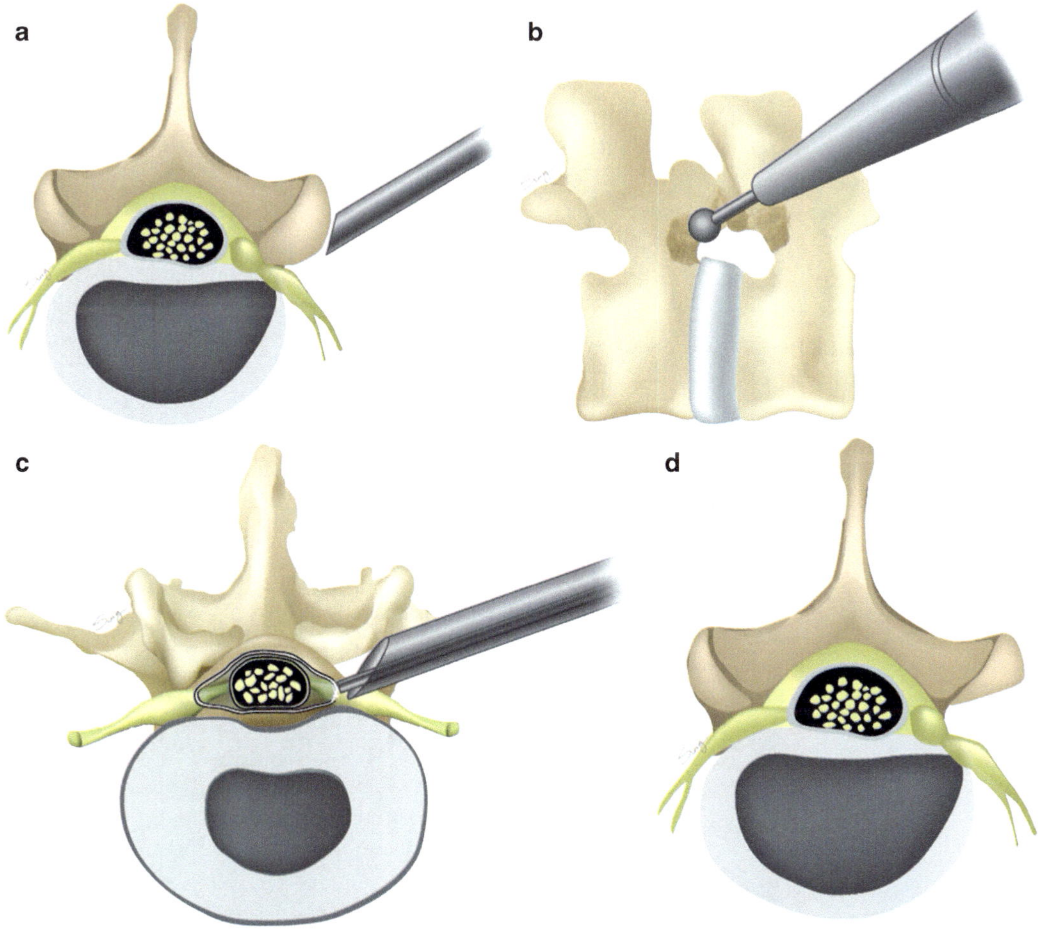

Fig. 2 Schematic illustrations of endoscopic foraminal decompression. (**a**) Extraforaminal landing of working cannula. (**b**) Undercutting of facet joint using endoscopic drill. (**c**) Selective foraminal decompression. (**d**) Confirmation of full decompression along the course of exiting nerve root

removed and wound closure is performed. After several hours of observation, the patient can be discharged.

Illustrated Cases

Case 1

A 54-year-old female patient presented with left leg pain. Preoperative magnetic resonance (MR) image demonstrated foraminal stenosis caused by hypertrophied ligamentum flavum and facet joint (Fig. 3a). After endoscopic foraminotomy, the patient's symptom improved and postoperative MR image showed complete decompression of foramen (Fig. 3b) (Video 1).

Case 2

A 58-year-old male patient presented with right leg pain. Preoperative magnetic resonance (MR) image demonstrated foraminal stenosis caused by osteophytic spur (Fig. 4a). After endoscopic foraminotomy, the patient's symptom improved and postoperative MR and CT images showed complete decompression of foramen (Fig. 4b) (Video 2).

Complication and its Management

Excessive manipulation or irritation of the dorsal root ganglion during foraminal decompression can lead to postoperative dysesthesia.

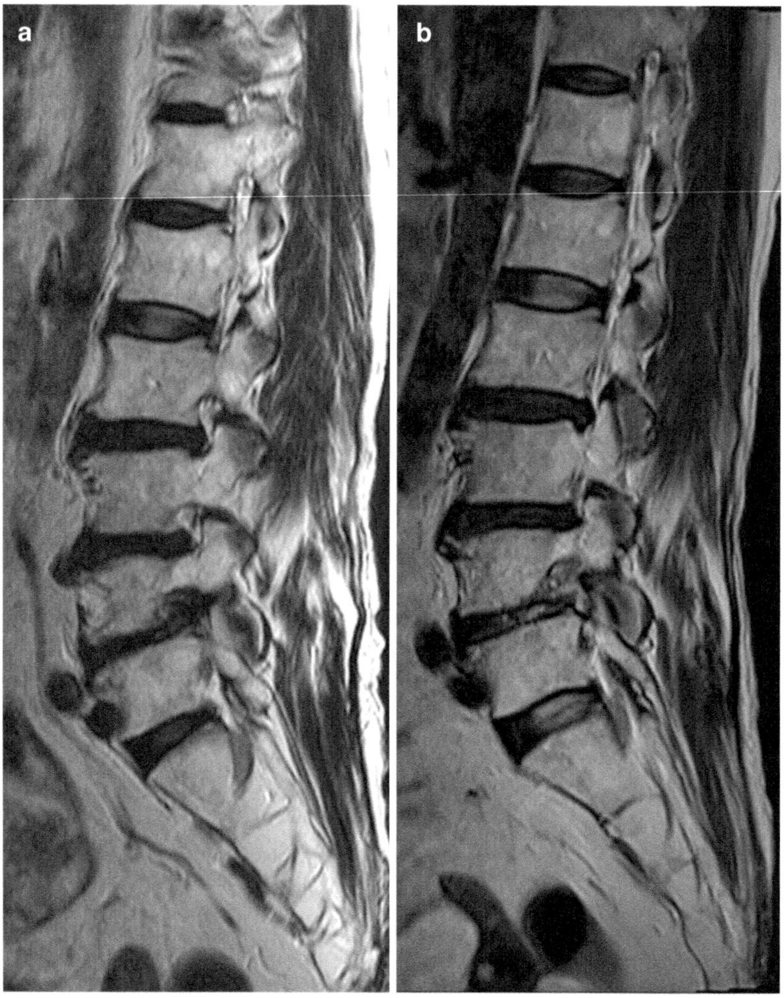

Fig. 3 (**a**) Preoperative magnetic resonance (MR) image showing foraminal stenosis caused by hypertrophied ligamentum flavum and facet joint. (**b**) Postoperative MR image showed complete decompression of foramen

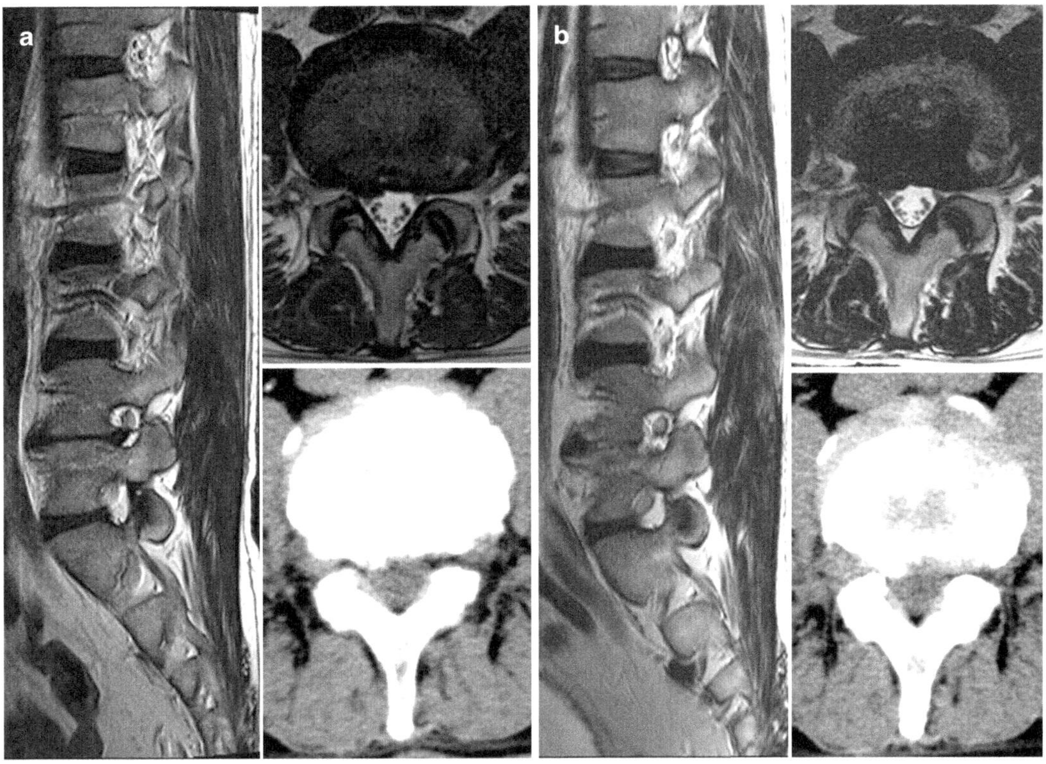

Fig. 4 (**a**) Preoperative MR image showing foraminal stenosis caused by osteophytic spur. (**b**) Postoperative MR and computed tomography images showing complete decompression of foramen

Postoperative dysesthesia can occur from 6.5% to 24% [1, 2]. Most patients improve gradually with conservative treatments such as nerve root blocks or medication therapy.

The posterior lateral transforaminal approach has limited working mobility and narrower vision than the open paraspinal approach. Thus, incomplete decompression may occur. In patients with pain that persists after endoscopic decompression, fusion surgery is usually needed.

Postoperative hematoma can also occur after endoscopic decompression. This can be reduced by the use of meticulous bleeding control and hemostatic agents during the procedure. Bone bleeding may occur after bone resection, which is difficult to control using endoscopic instruments. If there is uncontrolled bone bleeding, a drainage tube can be inserted and removed when the volume of blood decreases during the postoperative period [7].

Brief Discussion: Surgical Tip and Pitfall

The main target of decompression of endoscopic foraminotomy is the structures that compress the exiting nerve root. Therefore, the surgeon needs to identify the exiting nerve root and proceed with decompression along its course. For safe foraminal decompression, it is important to approach the foramen after a partial resection of the superior articular process after landing into the superior articular process of the extraforaminal area. In patients with foraminal stenosis, the working zone is very narrow, and there is a risk of nerve damage when the working cannula is inserted directly into the foramen without partial decompression of the facet. When working on the bone, use a drill or reamer to fully expose the lower margin of the upper pedicle and the upper margin of the lower pedicle under the guidance of fluoroscope and endoscope. Partial resection of the superior articular process only at the disc level may be insufficient to expose the proximal part of the exiting nerve root.

After access to the foramen, full-scale foraminal decompression along the exiting nerve root can be performed using a variety of surgical instruments. Instruments such as endoscopic burrs, bone reamers, punches, forceps, and lasers can be used for selective decompression under high-resolution endoscopic vision.

References

1. Shin S-H, Choi W-G, Hwang B-W, et al. Microscopic anterior foraminal decompression combined with anterior lumbar interbody fusion. Spine J. 2013;13:1190–9.
2. Ahn Y, Oh HK, Kim H, et al. Percutaneous endoscopic lumbar foraminotomy: an advanced surgical technique and clinical outcomes. Neurosurgery. 2014;75:124–33. discussion 32-3
3. Nellensteijn J, Ostelo R, Bartels R, et al. Transforaminal endoscopic surgery for lumbar stenosis: a systematic review. Eur Spine J. 2010;19:879–86.
4. Wiltse L, Spencer C. New uses and refinements of the paraspinal approach to the lumbar spine. Spine. 1988;13:696–706.
5. Shin S-H, Hwang B-W, Keum H-J, et al. Epidural steroids after a percutaneous endoscopic lumbar discectomy. Spine. 2015;40:E859–E65.
6. Ahn Y. Percutaneous endoscopic decompression for lumbar spinal stenosis. Expert Rev Med Devices. 2014;11:605–16.
7. Shin S-H, Bae J-S, Lee S-H, et al. Transforaminal endoscopic decompression for lumbar spinal stenosis: a novel surgical technique and clinical outcomes. World Neurosurg. 2018;114:e873–e82.
8. Evins AI, Banu MA, Njoku I Jr, et al. Endoscopic lumbar foraminotomy. J Clin Neurosci. 2015;22:730–4.
9. Li ZZ, Hou SX, Shang WL, et al. Percutaneous lumbar foraminoplasty and percutaneous endoscopic lumbar decompression for lateral recess stenosis through transforaminal approach: technique notes and 2 years follow-up. Clin Neurol Neurosurg. 2016;143:90–4.
10. Wen B, Zhang X, Zhang L, et al. Percutaneous endoscopic transforaminal lumbar spinal canal decompression for lumbar spinal stenosis. Medicine (Baltimore). 2016;95:e5186.

Full Endoscopic Paraspinal Approach for Lumbar Foraminal Stenosis

Chul Woo Lee, Dong-Chan Lee, and Yadhu Kasetti Lokanath

Introduction

Lumbar foraminal stenosis (LFS) is one of the common pathological conditions presenting as radicular leg pain. LFS is defined as the narrowing of bony exit of the nerve root caused by several pathological conditions such as diminishing disc height, osteoarthritis of the facet joint, buckling of the ligamentum flavum (LF), spondylolisthesis or protrusion of the annulus fibrosus [1].

Decompressive surgery for symptomatic foraminal stenosis can be performed in many ways.

The gold standard approaches to treat LFS include simple decompression via classic Wiltse approach [2] or lumbar interbody fusion. To overcome the limitations of these techniques, minimally invasive techniques were adopted as an alternative procedure such as tubular or endoscopic decompression [3, 4]. The ideal approach should provide direct access to the foramen with maximal benefit to patient by minimal facet resection and reduced muscle injury. Endoscopic approaches are said to have many merits such as less postoperative pain, short hospital stay and early return to normal life due to its minimal invasiveness [5]. However, it has certain challenges like feasibility of approaches and limitation in manoeuvring the instruments and achieving direct complete adequate decompression for LFS. Endoscopic decompressive surgery uses three different approaches (transforaminal, contralateral interlaminar and paraspinal) [4, 6, 7]. Each approach has its pros and cons.

Endoscopic paraspinal approach follows the same anatomical principle of classic Wiltse approach which provides thorough decompression of whole length of exiting nerve root from pedicle to extraforaminal area. However, minimal invasiveness of endoscope goes on to have more favorable outcome than traditional approach. More easy and comfortable handling of endoscopic instruments due to relative short surgical corridor and various operative angles is also another advantage of endoscopic paraspinal approach compared to other endoscopic approaches. We describe the whole concept and practical details of endoscopic paraspinal approach.

Electronic Supplementary Material The online version of this chapter (https://doi.org/10.1007/978-981-15-8253-0_8) contains supplementary material, which is available to authorized users.

C. W. Lee
Department of Neurosurgery, St. Peter's Hospital, Seoul, South Korea

D.-C. Lee (✉)
Department of Neurosurgery, Anyang Wiltse Memorial Hospital, Anyang-Si, Gyeonggi-Do, South Korea

Y. K. Lokanath
Department of Neurosurgery, Aster RV Hospital, Bangalore, Karnataka, India

H. S. Kim et al. (eds.), *Advanced Techniques of Endoscopic Lumbar Spine Surgery*, https://doi.org/10.1007/978-981-15-8253-0_8

Indication and Contraindication

Indication

1. Unilateral radiculopathy correlated with pure foraminal stenosis (bone spur, facet hypertrophy, flavum hypertrophy, spondylolisthesis).
2. Extraforaminal or foraminal disc herniations.

Contraindication

1. Relative contraindication.
   (a) Low-grade listhesis (grade I).
   (b) Combined spinal canal pathology (central canal and paracentral disc herniations, lateral recess stenosis).
   (c) Foraminal stenosis in adjacent segment disease.
   (d) Scoliosis and coronal plane deformity.
2. Definitive contradictions.
   (a) Dynamic instability.
   (b) Infection.
   (c) Tumours.
   (d) High-grade listhesis (grade II or more).

Anaesthesia and Position

1. General anaesthesia.
   - The primary option.
   - Easy control of patient's vital parameters (such as blood pressure, heart rate, and repiration).
   - Avoid patient's unexpected response.
2. Epidural anaesthesia with sedation.
   - Medically compromised, old-aged patients.
3. The patient is placed in prone position on a bolster (Fig. 1).
4. Special surgical instruments (Fig. 2).

Surgical Steps

Preoperative Targeting by Needle

1. Preoperative use of fluoroscopy to check the operative level and *planning the working trajectory.*
2. Initial approach target is the junction of pars and inferior margin of transverse process (TP). The tip of the needle should be located at the dorsal part of pars in lateral X-ray image and at the inferolateral margin of the pedicle in AP (anteroposterior) X-ray (Fig. 3).

Skin Incision

1 cm vertical skin incision on the symptomatic side 6 to 7 cm lateral from the midline, targeting lateral 1/third of transverse process (TP) (Fig. 4) which provides a trajectory angle of 60–70°.

Sequential Dilation and Working Cannula Insertion

1. Palpating the TP by first dilator and then sliding down to trace the inferior margin of the TP to find the junction between TP and pars by probing in semicircular fashion (Fig. 5a).

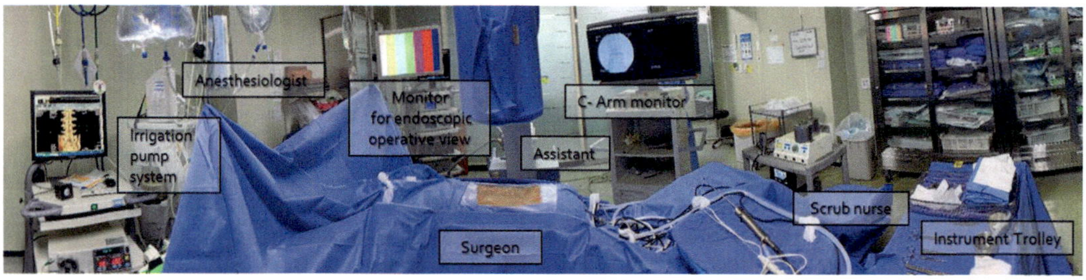

Fig. 1 Operative position and set-up in operating room

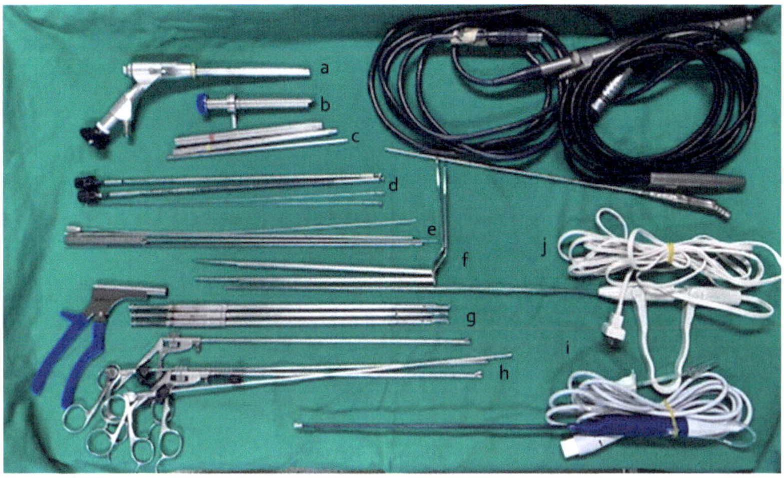

Fig. 2 Instruments for endoscopic paraspinal approach. (**a**) Endoscopy (whole length, 125 mm; outer diameter, 10 mm; working channel diameter, 6 mm). (**b**) Working cannula (outer diameter: 11.5 mm). (c) Serial dilators (3, 7, 10 mm). (**d**) Endoscopic burrs and drills—RPM 16,000–20,000, burr diameter 2.5–5.0 mm, cutting and diamond types. (**e**) Endoscopic hooks and flexible dissector probe. (**f**) Nerve root retractor. (**g**) Kerrison punches (variable sizes). (**h**) Endoscopic forceps and cutter. (**i**) Radio frequency probe. (**j**) Ellman RF coagulator

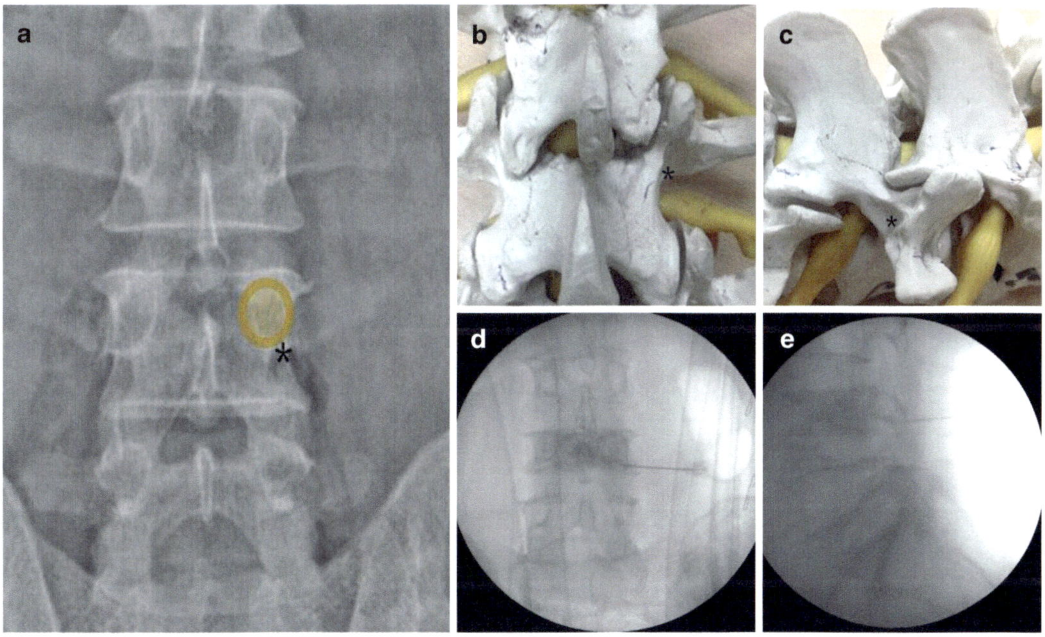

Fig. 3 Targeting by needle: yellow circle, pedicle; asterisk, target at the junction of pars and transverse process in (**a**) X-ray AP and (**b**, **c**) 3D spine model. The tip of the needle was placed at the initial target in (**d**, **e**) C-arm AP and Lat(lateral) images

2. Avoid aggressive scraping or dissection around the TP and pars to prevent undue aggressive bleeding from the branch of the radicular artery.
3. Once the working cannula position is confirmed on C-arm images (Fig. 5b, c), endoscopy is introduced under water irrigation system.

Confirmation of Anatomical Landmark and Initial Circumferential Bony Decompression

1. Using radio frequency (RF) probe, soft tissue is dissected to expose the TP and pars of superior vertebrae and lateral part of superior articular process (SAP) of inferior vertebrae.

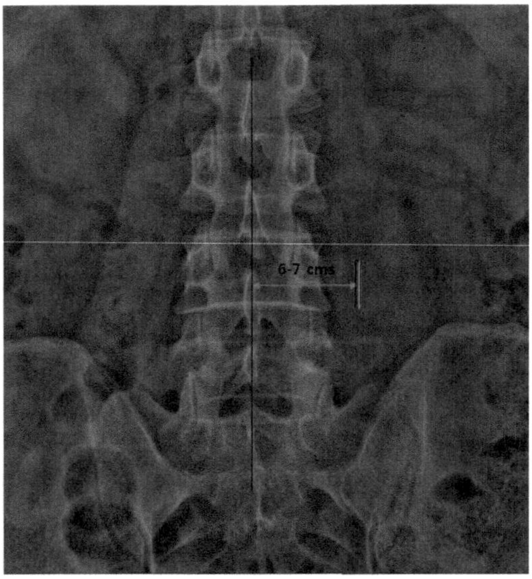

Fig. 4 Skin incision (red line) in X-ray AP image

2. Circumferential decompression around TP, pars lastly cranial tip of SAP is performed by endoscopic drill under direct endoscopic vision (Fig. 6).

The Removal of LF and Peri-eural Adhesiolysis

En bloc or piece meal removal of the intertransverse membrane and the ligamentum flavum to expose the exiting root (ER) (Fig. 7a). Soft tissue dissection and adhesiolysis around ER are performed (Fig. 7b).

Additional Decompression

Additional decompression including redundant disc material/additional removal of flavum in the axial area of the exiting root (Fig. 8a); if required, pediculotomy or bone spur or superior part of the vertebral body can be resected. The entire length of the ER should be decompressed from distal to proximal and from pedicle to extraforaminal area (Fig. 8b).

Haemostasis and Closure

Complete haemostasis should be achieved. Drain insertion in all cases followed by closure (Fig. 9).

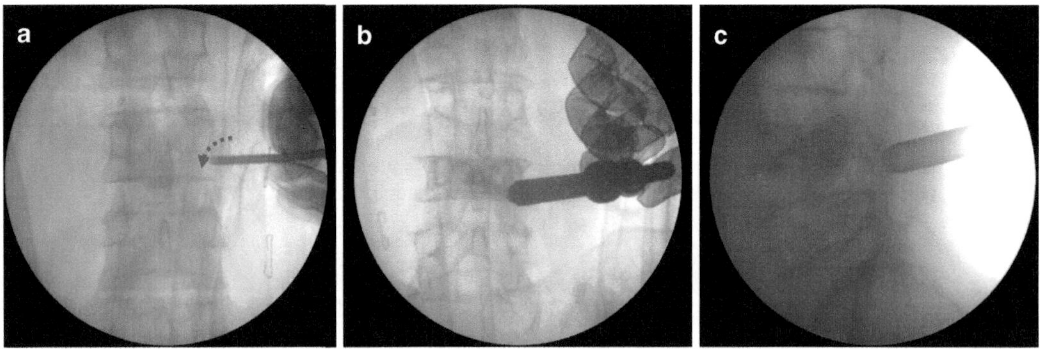

Fig. 5 (**a**) Initial first dilator was docked with scraping manoeuvre (blue dotted arrow). (**b, c**) Final position of working cannula in C-arm AP and Lat images

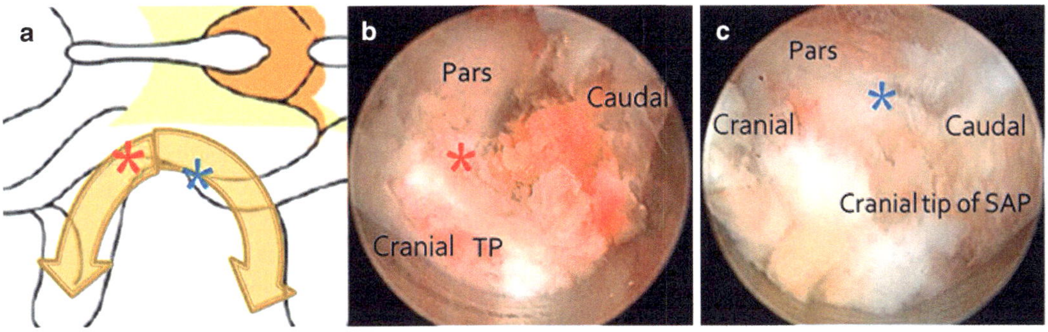

Fig. 6 Circumferential drilling on initial key structures such as transverse process (TP), pars and superior articular process (SAP) is performed. (**a**) Schematic drawing. (**b**, **c**) Endoscopic view. Red asterisk: junction of TP and pars. Blue asterisk: junction of superior and inferior articular process

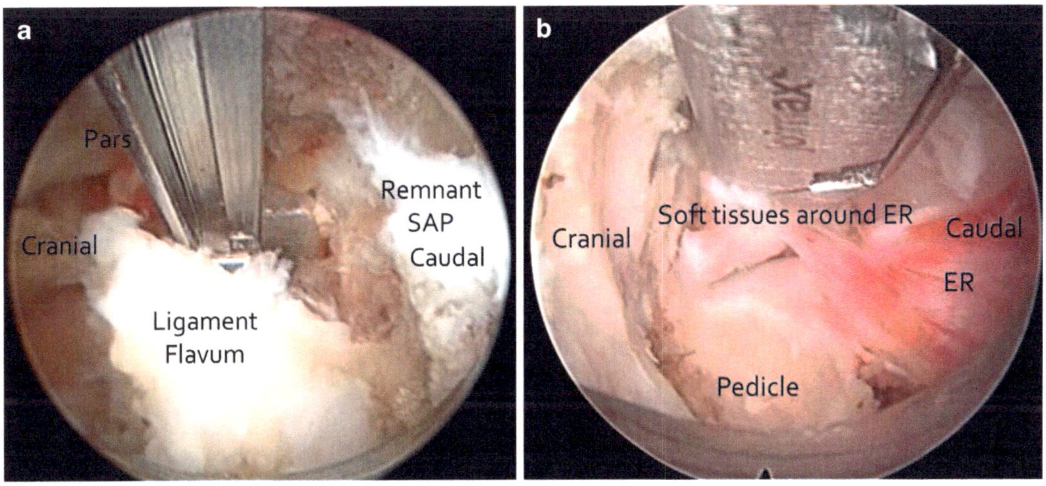

Fig. 7 (**a**) (Video 1) Removal of the ligamentum flavum and (**b**) (Video 2) adhesiolysis of the exiting nerve root (ER) from around soft tissues

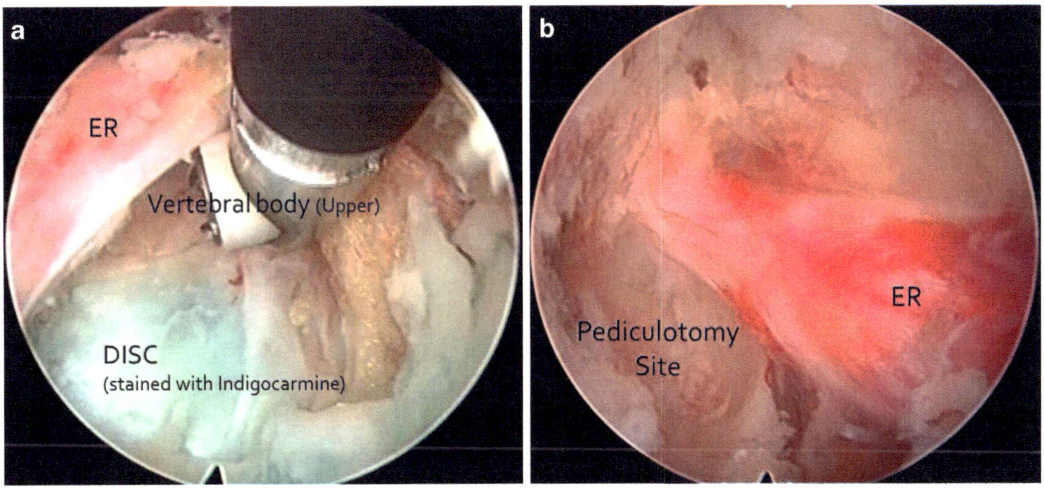

Fig. 8 (**a**) (Video 3) Decompression under the axilla area of the exiting root is examined with the shrinkage of redundant disc. (**b**) (Video 4) Fully decompressed exiting root is exposed from pedicle to extraforaminal area

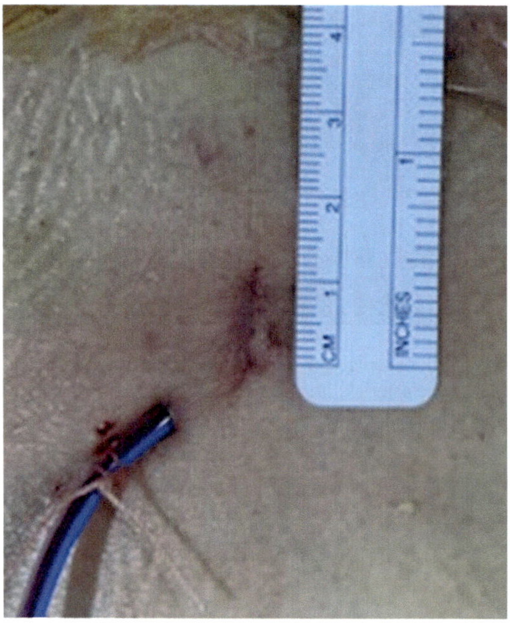

Fig. 9 Skin closure and drain

Illustrated Cases

Case 1: Extraforaminal Disc Herniation

A 49-year-old, man who had previous surgical history of laminectomy and discectomy at L4–L5 presented with back pain and right anterior thigh pain. He was unable to walk due to severe pain. On examination, VAS score was 5 and 8 for back and leg pain, with hip flexion weakness of grade 3 on right side. Routine X-ray revealed no evidence of instability and MRI showed right extraforaminal disc compressing the exiting nerve root on L3–4 level (Fig. 10a, b). Patient underwent endoscopic paraspinal decompression with discectomy (Fig. 10c, d). Postoperatively, the patient had resolution of leg pain, ambulating with no features of immediate postoperative instability on X-rays, and

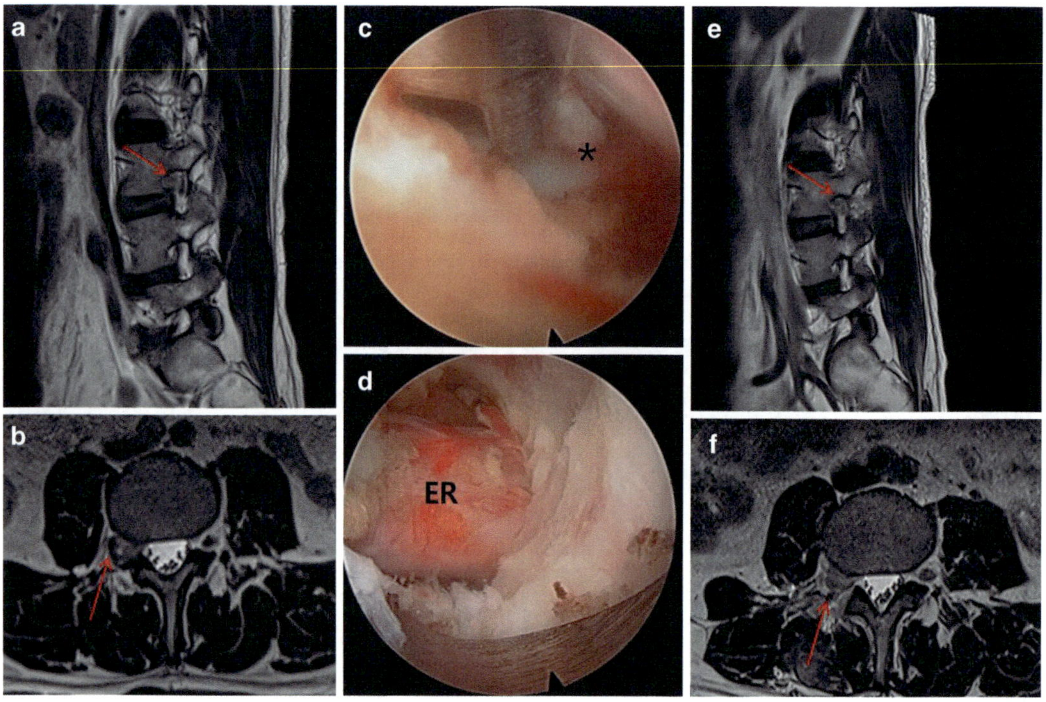

Fig. 10 (**a**, **b**) MRI T2 sagittal and axial images demonstrating extraforaminal disc herniation compressing the exiting nerve root (red arrow). (**c**, **d**) Intraoperative endoscopic view showing ruptured disc and decompressed exiting root. (**e**, **f**) Postoperative MRI showing resection of part of SAP and decompressed nerve by removal of herniated disc (red arrow). Asterisk, ruptured disc material; ER, decompressed exiting nerve root

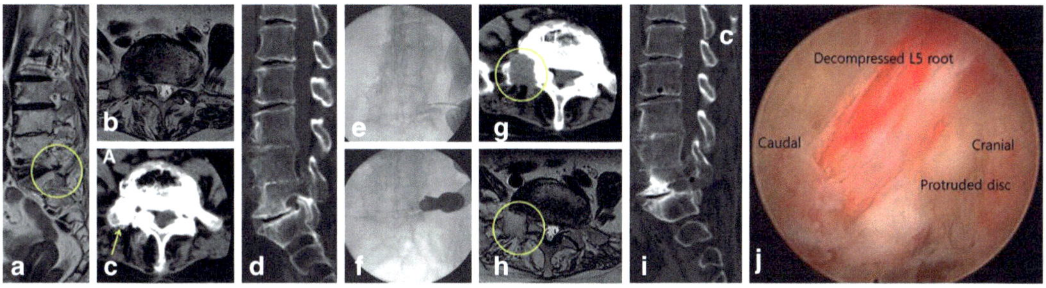

Fig. 11 (**a**, **b**) MRI T2 sagittal and axial image showing compressed root at L5–S1 right foramen with severe degenerative changes (yellow circle). (**c**, **d**) CT axial and sagittal images showing hypertrophied facet and sacral ala encroaching foramen to compress the nerve (yellow arrow) with multilevel vacuum disc phenomenon. (**e**) Intraoperative fluoroscopic image showing needle targeting. (**f**) Final position of working cannula on X-ray. (**g**, **h**) Postoperative axial CT and T2 MRI and sagittal reconstruction images showing partial facetectomy and pediculotomy on right side at L5–S1 to decompress the nerve (yellow circle). (**j**) Decompressed root and protruded disc

MRI revealed partial resection of SAP, removal of herniated disc and decompressed nerve root.

Case 2: Far out Syndrome

A 63-year-old woman presented with long-standing lower back pain and right lower limb pain, aggravated since 2 months. She had failed conservative management and had temporary relief by root block. X-ray lumbosacral spine showed coronal deformity with vacuum disc phenomenon at multiple levels with no features of instability. MRI and CT showed severely narrowed right side foramen with compressed root at L5–S1 with severe degenerative changes at multiple lumbar levels (Fig. 11a–d). The patient underwent endoscopic paraspinal decompression (Fig. 11e, f). The patient was ambulated 6 h after surgery with reduction of VAS score of leg from 9 to 2 with no neurological deficits. Postoperative X-ray showed no evidence any immediate instability with MRI and CT suggestive partial facetectomy and pediculotomy on right side at L5–S1 to decompress the nerve (Fig. 11g–j).

Case 3: Severe Foraminal Stenosis

A 60-year-old man presented with back pain and left lower limb radicular pain for 6 months. On examination, VAS score of the patient was 4 for back pain and 8 for leg pain. X-ray of lumbosacral spine revealed reduced disc space height at L4–L5, L5–S1 with vacuum disc at L5–S1 and no evidence of instability on dynamic X-rays. Computed tomography (CT) showed severely narrowed foramen with hypertrophy of the superior articular facet (Fig. 12a, c). MRI revealed severely narrowed foramen with fat signal barely seen within the foramen with hypertrophied facet narrowing the foramen at L4–L5 (Fig. 12e). The patient underwent diagnostic root block to confirm the pain generator, which offered temporary relief. In this case, the surgical anatomy was obscure due to severe degenerative change. Bulky mammillary process was used as an anatomical landmark under C-arm control to have initial surgical orientation (Fig. 12b). After placement of working cannula on mammillary process, decompression of exiting root was performed along it's pathway with the following tehnique. Hypertorophied and thickend bony structure encasing exiting root was drilled out until only thin bony egg shell on ER was left and the thinned bony crust was removed by forcep and currette. Intraoperative fluoroscopic image showed pedicle to extraforaminal decompression (Fig. 12f, g). The patient was ambulated 6 h post-surgery with reduction in VAS scores of 3 and 2 for back and leg, respectively, and discharged on the first postoperative day. Postoperative imaging showed no immediate postoperative instability and decompressed foramen with pediculotomy and resected SAP (Fig. 12h–j).

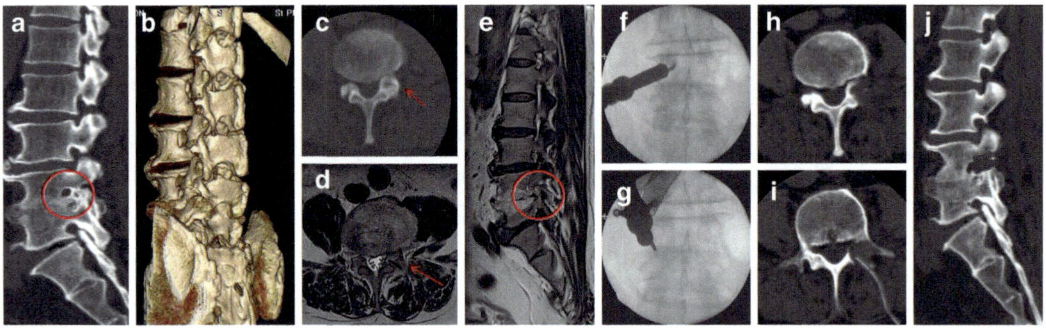

Fig. 12 (**a**) Computed tomography(CT) para-sagittal view showing nearly fused, severely narrowed foramen with hypertrophy of the superior articular facet at L4–L5 (red circle), reduced disc space and vacuum disc at L5–S1. (**b**) 3D reconstructed image showing narrowed foramen and bulky mammillary process. (**c**) CT axial view showing completely narrowed foramen with hypertrophy of the superior articular facet (red arrow). (**d**, **e**) MRI T2 axial image showing completely narrowed foramen (red arrow) and left para-sagittal image showing severely narrowed foramen with loss of fat signal (red circle) at L4–L5. (**f**, **g**) Intraoperative fluoroscopic image showing the extent of decompression from pedicle to extraforaminal area. (**h**, **i**) Postoperative axial CT showing resected cranial tip of SAP. (**j**) Sagittal CT showing decompressed foramen with pediculotomy and resection of cranial tip of SAP

Complications and Its Management

1. Incomplete decompression.
   - Incomplete decompression can lead to persistence of preoperative symptoms.
   - Target points of decompression should be determined by preoperative investigation (patient's neurologic symptom and radiologic images) before the operation.
   - The structures which can compress ER and evoke patient's symptom should be thoroughly decompressed and confirmed its decompressed status for successful postoperative outcome.
   – Bony compression at the area of junction between the inferior margin of TP and pars.
   – Pedicle kinking: pediculotomy is needed.
   – Ligament flavum at the axilla area of ER.
   – Bony spur of caudal margin of the upper vertebral body.
   – Redundant disc.
2. Facet violation.
   - The facet joint plays an important role in maintaining stability, but in certain cases, resection of the facet joint is inevitable for adequate decompression.
   - To avoid such complications, after initial exposure of ER, tailored, limited removal of bony structure along just the ER pathway in direct endoscopic view is recommended.
   - The intraoperative modification of flatter operative angle is also helpful to obliquely undercut SAP, to preserve the facet joint more than 50% and to prevent iatrogenic instability.
3. Neurological complications.
   - These complications can manifest in the form of dysthesia and motor weakness caused by direct manipulation of the exiting root or inappropriate usage of RF probe.
   - Delicate dissection of perineural structures from the ER is necessary in order to prevent neural injury. The manipulation of ER should be preceded by initial decompression (such as discectomy and bony unroofing of the ER) and adequate adhesiolysis of ER from around soft tissues. The excessive manipulation with the use of sharp instrument should be avoided.
   - RF bipolar should be used with adequate power (soft tissue ablation and bone bleeding control : 250 Watts, but around the neural structures : below 90 Watts) and toward proper direction. Posterior end of RF probe

should be directed against the nerve root so that discharge RF current is away from the neural structure not directly on it.

4. Bleeding.
   - Intraoperative bleeding is usually from the radicular artery or its branches.
   - Such an unexpected bleeding can be troublesome leading to longer operative time interrupting the operative flow.
   - Tips to prevent intraoperative bleeding includes beforehand coagulation of vessels which is easy to cause bleeding around the radicular artery. when uncontrollable intraoperative bleeding occurs, temporary elevation of irrigative pressure and the use of hemostatic agent (Floseal®) are useful.
5. Intra-abdominal fluid collection.
   - Intra-abdominal fluid collection can occur in certain cases.
   - It usually occurs with dissection at far lateral region of L5–S1 level. Aggressive long time dissection should be avoided to prevent inadvertent entry of irrigative water into retroperitoneal space. Decompressin of distal portion of ER should be delayed as a a last part of surgery and try to shorten the operative time for distal decompression.

Discussion (Surgical Tips and Pitfalls)

1. Importance of preoperative diagnosis for endoscopic foraminal decompression.
   - Symptoms and sign: history and neurological examination.
   - Identify the pathological area and rule out other causes.
   - Imaging—target pathology, rule out candidates for other kinds of operation (interbody fusion, other endoscopic approaches).
   - Diagnostic selective nerve root block.
2. Anatomical landmark.
   - Initial target: inferolateral margin of the pedicle in X-ray AP image, junction between pars and TP.
   - If a patient has obscure anatomy due to severe degenerative changes or deformity, identify patient's unique anatomy such as bony prominence or indentation around usual target area using 3D reconstructed CT and using it as an alternative landmark.
   - Key landmarks for surgical orientation during operation: cranial tip of SAP, TP and pars.
3. Complete decompression.
   - The most common cause of unfavourable outcome is incomplete decompression.
   - Based on preoperative planning, adequate decompression of key structure must be ensured.
   - In cases of L5–S1, sacral ala acts as a compressive element. Decompress ER with enough resection of alar and trace ER along its pathway far distally beyond lateral margin of L5–S1 disc. But be cautious not to do aggressive dissection and spend much time for decompression in far lateral area to avoid abdominal fluid collection.
4. Facet joint preservation.
   - Biomechanically, the facet joint limits the movement of the spinal motion segment, but excessive bone resection which can occur during unroofing of the ER for complete decompression could lead to postoperative instability or pars fracture.
   - Endoscopic paraspinal approach has relative short working trajectory and vertical approach angle compared to other endoscopic approaches (transforaminal and contralateral), which provide multidirectional variable operative angle and allow the surgeon to use endoscopic instruments without any difficulty enabling tailored facet resection.
5. Intraoperative bleeding.
   - Abrupt and massive bleeding during the operation is not rare in endoscopic paraspinal approach.
   - Most of intraoperative bleeding is from the radicular artery or its branches. Surgeons who perform endoscopic paraspinal

approach should know and understand the anatomy of the radicular artery and its course.

- Beforehand coagulation of vessel with RF bipolar or clips is essential for a bloodless endoscopic view and to prevent any haemorrhage and maintain stable operation without ceasement.
- Most of bleeding is confined to endoscopic operative field. When active bleeding occurs and operative view become blurred, the scope and working cannula complex shoud not be moved, instead, fixed temporarilly. The origin of bleeding is usually confined in small endoscopic working view. Temporary elevation of irrigative water pressure and intermittent compression by the blunt tip of RF coagulator in blind fashion, which can help the surgeon find bleeding focus and control it even in blurred operative vision.
- Haemostatic agents (Floseal®) are also useful to control intraoperative bleeding.

6. Neural injury.
   - Most common form of neural injury which can occur during the procedure is a dysthesia and motor weakness.
   - Initial bony decompression and adhesiolysis from around soft tissues should precede the manipulation of the root. Aggressive manipulation of the root should be avoided. Redundant root which was partially decompressed and freed from around structures should be dealt with careful and delicate manner.
   - The RF bipolar should be used with much caution. The surgeon should adhere to adequate power and direction in usage of RF.

References

1. Hasegawa T, An HS, Haughton VM, Nowicki BH. Lumbar foraminal stenosis: critical heights of the intervertebral discs and foramina. A cryomicrotome study in cadavera. J Bone Jt Surg. 1995;77(1):32–8.
2. Wiltse LL, Spencer CW. New uses and refinements of the paraspinal approach to the lumbar spine. Spine. 1988;13:696–706.
3. Kim HJ, Jeong JH, Cho HK, Chang BS, et al. Comparative observational study of surgical outcomes of lumbar foraminal stenosis using minimally invasive microsurgical extraforaminal decompression alone versus posterior lumbar interbody fusion: a prospective cohort study. Eur Spine J. 2015;24:388–95.
4. Ahn Y, Oh HK, Kim H, Lee SH, Lee HN. Percutaneous endoscopic lumbar foraminotomy: An advanced surgical technique and clinical outcomes. Neurosurgery. 2014;75(2):124–32.
5. McGrath LB, White-Dzuro GA, Hofstetter CP. Comparison of clinical outcomes following minimally invasive or lumbar endoscopic unilateral laminotomy for bilateral decompression. J Neurosurg Spine. 2019;30(4):491–9.
6. Kim HS, Patel R, Paudel B, Jang J, Jang IT, Oh SH, et al. Early outcomes of endoscopic contralateral foraminal and lateral recess decompression via an interlaminar approach in patients with unilateral radiculopathy from unilateral foraminal stenosis. World Neurosurg. 2017;108:763–73.
7. Nam HGW, Kim HS, Lee DK, Park CK, Lim KT. Percutaneous Stenoscopic lumbar decompression with Paramedian approach for Foraminal/Extraforaminal lesions. Asian Spine J. 2019;13(4):672–81.

Contralateral Sublaminar Approach for Lumbar Foraminal Stenosis Using Biportal Endoscopic Surgery

Dong Hwa Heo, Su Gi Jun, and Cheol Woong Park

Introduction

Endoscopic contralateral sublaminar approach was commonly performed for decompression of contralateral traversing nerve root in lumbar lateral recess stenosis [1, 2]. Modification of routine contralateral sublaminar approach can expose and decompress contralateral side traversing nerve root as well as traversing nerve root [3–5]. Biportal endoscopic lumbar surgery may be powerful methods for contralateral approach.

Indication and Contraindication

Indications [5, 6]

- Lumbar foraminal stenosis.
- Central stenosis combined with foraminal stenosis.
- Foraminal ruptured disc herniation.
- Lumbar juxta-facet cyst such as synovial cyst and ligamentum flavum cyst.

Contraindications

- Extraforaminal disc herniation.
- Infectious disease.
- Significant instability.

Surgical Instruments

Basic setting of contralateral sublaminar approach was the same as routine biportal endoscopic spine surgery. Specialized toolkit set of biportal endoscopic surgery was necessary. Generally, 0° endoscope was used. Sometimes 30° endoscope was used for exploration of contralateral exiting nerve root. Various kinds of curved curettes and partially curved foraminal Kerrison punch (2 and 3 mm diameter) were useful for decompression of contralateral nerve roots.

Surgical Steps (Videos 1 and 2)

1. Making two channels: Two stab wounds should be made for endoscopic portal and working portal. Generally, endoscopic portal was made for left hand (nondominant), and

Electronic Supplementary Material The online version of this chapter (https://doi.org/10.1007/978-981-15-8253-0_9) contains supplementary material, which is available to authorized users.

D. H. Heo
Department of Neurosurgery, Seoul Bumin Hospital, Seoul, South Korea

S. G. Jun · C. W. Park (✉)
Spine Center, Neurosurgery, Daejeon Woori Hospital, Daejeon, South Korea

H. S. Kim et al. (eds.), *Advanced Techniques of Endoscopic Lumbar Spine Surgery*,
https://doi.org/10.1007/978-981-15-8253-0_9

the other working portal was made for right hand (dominant) in right-handed spine surgeon. In some cases, the location of two portals should be modified for optimal decompression of exiting nerve root. We need to make the two channels a little bit lower (Figs. 1 and 2). Endoscopic portal is made below the lower border of pedicle of upper lumbar on lateral C-arm fluoroscopic view for well visualization of exiting nerve root and around structures (Fig. 1). Endoscopic sheath and working sheath were applied through skin incision sites (Fig. 2). Continuous saline irrigation was necessary for maintenance of clear vision and bleeding control (pressure: 25 to 50 mmHg). Continuous saline should be well drained from endoscopic portal to working portal.

2. Bone working and removal of the ligamentum flavum: Midline ipsilateral laminotomy of cranial lamina was performed around spinolaminar junction (Fig. 3). Basement of spinous process was partially removed by drill for approach to contralateral side (Fig. 3). Firstly, proximal end of contralateral ligamentum flavum was exposed. And then, contralateral ligamentum flavum was detached from sublaminar area using blunted dissectors. Contralateral sublaminar bony drilling was performed over the contralateral ligamentum flavum. Superficial layer of contralateral ligamentum flavum was removed using Kerrison punch and pituitary forceps. Distal end of deep layer of contralateral ligamentum flavum was detached from contralateral caudal laminar and superior articular process. Deep layer of the ligamentum flavum was removed with curettes, Kerrison punches, and pituitary forceps. After removal of contralateral ligamentum flavum, contralateral superior articular process and foraminal ligament were exposed. When the foraminal ligament was removed, contralateral exiting nerve root and epidural fat tissue were visible. In some cases with upward migration or hypertrophy of superior articular process, the tip of contralateral superior articular process was removed for decompression of contralateral exiting nerve root. If patients have foraminal ruptured disc herniation, ruptured disc particles can be easily removed by contralateral approach. If patients have lateral recess stenosis of compression of traversing nerve roots, decompression of traversing nerve roots was performed additionally like routine endoscopic decompressive procedures.

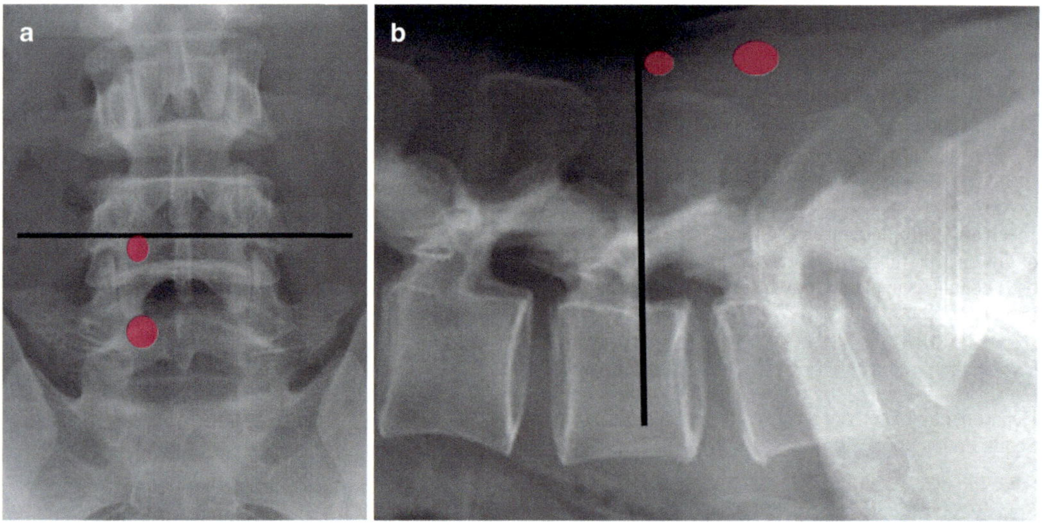

Fig. 1 Location of two portals. Endoscopic portal was usually made at the lower border of upper pedicle ((**a**) anteroposterior view; (**b**) lateral view)

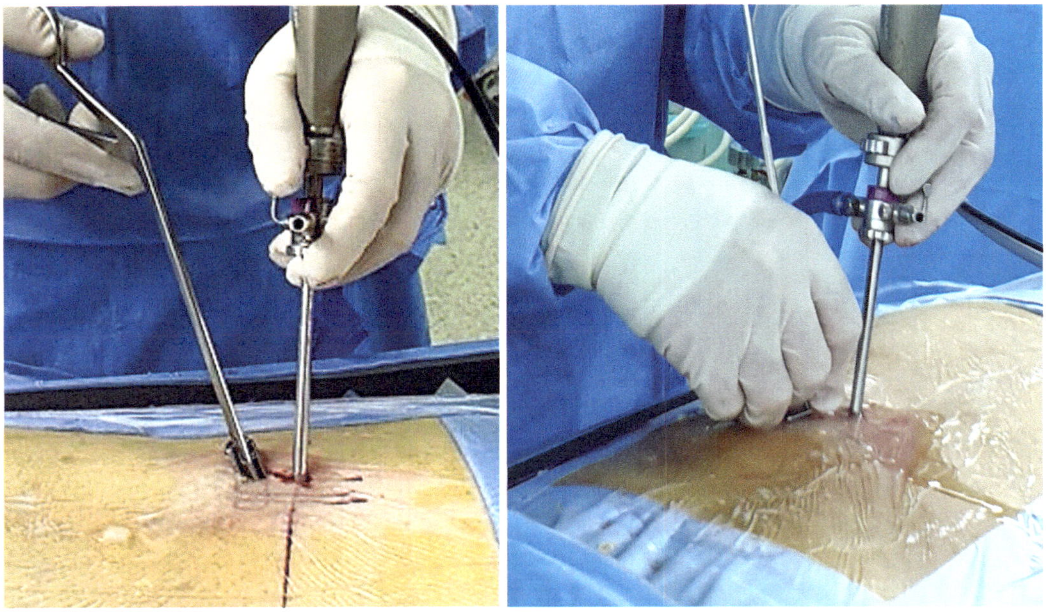

Fig. 2 Overview of biportal endoscopic surgery

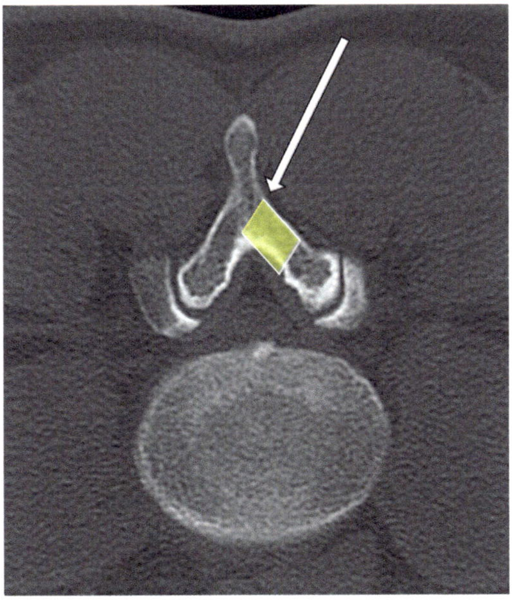

Fig. 3 Laminotomy area of contralateral sublaminar approach. The base of spinous process should be removed. Ipsilateral facet joint is preserved

Illustrated Cases

Case 1 (Video 1). A 65-year-old male patient complained of both leg pain and neurological intermittent claudication. Preoperative MR images show bilateral lateral recess stenosis with left side concomitant foraminal stenosis at L4–5 level (Fig. 4). This patient received right sided biportal endoscopic surgery for three nerve root decompression (bilateral L5 nerve roots and left side L4 nerve root). Left sided foraminal stenosis of L4–5 was decompressed by contralateral sublaminar approach (Fig. 4). Postoperative MR images reveal completely decompressive status of lateral recess stenosis and left side foraminal stenosis at L4–5 (Fig. 4). Patient's symptoms were significantly improved after biportal endoscopic treatment.

Case 2 (Video 2). A 72-year-old female patient complained of right leg pain of L4 dermatome. Preoperative MR images reveal lateral recess stenosis with right foraminal stenosis at L4–5 (Fig. 5). We did endoscopic decompression of right side L4 and L5 nerve roots via contralateral sublaminar approach using biportal endoscopic surgery (Fig. 5). Postoperatively, this patient's pain was significantly improved. Postoperative MR images show that right lateral recess and foraminal stenosis of L4–5 were decompressed after biportal endoscopic approach (Fig. 5).

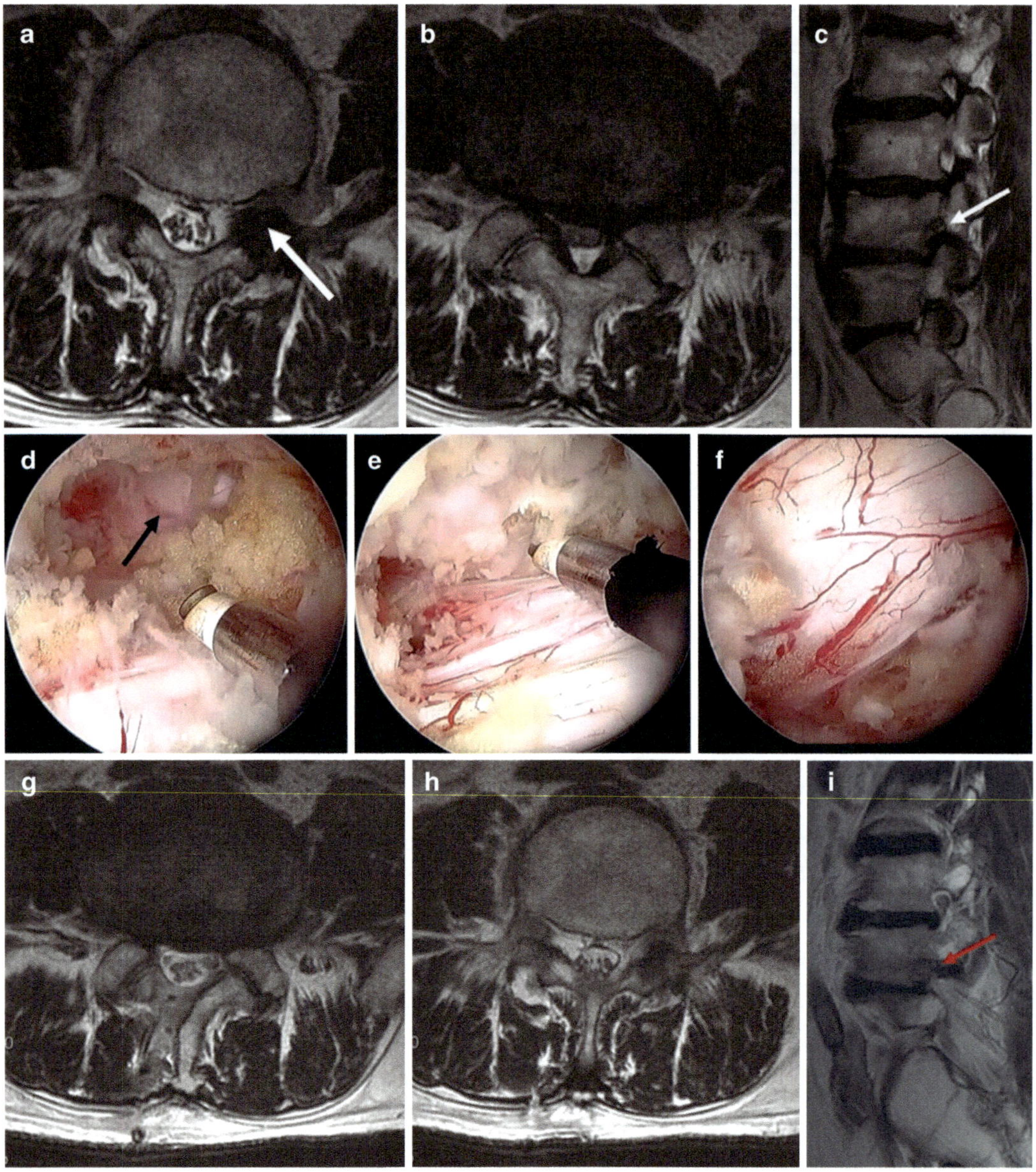

Fig. 4 A 65-year-old male patient presented with radicular pain of both legs and claudication. He complained of severe pain in the left leg compared to the right leg. Preoperative MR images show bilateral lateral recess stenosis with left side concomitant foraminal stenosis at L4–5 level (white arrow). Axial images (**a**, **b**) and sagittal image (**c**). Left L4 (black arrow) and L5 nerve roots were decompressed by contralateral sublaminar approach (**d**, **e**). Right L5 nerve root was also decompressed by ipsilateral approach (**f**). Postoperative MR images show that central canal was widened (**g**) and left side foraminal stenosis was resolved (H and I)

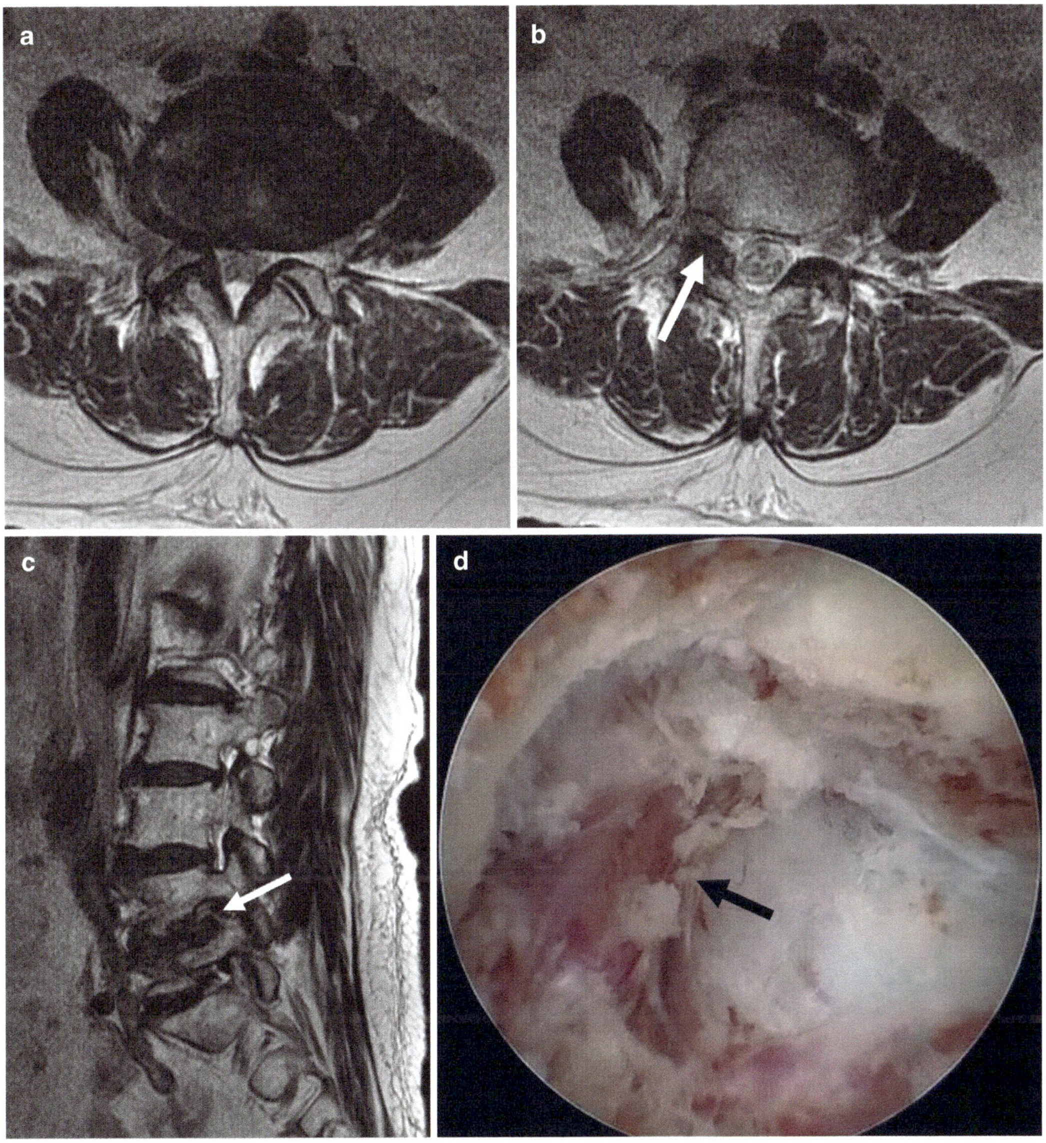

Fig. 5 A 72-year-old female patient presented with right leg pain (L4 dermatome) and claudication. Preoperative MR images show lateral recess stenosis (**a**) with right foraminal stenosis at L4–5 (white arrow, **b**, **c**). We did right side L4 and L5 nerve root decompression via contralateral sublaminar approach using biportal endoscopic surgery. Especially, right L4 exiting nerve root was completely decompressed (**d**). Postoperatively, this patient's pain was disappeared. Postoperative MR images show that right lateral recess (**e**) and foraminal stenosis of L4–5 (**f**, **g**) were decompressed after biportal endoscopic approach

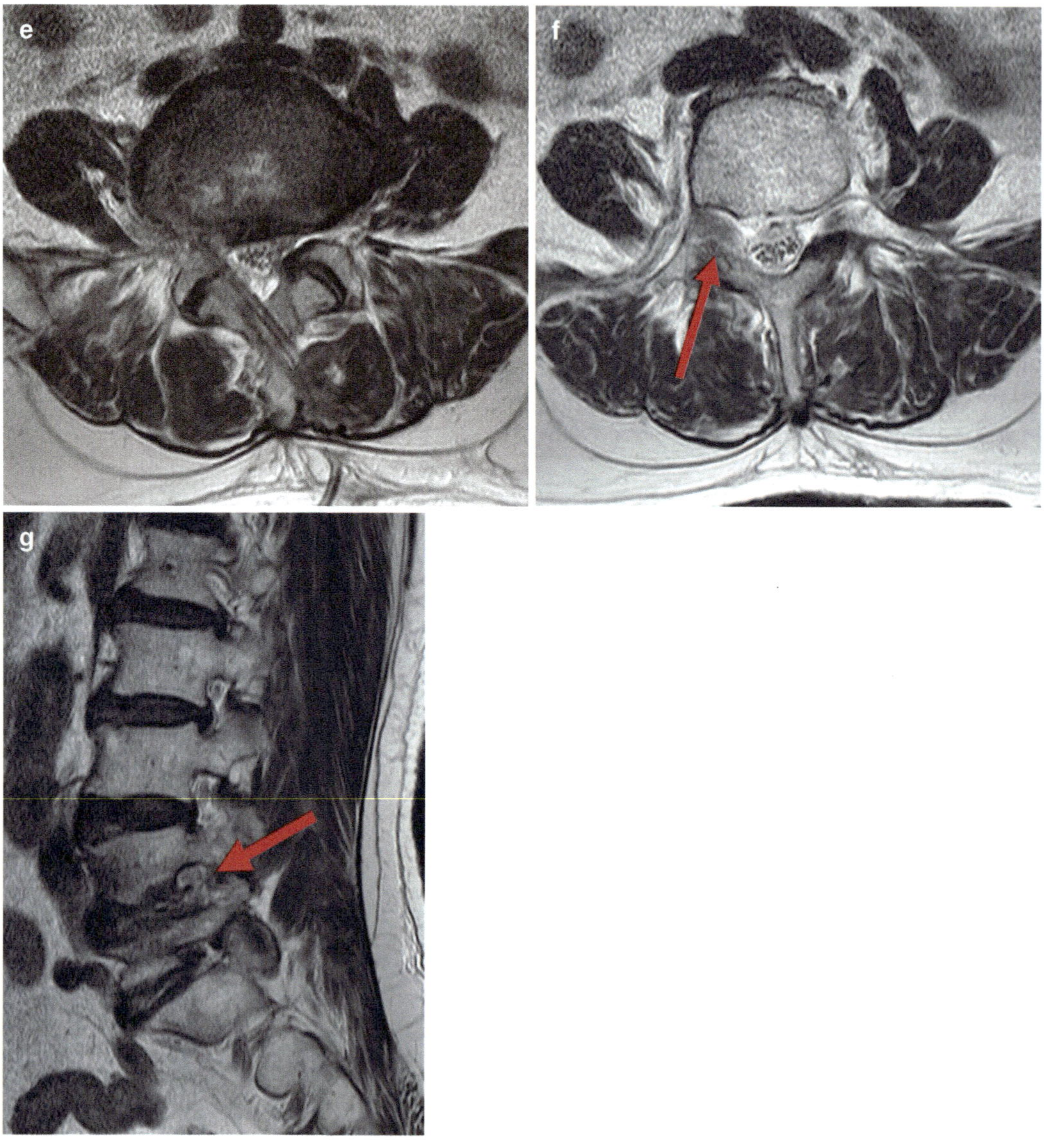

Fig. 5 (continued)

Complication and its Management

1. Dural tear: Incidental dural injury occurred when the ligamentum flavum was removed. Before removal of the ligamentum flavum, we have to check adhesion between dura and ligament. Small dura tear site can be repaired by TachoSil and clips [2, 7].
2. Neural tissue injury: Excessive retraction of dura and nerve root occur postoperative motor weakness. Sublaminar bone drilling of contralateral side is important for safety insertion of an endoscopy to contralateral side without dura compression. Usually, an endoscopy did not compress the central dura significantly during contralateral sublaminar decompression.
3. Postoperative epidural hematoma: It is recommended to insert a drainage catheter to prevent hematoma after surgery.

4. Incomplete decompression: Extraforaminal lesion decompression is difficult using contralateral sublaminar approach. Intraoperative C-arm fluoroscopic monitoring is useful for complete decompression. Especially, extraforaminal lesion was suitable for paraspinal approach or transforaminal approach.

Discussion

For exiting root decompression via contralateral approach, midline laminotomy should be necessary [5, 6]. Midline laminotomy should be performed until exposure over proximal end of the ligamentum flavum. There were two landmarks for exploration of a contralateral exiting nerve root. First is the contralateral foraminal ligament (Fig. 6). Foraminal ligament was inserted around superior pedicle and covered an exiting nerve root. The bone drilling of contralateral sublaminar area should be performed preservation of foraminal ligament. The other landmark of exiting nerve root is the tip of superior articular process. Sometimes, a superior articular process was upwardly migrated due to disc space narrowing in patients with foraminal stenosis. Therefore, an exiting root was placed around the tip of superior articular process (Fig. 6). Also, foraminal ligament was connected with superior articular process. The authors firstly explored the tip of superior articular process. And then, foraminal ligament was carefully removed using small size of Kerrison punches and pituitary forceps. Yellowish epidural fatty tissue was detected after removal of ligament. An exiting nerve root was fully exposed after removal of epidural fat. Sometimes, the authors removed the tip of contralateral superior articular process for decompression of distal part of exiting nerve root case by case. The authors suggested that two surgical landmarks are very useful for optimal decompression of exiting nerve root using contralateral sublaminar endoscopic approach.

Usually, there was abundant epidural vessel around nerve roots. Coagulation of vessels was necessary for optimal decompression of nerve roots. The energy power of RF should be decreased for prevention of dermal injury of neural tissue during preventive coagulation and bleeding control.

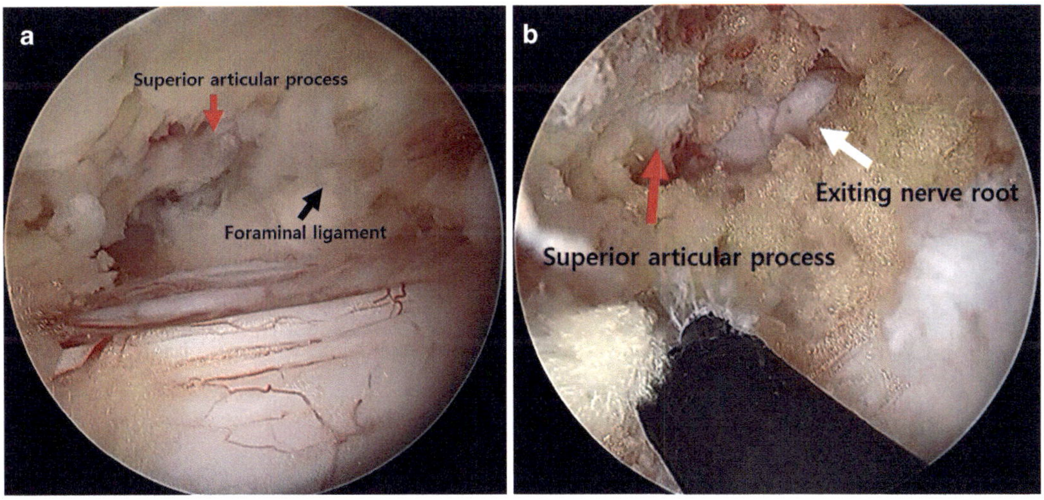

Fig. 6 Two surgical landmarks of exiting nerve root in contralateral sublaminar approach. First is the foraminal ligament (black arrow). Second is the tip of superior articular process (red arrow). Exiting nerve root was passed around two surgical landmarks

References

1. Heo DH, Lee DC, Park CK. Comparative analysis of three types of minimally invasive decompressive surgery for lumbar central stenosis: biportal endoscopy, uniportal endoscopy, and microsurgery. Neurosurg Focus. 2019;46(5):E9.
2. Heo DH, Quillo-Olvera J, Park CK. Can percutaneous Biportal endoscopic surgery achieve Enough Canal decompression for degenerative lumbar stenosis? Prospective case-control study. World Neurosurg. 2018;120:e684–9.
3. Hwang JH, Park WM, Park CW. Contralateral Interlaminar keyhole percutaneous endoscopic lumbar surgery in patients with unilateral radiculopathy. World Neurosurg. 2017;101:33–41.
4. Krzok G, Telfeian AE, Wagner R, Hofstetter CP, Iprenburg M. Contralateral facet-sparing sublaminar endoscopic foraminotomy for the treatment of lumbar lateral recess stenosis: technical note. J Spine Surg. 2017;3(2):260–6.
5. Akbary K, Kim JS, Park CW, Jun SG, Hwang JH. Biportal endoscopic decompression of exiting and traversing nerve roots through a single Interlaminar window using a contralateral approach: technical feasibilities and morphometric changes of the Lumbar Canal and foramen. World Neurosurg. 2018;117:153–61.
6. Heo DH, Kim JS, Park CW, Quillo-Olvera J, Park CK. Contralateral sublaminar endoscopic approach for removal of lumbar Juxtafacet cysts using percutaneous Biportal endoscopic surgery: technical report and preliminary results. World Neurosurg. 2019;122:474–9.
7. Heo DH, Son SK, Eum JH, Park CK. Fully endoscopic lumbar interbody fusion using a percutaneous unilateral biportal endoscopic technique: technical note and preliminary clinical results. Neurosurg Focus. 2017;43(2):E8.

Biportal Endoscopic Paraspinal Approach for Foraminal and Extraforaminal Disc Herniations

Man Kyu Park and Dong Hwa Heo

Introduction

Lumbar radiculopathy caused by lumbar foraminal or extraforaminal stenosis is a common pathology of degenerative lumbar spine disease [1, 2]. Traditionally, microsurgical decompression of foraminal lesions using a paraspinal approach, introduced by Wiltse, has been considered as the gold standard for the surgical treatment of lumbar foraminal stenosis [3]. In addition, a combination of total facetectomy and spinal fusion surgery has generally been performed for lumbar foraminal stenosis. However, excessive manipulation of the dorsal root ganglion can cause postoperative leg pain or dysesthesia, and the deep location of the foraminal lesions makes the surgery technically challenging and more invasive [4]. Recently, as a result of advancements in endoscopic spine surgery, the biportal endoscopic technique has come to be applied in various degenerative spine diseases [5–7]. Biportal endoscopic approaches were also widely known as unilateral biportal endoscopy (UBE). For lumbar foraminal stenosis, the biportal endoscopic technique, which can reach deeper into the foramen less invasively, is becoming widespread and surpassing microscopic surgery in popularity. The purpose of this chapter is to describe the surgical decompression of foraminal stenosis with the biportal endoscopic paraspinal approach. The surgical anatomy is first identified as a landmark, including the lateral part of the isthmus, the lower part of the TP, and the top of the SAP. After completion of bone working, the proximal portion of the foraminal ligament is detached from the transverse process and SAP using a freer elevator and Kerrison rongeur. After confirmation of the compressed root, careful and thorough decompression of the root is performed through the entire passage in the foraminal area.

Electronic Supplementary Material The online version of this chapter (https://doi.org/10.1007/978-981-15-8253-0_10) contains supplementary material, which is available to authorized users.

M. K. Park
Department of Neurosurgery, ParkWeonWook Hospital, Busan, South Korea

D. H. Heo (✉)
Department of Neurosurgery, Seoul Bumin Hospital, Seoul, South Korea

Indication and Contraindication

The indications of the biportal endoscopic paraspinal approach for foraminal and extraforaminal lesions are the same as those for microsurgical decompression via the Wiltse approach.

Indications

- Foraminal/extraforaminal disc herniation or stenosis confirmed on CT or MRI.
- Unilateral lumbar radicular pain refractory to conservative management.

H. S. Kim et al. (eds.), *Advanced Techniques of Endoscopic Lumbar Spine Surgery*,
https://doi.org/10.1007/978-981-15-8253-0_10

Relative contraindications

- Degenerative spondylolisthesis.
- Spondylolysis.
- Isthmic spondylolisthesis.
- Bilateral symptomatic foraminal stenosis.

If the patients were old age and had a serious illness that makes it difficult to undergo major surgery, the authors have selectively attempted the biportal endoscopic approach for foraminal stenosis in patients with spondylolysis or spondylolisthesis.

Contraindications

- Segmental instability.
- High-grade spondylolisthesis.
- Pathological conditions such as infection and tumor.

Anesthesia and Position

Under general or epidural anesthesia, a patient is placed in the prone position on a radiolucent table. Severe flexed posture in the Wilson frame is not recommended to avoid an increase in epidural pressure resulting in more epidural bleeding during the operation. The operator stands on the ipsilateral side of the pathology of the foraminal and extraforaminal lumbar stenosis.

Special Surgical Instruments

For the equipment, a camera system and endoscope, a shaver system, a radiofrequency system, and conventional spine instruments such as a Kerrison rongeur, pituitary forceps, and a freer elevator should be prepared. During the procedure, we commonly used 0°, 4-mm rigid arthroscope, 4-mm round cutting burr, 3.5-mm radiofrequency (RF) ablation probe, serial dilators, and a periosteal dissector. Sometimes, we used 30° endoscope for exploration of medical foraminal area (preganglionic area). Partially curve punch and curette were useful for undercutting of SAP and isthmus for decompression of preganglionic lesion.

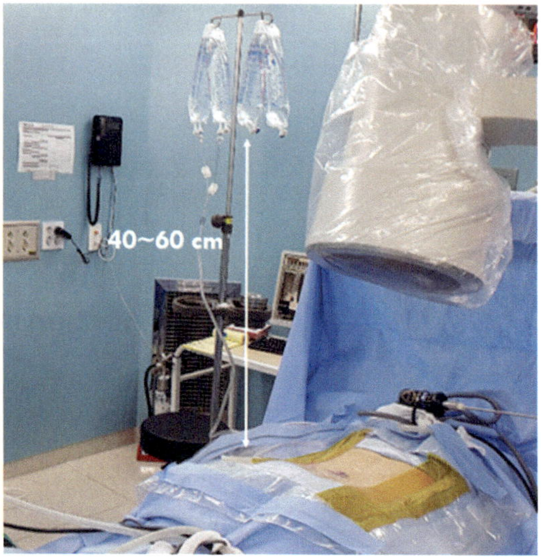

Fig. 1 The proper height of the fluid back is about 40–60 cm from the patient's back

Using pressure irrigation pump systems is not recommended as saline can be sufficiently infused by gravity, which is enough to achieve a clear view while minimizing epidural bleeding. The proper height of the fluid back is about 40–60 cm from the patient's back (Fig. 1). If pressure pump irrigation was used, recommended irrigation pressure was from 25 to 50 mmHg.

Surgical Steps (Illustration, Photos, and Video)

Skin Marking

The target point is below the pedicle, which is located on top of the superior articular process (SAP) and lateral to the isthmus on an anteroposterior (AP) view of the C-arm fluoroscopy. For right-handed surgeons, a left-side incision is used for the scopic portal for endoscopic viewing, and a right-side incision is used for a working portal for insertion and manipulation of the surgical instruments. The two incisions are about 3 cm apart, where the center of each incision is placed at 1 cm lateral to the target point (Fig. 2). In the case of a L5–S1 level, where caudal incision is blocked by the iliac crest, a caudal incision could be made medially avoiding the iliac crest.

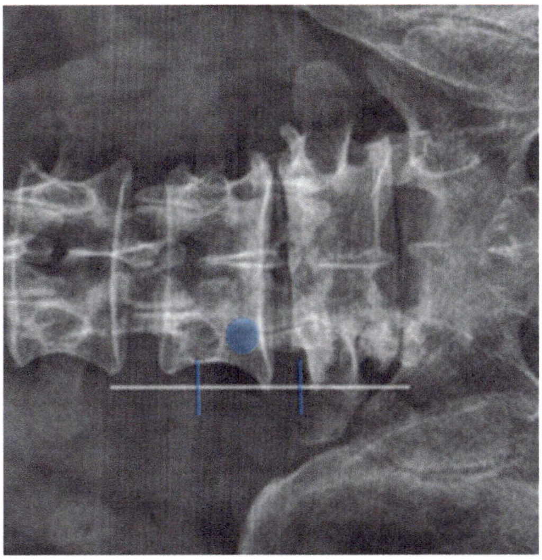

Fig. 2 Skin incision and target point on the fluoroscopic AP view. Target point (blue circle) is below the pedicle. The two incisions (blue line) are about 3 cm apart, where the center of each incision is placed at 1 centimeter lateral to the target (white line). A scope through the left incision and a retractor and a working tool through the right incision

Making a Portal

Under fluoroscopic guidance, serial dilators are introduced through the working portal and obturator, and a scopic sheath is inserted to the targeting point through the scopic portal. It is important to make a triangular position of the endoscopic sheath and serial dilator at just below the pedicle on the C-arm fluoroscopic view (Fig. 3). Continuous saline irrigation through two portals (inflow through the scopic portal and outflow through the working portal) makes a clear surgical view during surgery.

Making the Working Space (Video 1)

After confirming the correct positioning of both portals, a radiofrequency coagulator is used to clean the surrounding soft tissues and muscles to identify the target point. When osteophytes from the transverse process (TP) or SAP grow over the target point, the bony landmark should be identified by drilling the osteophytes. After drilling these osteophytes, the surgical anatomy is first identified as a landmark, including the lateral part of the isthmus, the lower part of the TP, and the top of the SAP (Fig. 4).

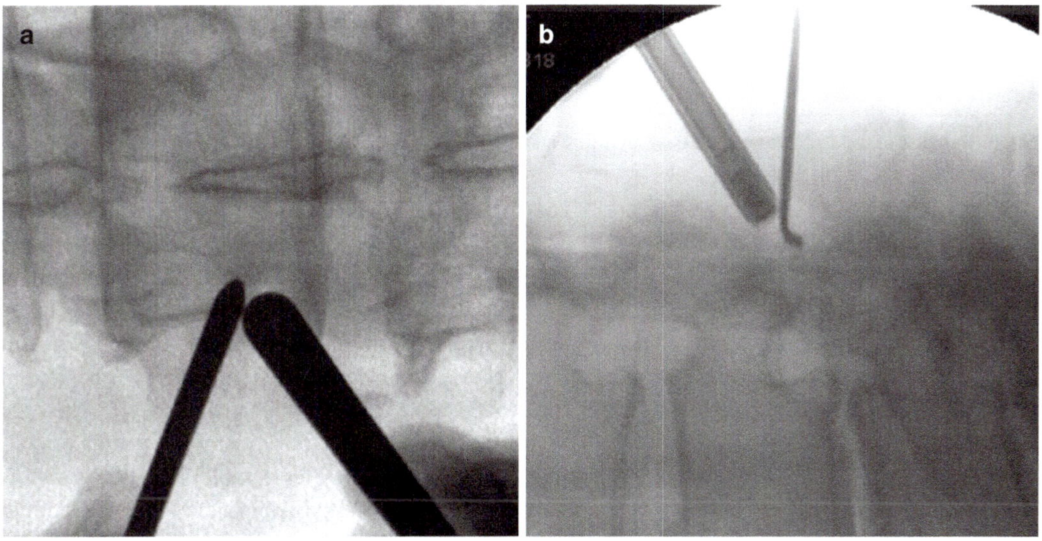

Fig. 3 Portal placement for paraspinal approach, intraoperative anteroposterior (**a**) and lateral (**b**) fluoroscopic views

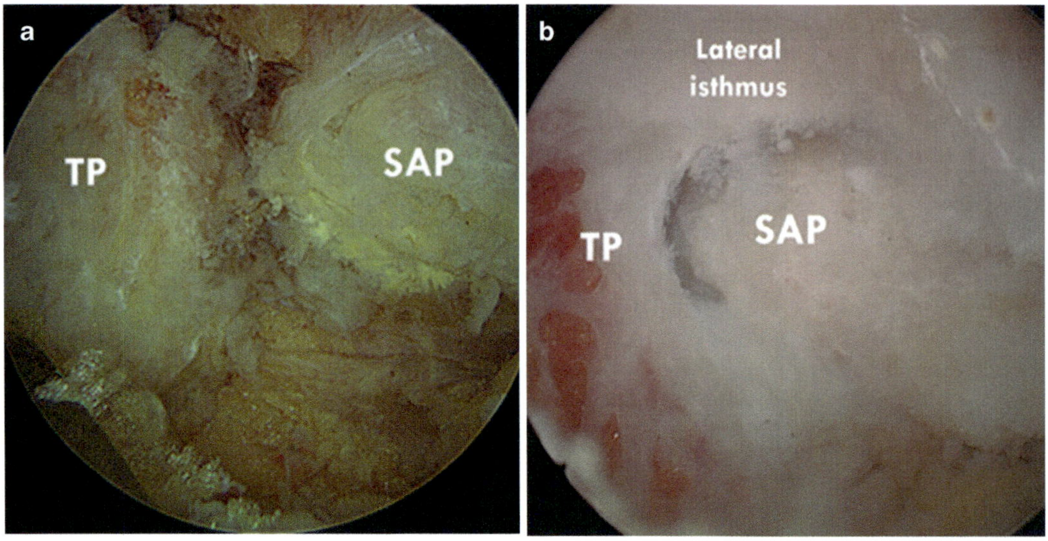

Fig. 4 (**a**) The first step is to expose the lower part of the TP and the top of the SAP using a radiofrequency coagulator. (**b**) After drilling these osteophytes, the surgical anatomy is first identified as a landmark, including the lateral part of the isthmus, the lower part of the TP, and the top of the SAP

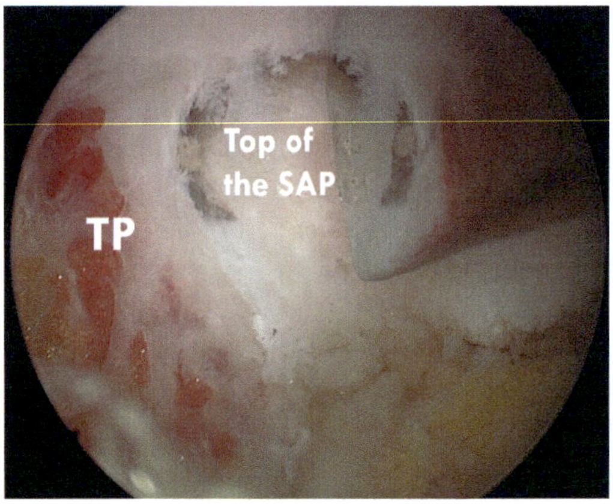

Fig. 5 Partial removal of the top of the SAP by using an osteotome

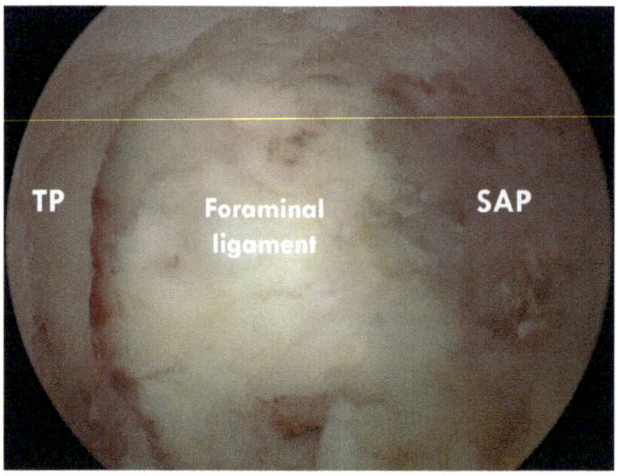

Fig. 6 After bone working, the foraminal ligament is identified

Bone Working (Video 2) **and Removal of the Foraminal Ligament** (Video 3)

Removal of the top of the SAP should be performed using an osteotome or Kerrison rongeur to make space for bone working (Fig. 5). The lower part of the TP, the lateral portion of the isthmus, and the SAP were partially removed with a high-speed drill and Kerrison rongeur. This bony landmark was removed until the ligament was released from the bony structures (Fig. 6). A bone working is dangerous after removal of the foraminal ligament, so make sure you have adequate bony resection before removal of the ligament. The lower part of the TP is removed from medial to lateral until detachment of the foraminal ligament (Fig. 7). The lateral isthmus and proximal transverse process are removed until the lower margin of the upper pedicle is touched. After completion of bone working, the proximal portion of the foraminal ligament is detached from the transverse process and SAP using a freer elevator and Kerrison ron-

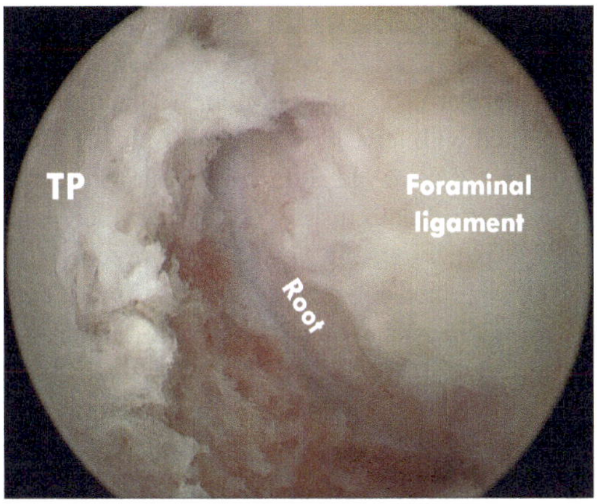

Fig. 7 The lower part of the TP is removed from medial to lateral until detachment of the foraminal ligament

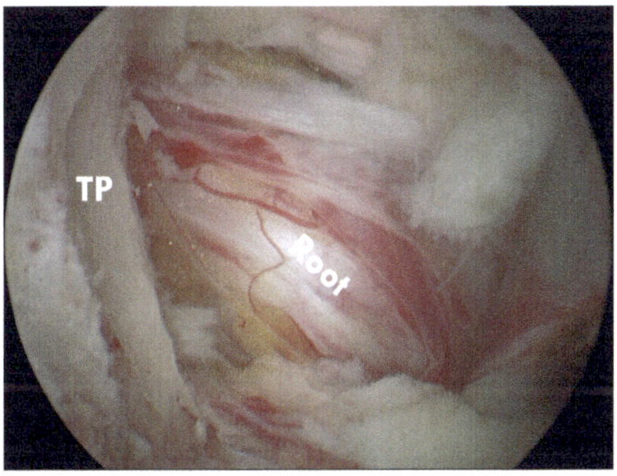

Fig. 8 The proximal portion of the foraminal ligament is detached from the transverse process and SAP using a freer elevator

geur (Fig. 8). After removal of the ligament, the underlying exiting nerve root could be identified.

Removal of Disc/Osteophytes (Video 4)

After confirmation of the compressed root, careful and thorough decompression of the root is performed through the entire passage in the foraminal area. It is critical to thoroughly remove the bulging disc and osteophytes of the vertebral body that compress the exiting root ventrally. After completion of the flavectomy, the annulus

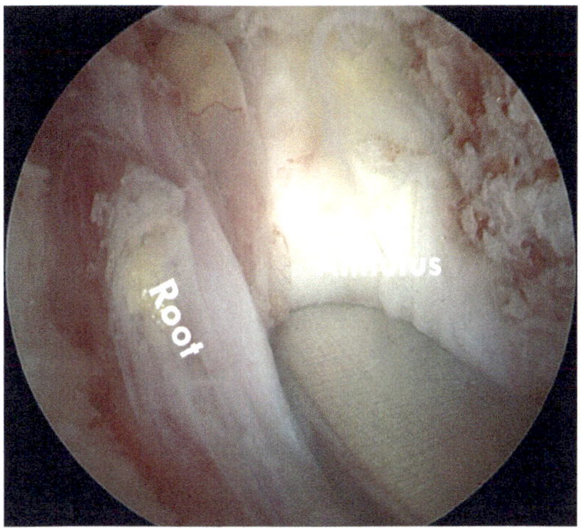

Fig. 9 The annulus is exposed just below the root

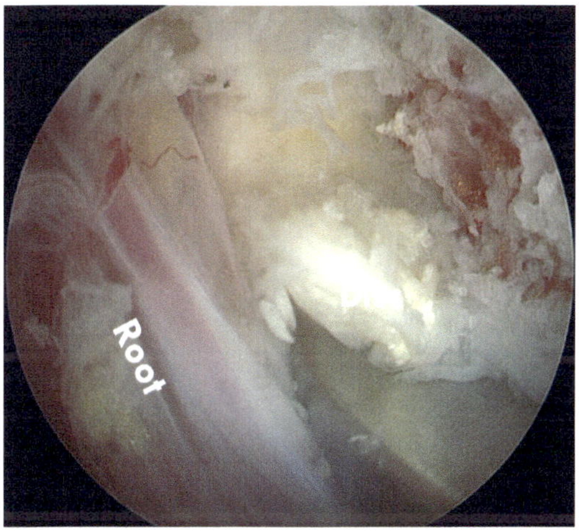

Fig. 10 Removal of disc fragment

is exposed just below the root (Fig. 9). Then we used a RF to perform the annulotomy and insert straight or curved pituitary forceps to remove disc fragments or osteophytes (Fig. 10). After removal of ventral lesions, lateral decompression is continued laterally towards the point the exiting root enters the pelvic cavity. The endpoint of foraminal decompression is free mobilization of the nerve root, which can be confirmed with endoscopic viewing (Fig. 11). After optimal decompression, we usually inserted small diameter of a drainage catheter through the working channel for the prevention of postoperative hematoma.

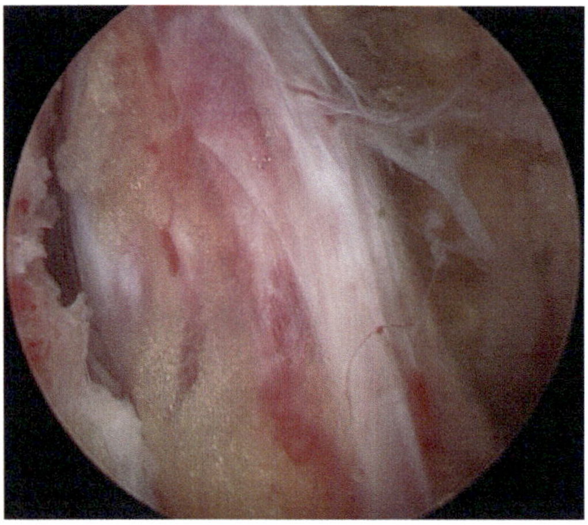

Fig. 11 Foraminal decompression is free mobilization of the nerve root, which can be confirmed with endoscopic viewing

Illustrated Case or Cases

1. Case 1: A 65-year-old female patient presented with left-sided leg pain (Fig. 12).

   A 65-year-old female patient presented with a 5-month history of left-sided leg pain. The patient's sagittal and axial preoperative T2-weighted magnetic resonance image was shown in (a) and (b). There was foraminal stenosis at L4–5, left. She underwent the biportal endoscopic paraspinal approach for foraminal stenosis. Postoperative magnetic resonance image confirmed that left exiting root of L4 was well decompressed (c,d). She had significant reduction of radicular leg pain.
2. Case 2: A 58-year-old male patient complained of left-sided leg pain (Fig. 13).

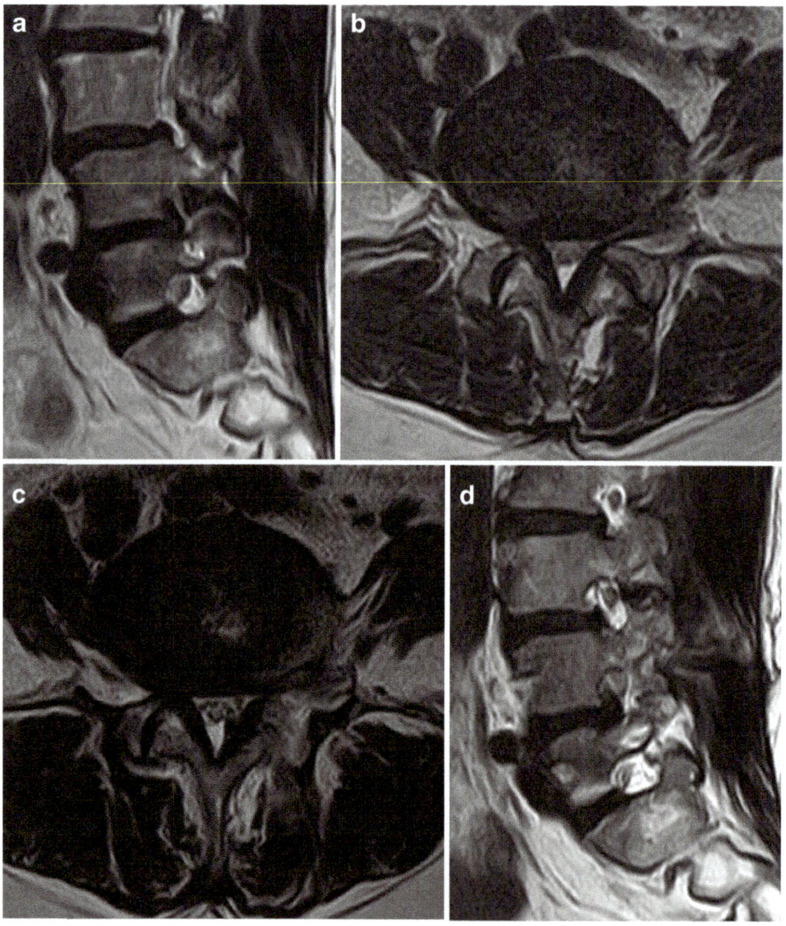

Fig. 12 Case 1. Preoperative T2-weighted magnetic resonance image of a patient with foraminal stenosis at L4–5, left; sagittal plane (**a**) and axial plane (**b**). Postoperative magnetic resonance image; sagittal plane (**c**) and axial plane (**d**)

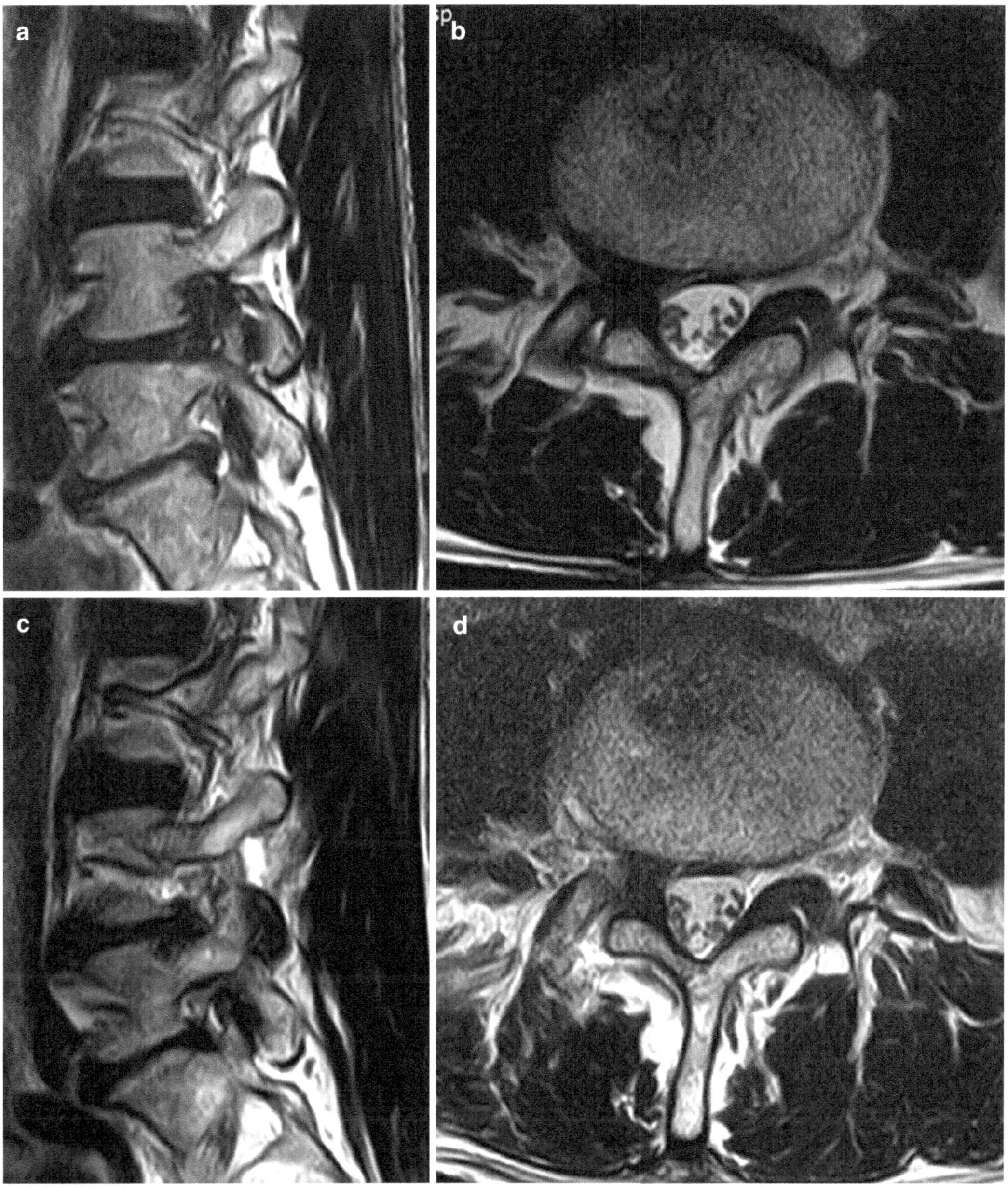

Fig. 13 Case 2. Preoperative T2-weighted magnetic resonance image of a patient with foraminal HNP at L4–5, right; sagittal plane (**a**) and axial plane (**b**). Postoperative magnetic resonance image; sagittal plane (**c**) and axial plane (**d**)

A 58-year-old man had radiating pain in his left leg for 2 months. Preoperative T2-weighted magnetic resonance image of a patient showed a foraminal HNP at L4–5, right (a, b). The biportal endoscopic paraspinal approach for foraminal HNP was successfully performed. Postoperative magnetic resonance image confirmed removal of foraminal HNP (c, d). The patient had complete resolution of radicular symptoms.

Complication and its Management

Postoperative Hematoma

Epidural bleeding can be coagulated using a radiofrequency probe at the lowest power, and uncontrolled epidural bleeding even after coagulation can be controlled by packing hemostatic materials such as gel foam and soluble hemostatic gauze (WoundClot™, Core Scientific Creations, Israel). Bleeding from a bone resection site can be effectively controlled by applying bone wax. A suction drain is inserted in the dorsal space of the nerve root to prevent postoperative hematoma. On postoperative day 2, postoperative MRI should be checked and the drainage should be removed.

Dural Tear

Durotomy is not common but can occur mostly during working blindly with the Kerrison rongeur. However, the sizes of most durotomies are not big enough to suture directly, and dural tear is controlled by attaching a fibrin collagen patch (TachoComb) and by maintaining lumbar drain for 5 to 7 days. However, if the size of durotomy is big, we recommend direct dural repair.

Abdominal Fluid Collection

Special care should be taken to not proceed ventrally farther than where the psoas muscle is. Otherwise, there is a possibility of fluid accumulating into the retroperitoneal space. That is why we need to pay more attention to fluid coming out in the biportal endoscopic paraspinal approach. Surgical landmarks are important for prevention of abdominal fluid collection. The surgeon always checks the SAP and isthmus and foraminal ligament structure during this approach. If muscle structures were only seen under endoscopic view during surgery, there was high possibility of lateral location of an endoscopy and instruments. Moreover, there was high possibility of abdominal fluid collection. Medial location of an endoscopy and surgical instruments around SAP and isthmus is important for prevention of abdominal fluid collection. C-arm fluoroscopic monitoring was also helpful to optimal location of an endoscopy and instruments.

Discussion

The best advantage of the biportal endoscopic paraspinal approach is that it can reach deep into the foramen less invasively with relatively free angles. This technique also facilitates decompression of the foraminal area, without sacrificing too much of the facet joint and paraspinal muscles. As a result, this approach carries little risk of postoperative instability. Further, this technique provides a good field of vision in a high magnification endoscopic view and a clearing view by continuous irrigation for good decompression of foraminal stenosis. Biportal surgery can provide the same surgical magnifying endoscopic view with a microsurgical view, which is familiar to most spine surgeons, which may help in learning the technique.

There are several potential technical pitfalls about the biportal endoscopic paraspinal approach. First, the tip of the two portals must be located below the pedicle. Second, the top of the SAP must be removed to provide space for additional bone working. Third, if the top of the SAP can be removed by using an osteotome, it is important to check the preoperative image to see whether there is calcification of the foraminal ligament. This is because when the foraminal ligament is calcified, there is a possibility of root injury. Fourth, if removal of the SAP medial part is enough, the disc can be removed without much root retraction. Finally, taking great care to maintain fluid output is important to prevent increasing intracranial pressure and retroperitoneal fluid collection.

References

1. Hasegawa T, Mikawa Y, Watanabe R, An HS. Morphometric analysis of the lumbosacral nerve roots and dorsal root ganglia by magnetic resonance imaging. Spine (Phila Pa 1976). 1996;21(9):1005–9.
2. Kunogi J, Hasue M. Diagnosis and operative treatment of intraforaminal and extraforaminal nerve root compression. Spine (Phila Pa 1976). 1991;16(11):1312–20.

3. Wiltse LL, Spencer CW. New uses and refinements of the paraspinal approach to the lumbar spine. Spine (Phila Pa 1976). 1988;13(6):696–706.
4. Chang SB, Lee SH, Ahn Y, Kim JM. Risk factor for unsatisfactory outcome after lumbar foraminal and far lateral microdecompression. Spine (Phila Pa 1976). 2006;31(10):1163–7.
5. Kim JE, Choi DJ. Bi-portal arthroscopic spinal surgery (BASS) with 30 degrees arthroscopy for far lateral approach of L5-S1 - technical note. J Orthop. 2018;15(2):354–8.
6. Heo DH, Sharma S, Park CK. Endoscopic treatment of Extraforaminal entrapment of L5 nerve root (far out syndrome) by unilateral Biportal endoscopic approach: technical report and preliminary clinical results. Neurospine. 2019;16(1):130–7.
7. Park MK, Park SA, Son SK, Park WW, Choi SH. Clinical and radiological outcomes of unilateral biportal endoscopic lumbar interbody fusion (ULIF) compared with conventional posterior lumbar interbody fusion (PLIF): 1-year follow-up. Neurosurg Rev. 2019;42(3):753–61.

Part IV

Lumbar Disc Herniation

Full Endoscopic Approach with Foraminoplasty

Kyung-Chul Choi and Hyeong-Ki Shim

Introduction

Transforaminal endoscopic lumbar discectomy (TELD) gives results comparable to those of conventional open surgery for treatment of herniated discs (HDs). Since the introduction of contemporary endoscopic discectomy by Kambin and Sampson [1], remarkable advances in techniques and instruments have expanded its surgical application for various types of HDs. [2, 3] Nevertheless, the inability to place a working cannula near the disc fragment because of an anatomical barrier can lead to surgical failure and to the need for revision open surgery. The superior articular process (SAP) should be the chief obstacle to transforaminal endoscopic access to the dural sac and nerve root in the spinal canal. To overcome this hurdle, foraminoplasty can be considered, as it allows the working cannula to access the herniated disc. In this chapter, we describe our experience using foraminoplasty for HDs and propose indications for its use. [4]

Electronic Supplementary Material The online version of this chapter (https://doi.org/10.1007/978-981-15-8253-0_11) contains supplementary material, which is available to authorized users.

K.-C. Choi (✉) · H.-K. Shim
Department of Neurosurgery, Seoul Top Spine & Joint Hospital, Goyangsi, South Korea

Indications

- Decreased disc height.
- High-grade up/down migration.
- Sequestration.
- Recurrent disc herniation.
- Central disc herniation with wide lamina angle.
- Huge (large) disc herniation.
- L5-S1 disc herniation with high iliac crest.
- Disc herniation with foraminal stenosis & lateral recess stenosis.

Anesthesia and Position

- **Local**/regional/general anesthesia.
- **Prone position**/lateral decubitus.

Special Surgical Instruments (Fig. 1)

- Manual bone drills.
- Endoscopic drill.
- Endoscopic Kerrison punch.
- Curved semi-flexible forceps/probe.

H. S. Kim et al. (eds.), *Advanced Techniques of Endoscopic Lumbar Spine Surgery*,
https://doi.org/10.1007/978-981-15-8253-0_11

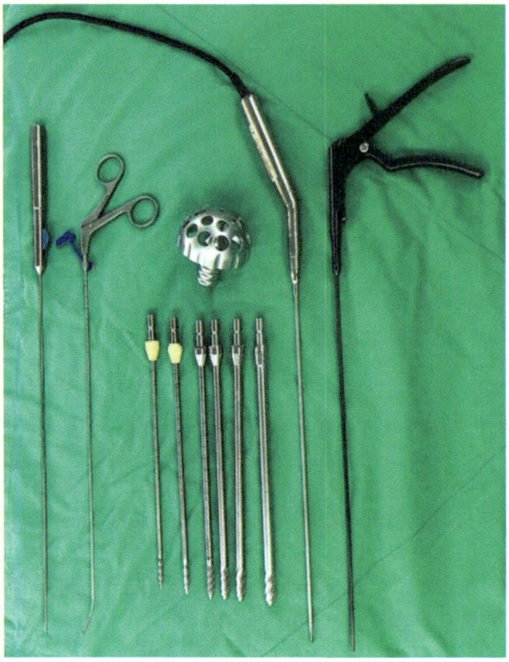

Fig. 1 Endoscopic instruments for foraminoplasty. Manual bone drills, endoscopic diamond drill, endoscopic Kerrison punch, semi-flexible forceps and probe

Surgical Steps

Initial Targeting

TELD was performed under local anesthesia with patients in the prone position. The entry point on the skin was generally 8–14 cm from the midline, with consideration of both body size and disc location (Fig. 2a). After infiltration of the entry point with local anesthetics, an 18-gauge spinal needle was introduced under the guidance of fluoroscopic imaging. Subsequently, an epidurography was performed using contrast media to confirm the location of the exiting and traversing roots (Fig. 2b). Then, 1–2 cc of 1% lidocaine was injected on the outer surface of the annulus. After inserting the spinal needle into the disc, the nucleus pulposus was stained blue with 1 mL of contrast media (Telebrix, Guerbet, France) and indigo carmine solution (Carmine, Korea United Pharmaceutical, Yoenki, Korea) for discography (Figs. 2c, d). The location of the spinal needle was checked at the medial pedicular line on the AP view and the posterior vertebral line on the lateral view. The final target point depended on the disc location and surgical level. In paramedian disc herniation, the final target point of the spinal needle was the medial pedicular line on the anteroposterior (AP) view and the posterior vertebral line on the lateral view. For central disc herniation, the spinal needle was targeted between the medial pedicle line and midline in the AP view and on the posterior vertebral line on the lateral view. For downward migrated disc herniation, the needle was located on the superior vertebral notch of the lower vertebra with a cranio-caudal inclinatory 20–30° angle (Fig. 2e). However, when the spinal needle was located close to the target point in the AP view and the needle tip was located within the disc space in the lateral view, foraminoplasty should be performed; using a bone reamer or endoscopic drill, the SAP was partially removed.

Foraminoplasty

Serial manual bone drills were advanced to the medial pedicular line under fluoroscopy in ascending order of size (Figs. 3a, b). After using the largest reamer, needle placement was re-attempted.

Final PELD Procedure

After foraminoplasty, a tapered cannulated obturator was inserted along the guidewire; after touching the annulus, an obturator was inserted into the disc using hammering; a bevel-ended and oval-shaped working cannula was inserted into the disc along the obturator, and the obturator was removed. Next, an endoscope (Vertebris system; Richard Wolf GmbH, Germany) was inserted through the cannula (Fig. 3c). The facet joint was partially removed using an endoscopic drill, cutting forceps, and endoscopic Kerrison punch, while engaging the

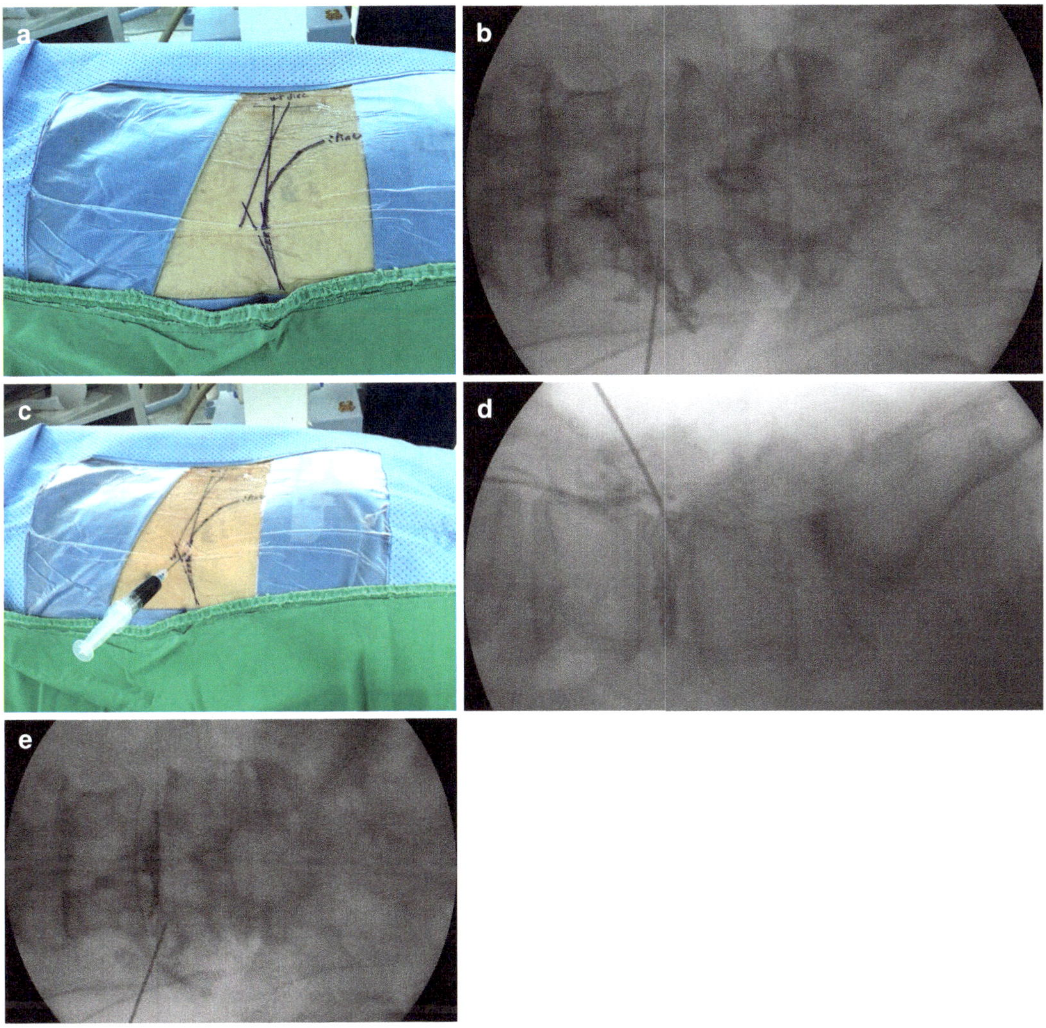

Fig. 2 Surgical steps (**a**) skin entry point, (**b**) epidurogram, (**c**, **d**) discography, and (**e**) intraoperative radiography revealing initial targeting for downward migrated disc herniation

working cannula. The yellow ligament was removed, and the traversing nerve root was exposed. Generally, the fragment is hidden under the traversing nerve root. Under endoscopic view, the disc fragment was pulled out with a curved probe and curved forceps. After removal of the fragment, the traversing nerve root became mobile. If disc protrusion was found in the disc space, the subannular disc was removed using the conventional method. After the herniated fragment was completely removed, the endoscope was removed.

High-Grade Migration/Downward Sequestration

Conventional TELD techniques may present difficulties in removing migrated HDs. Rigid instrumentation, poor visualization, and inability to reach or grasp herniated fragments render migrated discs inaccessible in conventional TELD. In particular, a rigid endoscope cannot be used to visualize the whole fragment for large migrated HDs. However, an inclinatory approach from the cranio-caudal or caudo-cra-

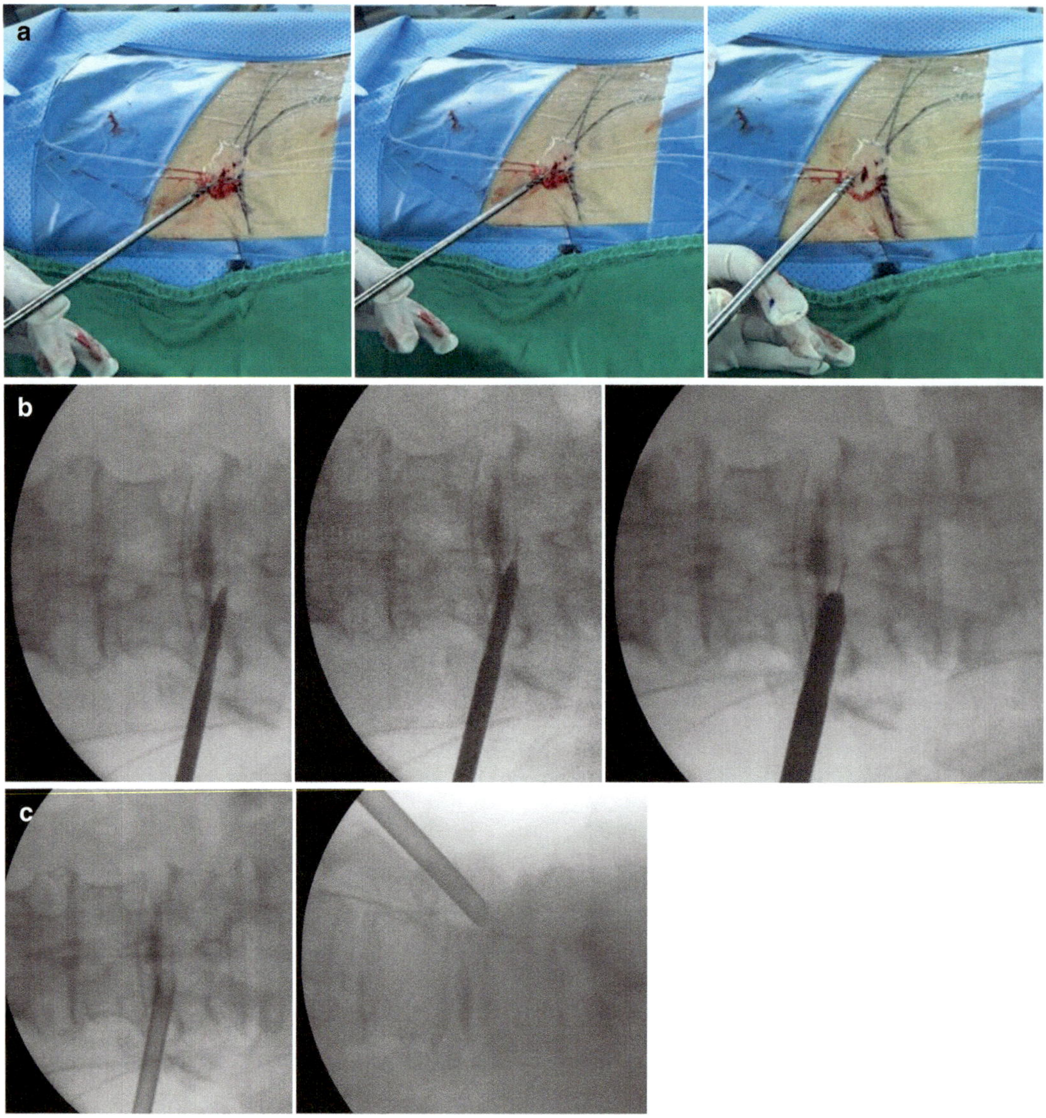

Fig. 3 Sequential reaming (**a**) intraoperative photos, (**b**) intraoperative radiographies and (**c**) the location of working cannula on the target point

nial direction can help extract and grasp the disc fragment using flexible curved forceps. For high-grade down migration or down-migrated sequestration, resection of the base of the superior facet and upper pedicle can aid in the visualization of hidden disc fragments in the anterior epidural space.

Illustrative Case

A 71-year-old woman had undergone microscopic discectomy at L4-L5 level 3 years prior. She complained of left leg pain and buttock pain. MR images revealed a large disc fragment that had migrated inferior to the level (Fig. 4a, b). The

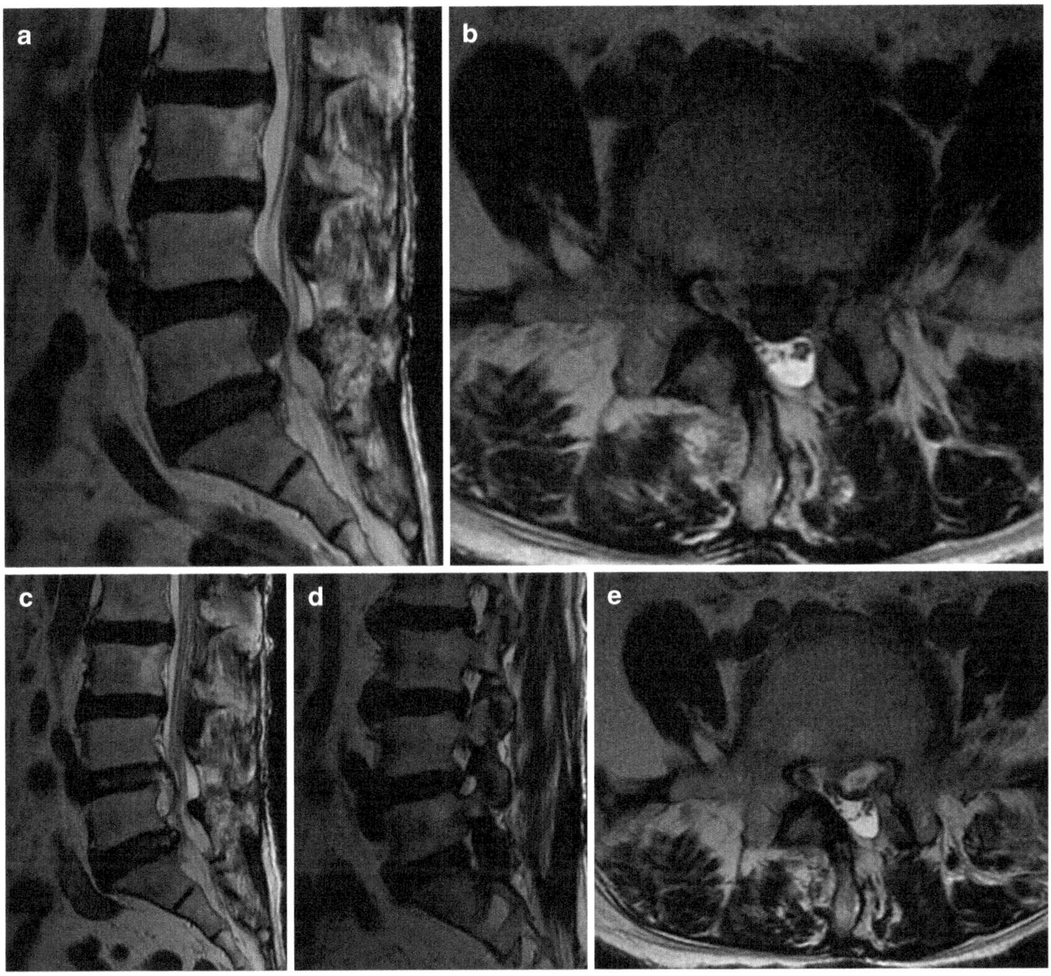

Fig. 4 Recurrent disc herniation with downward migration (**a**) Preoperative MR sagittal image revealing the HD extending downwardly at L4–5, (**b**) MR axial image, (**c**) postoperative MR sagittal image showing complete removal of HD, (**d**) MR sagittal image showing partial removal of the superior articular process (SAP) at the foraminal zone and (**e**) MR axial image

pain did not diminish after two epidural steroid injections. After endoscopic foraminoplasty, the disc fragment was removed using TELD (Video 1). MR images (Fig. 4c–d) showed complete removal of the HD and partial resection of the facet joint.

Recurrent Disc Herniation

TELD via the transforaminal route is effective for recurrent disc herniation and can reduce surgery-related complications and operation time. It can also facilitate rapid recovery using a virgin trajectory. After lumbar discectomy, disc height (DH) is significantly decreased and disc degeneration and facet arthropathy might progress. These changes can lead to foraminal narrowing, making it difficult for transforaminal endoscopic access to the epidural space and increasing the possibility of exiting nerve injury. If the working cannula is located far from the HD fragment due to facet hypertrophy, a disc fragment in the epidural space might remain if only the subannular disc or nucleus pulposus within the disc space is removed. Removing the middle part of the SAP

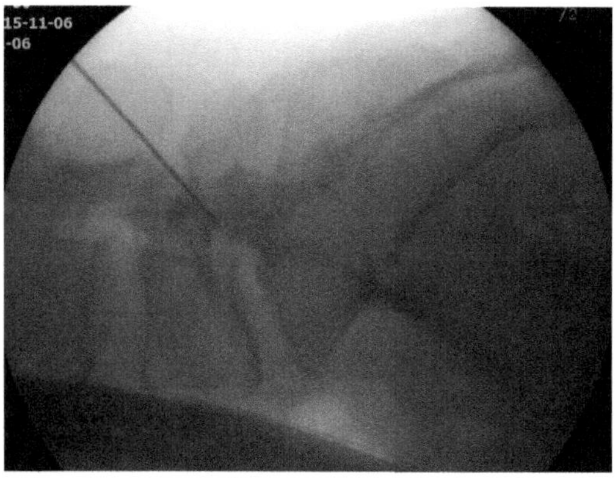

Fig. 5 For L5-S1 disc herniation, the trajectoy of the needle is cranio-caudal

can reduce the trajectory angle and facilitate working cannula access to the epidural space.

L5-S1 Intracanal Disc Herniation with a High Iliac Crest

The foraminal dimension decreases as the spinal level decreases; the L5-S1 level has a relatively shorter DH with larger facet joints than those of the other levels. These anatomical characteristics are barriers to performing TELD. Suprailiac entry, a cranio-caudal oblique trajectory, and widening of the posterior border (SAP) of the working zone can overcome anatomical barriers, allowing access near the epidural space (Fig. 5a). If the highest point of the iliac crest is located above the upper margin of the L5 pedicle in lateral radiography, foraminoplasty will be required [5].

Illustrative Case

A 36-year-old woman suffered from left posterior leg pain. The deep tendon reflex of ankle was diminished. Although she took medications and underwent physical therapy, the pain remained. A large central disc herniation compressed the thecal sac and left S1 nerve root (Fig. 6a, b). The iliac crest overlapped the intervertebral foramen of L5-S1 (Fig. 6c). To access near the HD, foraminoplasty was required. MR images (Fig. 6d, e) showed complete removal of HD and partial removal of SAP.

Central Disc Herniation with a Wide Lamina Angle

A conventional "inside-out technique" has an approach angle of approximately 25° and involves an intradiscal working channel that utilizes a cavity via an annulotomy opening using biting forceps. However, this technique is limited with respect to the removal of epidural disc fragments in the central portion of an HD. In cases of centrally located HDs, a bevel-ended cannula should be placed in the midline on the AP view and between the epidural space and intra-annular portion on the lateral view under intraoperative fluoroscopic guidance. The entry point is further from the midline than for a paramedian disc herniation, and the approach angle is shallower. When a central disc herniation is accompanied by a wide lamina angle (>100°), the working cannula will be far from the disc herniation with a steep approach angle (Fig. 7a) [4]. Partial removal of the superior facet joint (Fig. 7b) can reduce the approach angle, allowing the working cannula to be placed below the disc fragment (Fig. 7c).

Complications and their Management

TELD under local anesthesia potentially limits neural injury, although some authors perform PELD safely under general anesthesia [6]. The exiting nerve root (ENR) should be protected during the procedure. Irritation of the ENR and dorsal root ganglion can cause severe leg pain. In this situation, if irritation symptoms develop, the surgeon should try to adjust the entry point and trajectory, and then stop the procedure if the pain persists. Postoperative dysesthesia is one of the significant sequelae that negatively affects the quality of life. Considering the safety triangle, far from the ENR, a more caudal approach along the superior border of the inferior pedicle may be safe. Serial dilation and sequential reaming procedures

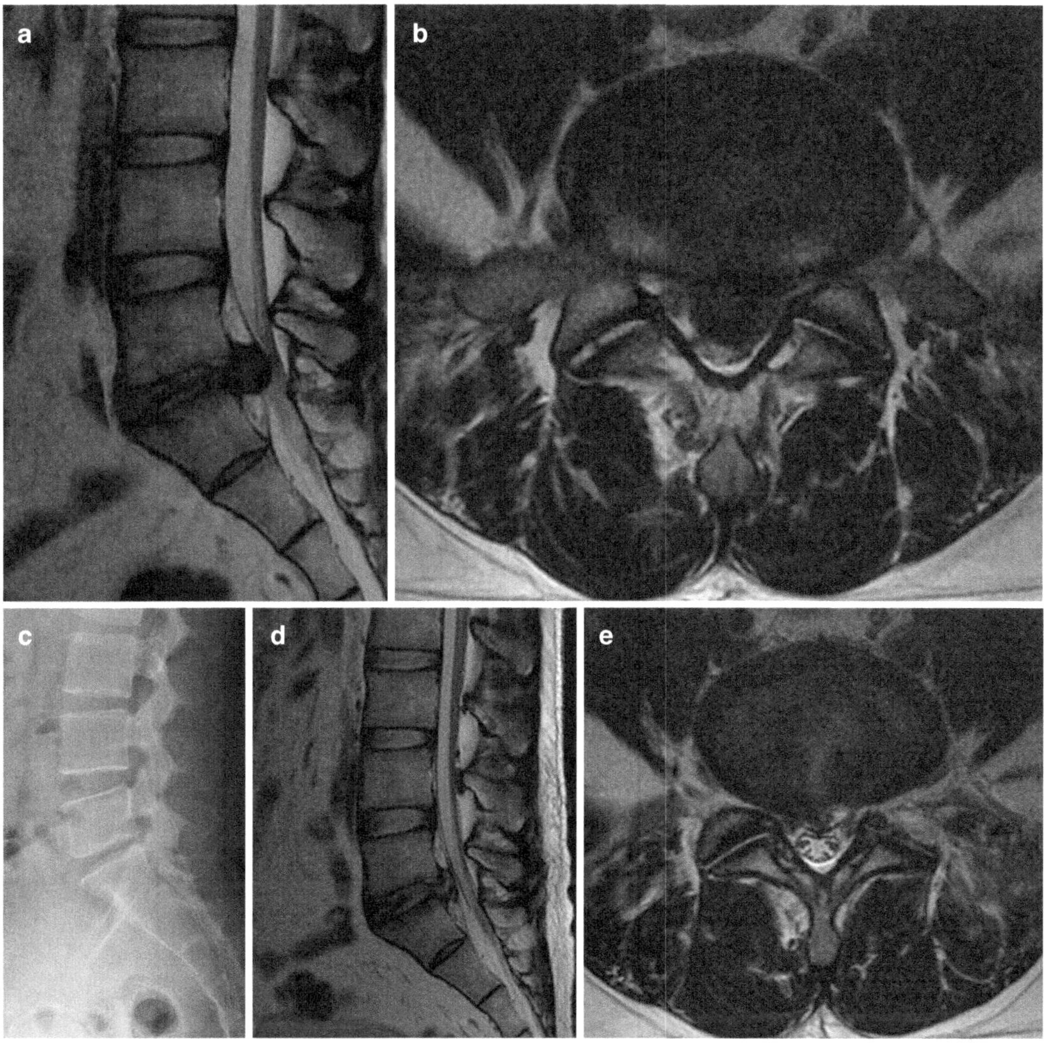

Fig. 6 L5-S1 disc herniation (**a**) preoperative MR sagittal image, (**b**) MR axial image showing large disc herniation compressed thecal sac and left S1 nerve root, (**c**) lateral radiography showing iliac crest overlapped the intervertebral foramen of L5-S1, (**d**) postoperative MR sagittal image and (**e**) MR axial image showing complete removal of HD with partial removal of the SAP

can reduce injury to the ENR. In severe foraminal stenosis, endoscopic foraminotomy using an endoscopic diamond drill from outside foramen to inside foramen is safer and more effective than using a manual bone drill. Reaming with too steep an approach angle, the disc space could be directly violated. Using fluoroscopic lateral imaging, the procedure can proceed appropriately.

Concomitant persistent pain is commonly caused by surgically unappreciated disc fragments, concurrent lateral recess stenosis, nerve root injury, epidural hematoma, and nerve root edema regardless of the appearance of complete removal of the herniated disc on postoperative MR. Concurrent lateral recess stenosis (Fig. 8a) is associated with poor prognosis. Lateral recess bony stenosis can be addressed with a separate decompression procedure. This requires partial removal of the SAP and ligamentum flavum (Fig. 8b).

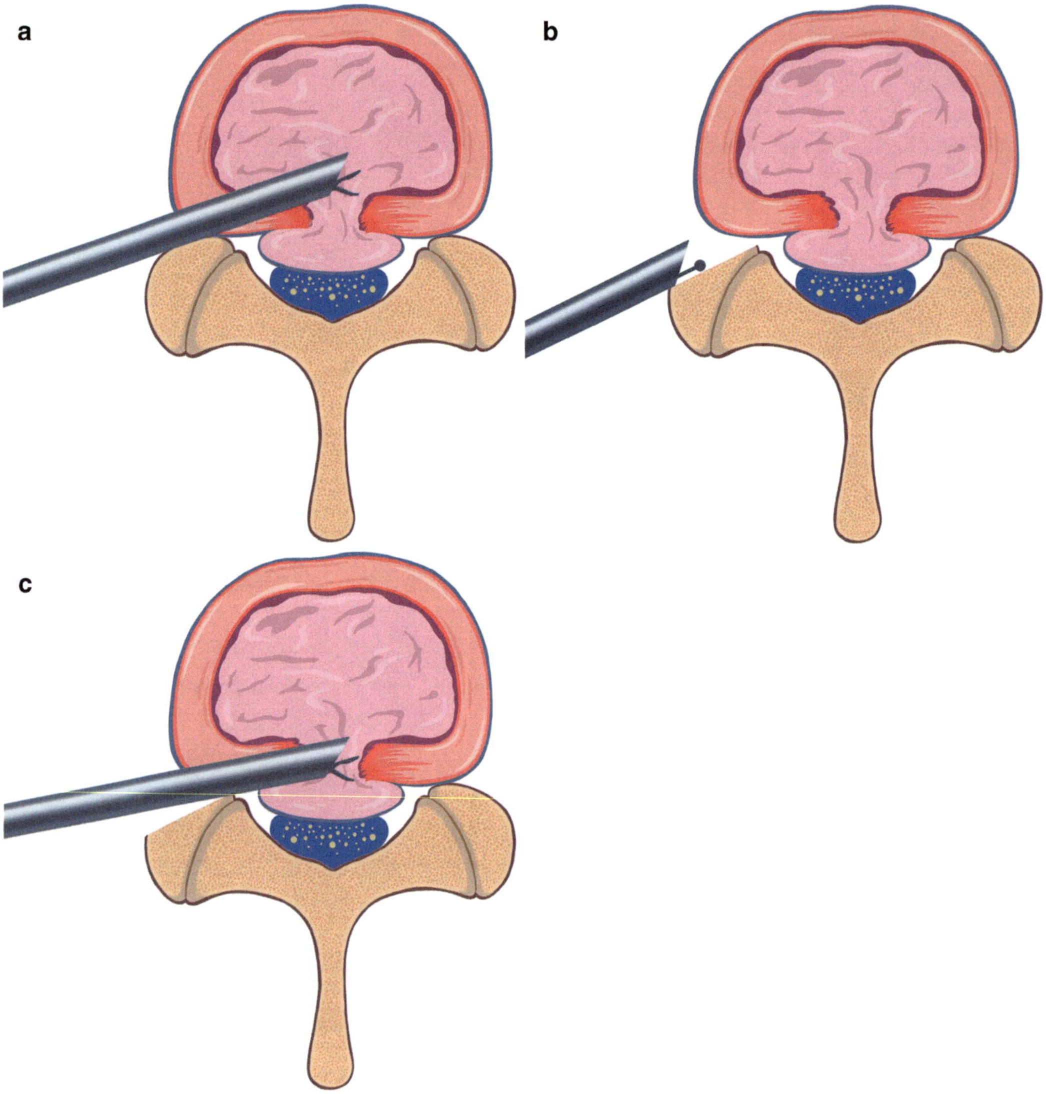

Fig. 7 Schematic illustration of transforaminal endoscopic lumbar discectomy (TELD) facilitated by endoscopic foraminoplasty for central disc herniation. (**a**) Conventional posterolateral TELD technique is shown with a herniated disc fragment in the epidural space inaccessible to the working cannula. (**b**) Removal of a SAP with an endoscopic drill is shown. (**c**) After foraminoplasty, the working cannula is located near the herniated disc fragment

Brief Discussion: Surgical Tip and Pitfall

Endoscopic foraminoplasty was first introduced by Knight et al. [7] Using a Holmium-Yag side-firing laser, undercutting of the facet joint, discectomy, mobilization of the exiting and traversing nerve roots, and ablation of osteophytes could be performed. Foraminal widening techniques, called "foraminoplasty," help surgeons access the epidural space, allowing visualization of hidden disc fragments and decompression of foraminal or lateral recess stenosis. Advances in endoscopic instruments, bone

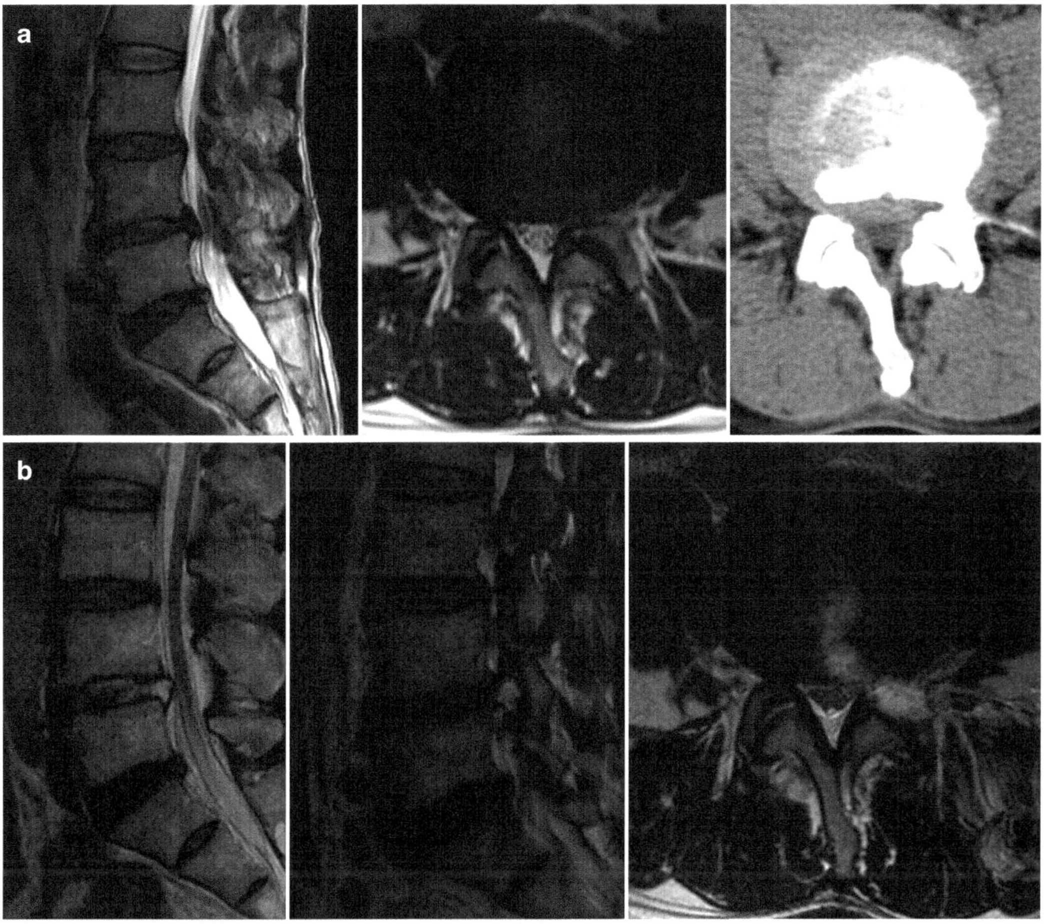

Fig. 8 HD with lateral recess stenosis (**a**) MR images and CT scan showing disc herniation with lateral recess stenosis at L4–5. (**b**) Postop MR images showing removal of HD and the SAP

Table 1 Clinical results of endoscopic foraminoplasty

Authors	No. of patients	Disease	Technique	Aim	Instruments	Success rate	Complication	Publication year
Knight et al. [7]	250	Foraminal stenosis	Endoscopic foraminoplasty	Decompression of exiting nerve root and traversing nerve root	Laser	73%	1 foot drop, 5% revision	1998
Schubert and Hoogland [8]	558	Disc herniation	Endoscopic foraminoplasty	Widening of foraminal zone	Reamer	95%	0.5% transient paresthesia, 3.6% revision	2005
Choi et al. [2]	59	Migrated disc herniation	Endoscopic foraminoplasty	Widening of foraminal zone and partial pediculectomy	Endoscopic drill	91%	8.5% revision	2008
Ahn et al. [9]	33	Foraminal stenosis	Endoscopic foraminotomy	Decompression of exiting nerve root	Endoscopic drill, laser, micropunch	82%	6.1% dysesthesia, 3% revision	2014
Choi and Park [5]	100	Disc herniation at L5–S1	Endoscopic foraminoplasty	Widening of foraminal zone	Reamer	92%	2% revision	2016

trephines, reamers, and endoscopic drills have occurred (Table 1). For example, an endoscopic diamond drill was used to undercut the superior facet in a study by Choi et al. [2] By contrast, a bone reamer under fluoroscopic guidance was used by Schubert and Hoogland. [8] Choi and Park also used reamers to engage the L5-S1 foramen [5]. Ahn et al. described a technique called "endoscopic foraminotomy" that achieves full decompression of the exiting nerve root in a foraminal stenosis using an endoscopic drill, side-firing laser, and endoscopic Kerrison punch. An endoscopic reamer or endoscopic drill was used for foraminal widening [9]. Sequential reaming using bone reamers or trephines is not a time-consuming technique and only depends on fluoroscopy. Nevertheless, sequential reaming can lead to neural injury and difficulties in controlling bone bleeding. To prevent neural injury, the reamer should not be advanced over the medial pedicular line, as suggested by Lee et al. [10] Furthermore, reaming is limited in terms of removal of a large portion of a large facet joint or hypertrophied facet joint. By contrast, an endoscopic drill can minimize neural injury under vision and a large amount of the facet joint can be removed. Finally, a diamond burr rarely causes bone bleeding. The downside of this procedure is that it is time-consuming.

The foraminoplasty target (Fig. 9) should be individualized for each situation. For a L5-S1 disc herniation in the spinal canal, removal of the cranial tip of the SAP through an oblique trajectory in the cranio-caudal direction can facilitate access to the disc fragment. For large central disc and recurrent disc herniation, the trajectory angle can be reduced by removing the mid-portion of the SAP at the mid-disc space level. For a downward-migrated disc, removing the base of the SAP and partially removing the upper pedicle can provide good visualization of a hidden disc.

Endoscopic lumbar foraminoplasty may be effective for small DH, high-grade downward migration, downward sequestration, recurrent HD, HD in L5-S1 with a high iliac crest, central HD with a wide lamina angle, and HD with lateral recess stenosis.

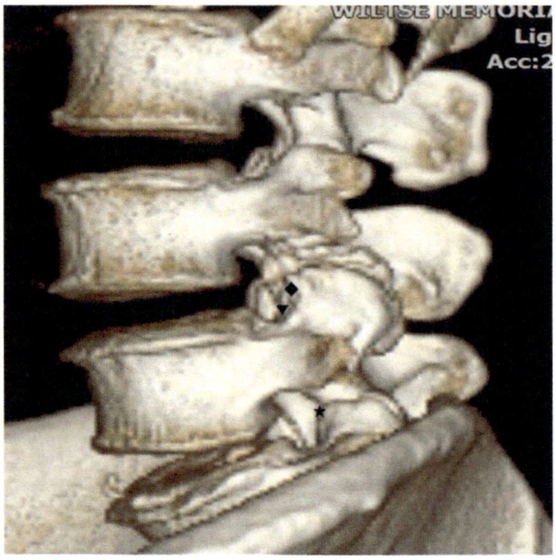

Fig. 9 Foraminoplasty target. For a L5-S1 disc herniation, the cranial tip (★) of the SAP through an oblique trajectory in the cranio-caudal direction. For large central disc and recurrent disc herniation, the mid portion (◆) of the SAP at the mid-disc space level. For a down-migrated disc, removing the base (▼) of the SAP and partially removing the upper pedicle

References

1. Kambin P, Sampson S. Posterolateral percutaneous suction-excision of herniated lumbar intervertebral discs. Report of interim results. Clin Orhtop Relat Res. 1986;207:37–43.
2. Choi G, Lee SH, Lokhande P, et al. Percutaneous endoscopic approach for highly migrated intracanal disc herniations by foraminoplastic technique using rigid working channel endoscope. Spine (Phila Pa 1976). 2008;33:E508–15.
3. Choi KC, Lee DC, Shim HK, et al. A strategy of percutaneous endoscopic lumbar discectomy for migrated disc herniation. World Neurosurg. 2017;99:259–66.
4. Choi KC, Shim HK, Park CJ, et al. Usefulness of percutaneous endoscopic lumbar Foraminoplasty for lumbar disc herniation. World Neurosurg. 2017;106:484–92.
5. Choi KC, Park CK. Percutaneous endoscopic lumbar discectomy for L5-S1 disc herniation: consideration of the relation between the iliac crest and L5-S1 disc. Pain Physician. 2016;19:E301–8.
6. Ruetten S, Komp M, Merk H, et al. Full-endoscopic interlaminar and transforaminal lumbar discectomy versus conventional microsurgical technique: a prospective, randomized, controlled study. Spine (Phila Pa 1976). 2008;33:931–9.
7. Knight MT, Vajda A, Jakab GV, et al. Endoscopic laser foraminoplasty on the lumbar spine--early experience. Minim Invasive Neurosurg. 1998;41:5–9.

8. Schubert M, Hoogland T. Endoscopic transforaminal nucleotomy with foraminoplasty for lumbar disk herniation. Oper Orthop Traumatol. 2005;17:641–61.
9. Ahn Y, Oh HK, Kim H, et al. Percutaneous endoscopic lumbar foraminotomy: an advanced surgical technique and clinical outcomes. Neurosurgery. 2014;75:124–33. discussion 132-123
10. Lee CW, Yoon KJ, Ha SS, et al. Foraminoplastic superior vertebral notch approach with reamers in percutaneous endoscopic lumbar discectomy : technical note and clinical outcome in limited indications of percutaneous endoscopic lumbar discectomy. J Korean Neurosurg Soc. 2016;59:172–81.

Full-Endoscopic Transpedicular Approach

Jin-Sung Kim, Kuo-Tai Chen, and Gun Choi

Introduction

Though full-endoscopic spine surgery has developed to treat nearly all kinds of lumbar disc herniation, removal of the high-grade down-migrated disc below the suprapedicular border and medial to the pedicle remains a challenge even to an experienced endoscopic surgeon. With the advent of the endoscopic technology, notably endoscopic drill and various articulated or navigable instruments, different techniques have been proposed to achieve fragmentectomy in this situation. Options presented in the previous literature included (1) transforaminal approach with foraminoplasty by removing the ventral part of superior articular process and partially superior portion of the inferior pedicle by reamer or burr [1]; (2) contralateral transforaminal route reaching the target under the thecal sac through the contralateral neural foramen [2]; and (3) interlaminar approach with inferior laminectomy including the pars interarticularis, medial facetectomy, and retraction of traversing nerve root and dural sac [3, 4]. However, the transforaminal technique might put the exiting root at risk. Retraction of traversing root and complicated procedures with longer operation time is mainly concerned with the interlaminar approach. Krzok et al. introduced the transpedicular technique to access the juxta-pedicular epidural space [5–7]. The surgical corridor is away from the exiting root, and the retraction of the traversing root is needless. These procedures have been followed by other spine surgeons [8, 9]. The following paragraphs will describe the full-endoscopic transpedicular approach in detail.

Electronic Supplementary Material The online version of this chapter (https://doi.org/10.1007/978-981-15-8253-0_12) contains supplementary material, which is available to authorized users.

J.-S. Kim
Department of Neurosurgery, Seoul St. Mary's Hospital, The Catholic University of Korea, Seoul, South Korea

K.-T. Chen
Department of Neurosurgery, Chang Gung Memorial Hospital, Chia-Yi, Taiwan

G. Choi (✉)
Department of Neurosurgery, Pohang Woori Hospital, Pohang, South Korea

Anatomy

The anatomical characteristics of the lumbar pedicle vary according to the different levels. The pedicular diameters and cranial-caudal length determine the feasibility of the transpedicular approach. According to the cadaveric study, the widest lumbar pedicle was measured at L5 as 17.1 ± 4.2 mm and the narrowest at L1 as 8.4 ± 1.8 mm. The longest lumbar pedicle was measured at L2 as 15.3 ± 2.2 mm and the shortest

H. S. Kim et al. (eds.), *Advanced Techniques of Endoscopic Lumbar Spine Surgery*,
https://doi.org/10.1007/978-981-15-8253-0_12

at L4 as 13.8 ± 2.3 mm [10]. These data indicated that the surface area of the L1 and L2 pedicles is approximately half of the surface area of the L5 pedicles. The diameter of the working cannula available on the market is usually 7.0–7.5 mm. Therefore, there is a risk of iatrogenic fracture at L1 and L2 levels for transpedicular trajectory due to the relatively smaller cross-sectional area.

Indication and Contraindication

Indication

- High-grade down-migrated disc herniations medial to the pedicle and located in the shoulder of the traversing nerve root.
- Facet cysts arising to the medial pedicle [6].

Contraindication/limitations

- Calcified disc fragment on preoperative image.
- Prolonged symptoms, more than 6 months.
- Disc fragment axillary in location to the traversing nerve root.
- Approach to L1 and L2 pedicles (when the size of the pedicle is less than 12 mm).
- Severe osteoporosis.
- Centrally down-migrated disc herniation.
- Hypoplastic pedicle at the index level.
- Severe canal compromise with high-grade migration with neurologic deficits.
- High iliac crest [7].

Surgical Instruments [8]

- Endoscope profile: angle of optics, 25°; length, 207 mm; working channel, 4.1 mm; 6.3-mm outer diameter (RIWOspine GmbH, Knittlingen, Germany).
- 18-gauge spinal needle
- Guidewire: 0.8 mm.
- Trephine or reamer: 3 mm, 5 mm.
- Obturator: 6.5 mm.
- Working cannula: 7 mm.
- Endoscopic drill: diamond tip (3 mm or 3.5 mm).
- Endoscopic forceps: working length (320 mm) and diameter (3.5 mm).
- Radiofrequency cautery (Trigger-Flex, Elliquence, LLC, Baldwin, USA).
- Dissection tools: blunt tip probe, curved nerve hook.

Surgical Techniques [8, 9]

1. Position
   The patient is placed prone with hips and knees in flexion posture on a radiolucent Jackson table.
2. Plan entry point
   The entry point is planned by preoperative imaging (CT scan and MRI) and is located approximately 12 cm lateral to the midline for L5 pedicle, 11 cm for L4, and 10 cm for L3.
3. Anesthesia and needle insertion
   Local anesthesia with conscious sedation is performed. The intravenous midazolam 0.05 mg/kg and fentanyl 0.8 mg/kg can be administered for conscious sedation initially and repeated intraoperatively if required. The skin is infiltrated with 1% lidocaine, and a 25-cm, 18-gauge spinal needle is advanced and placed on the lateral wall of the pedicle, behind the transverse process. The periosteum of the pedicle is also infiltrated with 1% lidocaine to avoid perioperative pain during the approach. The anteroposterior (AP) and lateral C-arm fluoroscopy confirms the correct location of the spinal needle (Fig. 1).
4. Docking working cannula
   After local anesthesia, the spinal needle is replaced by a K-wire. The obturator is placed through the wire to dilate paraspinal muscles. A tapered obturator with 6.5 mm in diameter is introduced through an 8-mm skin incision. The tip of the obturator should be placed on

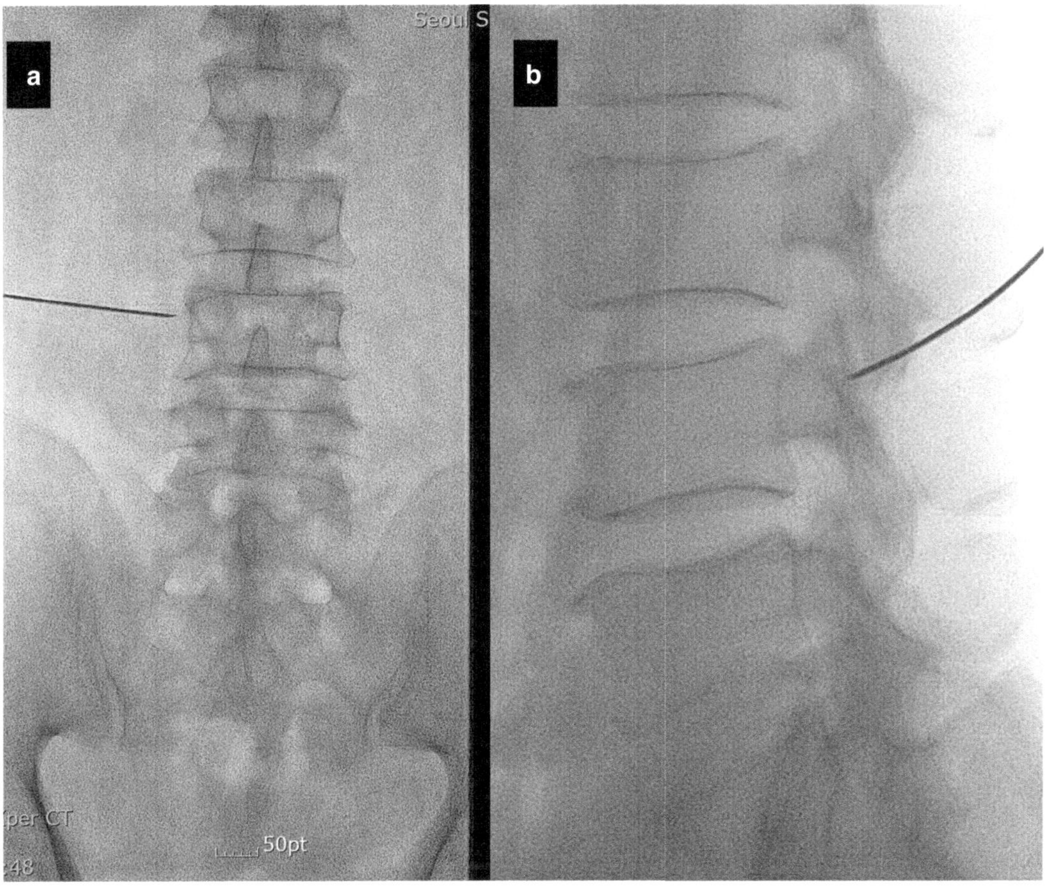

Fig. 1 The illustration of the ideal needle placement for left pedicular approach. (**a**) On the AP view fluoroscopy, the needle is placed at 9 o'clock on the lateral pedicle wall. (**b**) On the lateral view fluoroscopy, the needle is placed at the midpoint of the pedicle posterior to the transverse process

the lateral wall of the pedicle, for the right pedicle at 3 o'clock, and the left pedicle at 9 o'clock on the AP view (Fig. 2). The K-wire is removed, and a 7-mm diameter beveled working cannula is passed over the obturator.

5. Create a transpedicular tunnel

   A 25° rod-lens endoscope of 6.3-mm outer diameter is advanced through the beveled working cannula to visualize the lateral wall of the pedicle directly. Then, an 8-mm transpedicular tunnel is made with an endoscopic drill using a cutting or diamond tip depending on the surgeon's preference. The target point is always the medial wall of the pedicle to reach the juxta-pedicular disc fragment. Frequently intermittent intraoperative fluoroscopy is highly encouraged at this step. After transpedicular drilling, a thin layer of cortical bone from its medial wall is removed with endoscopic Kerrison punch. The endoscope is advanced through the tunnel to visualize the migrated disc herniation directly (Fig. 3). During drilling the pedicle, bleeding from the cancellous bone usually occurs and radiofrequency (RF) probe can help hemostasis.

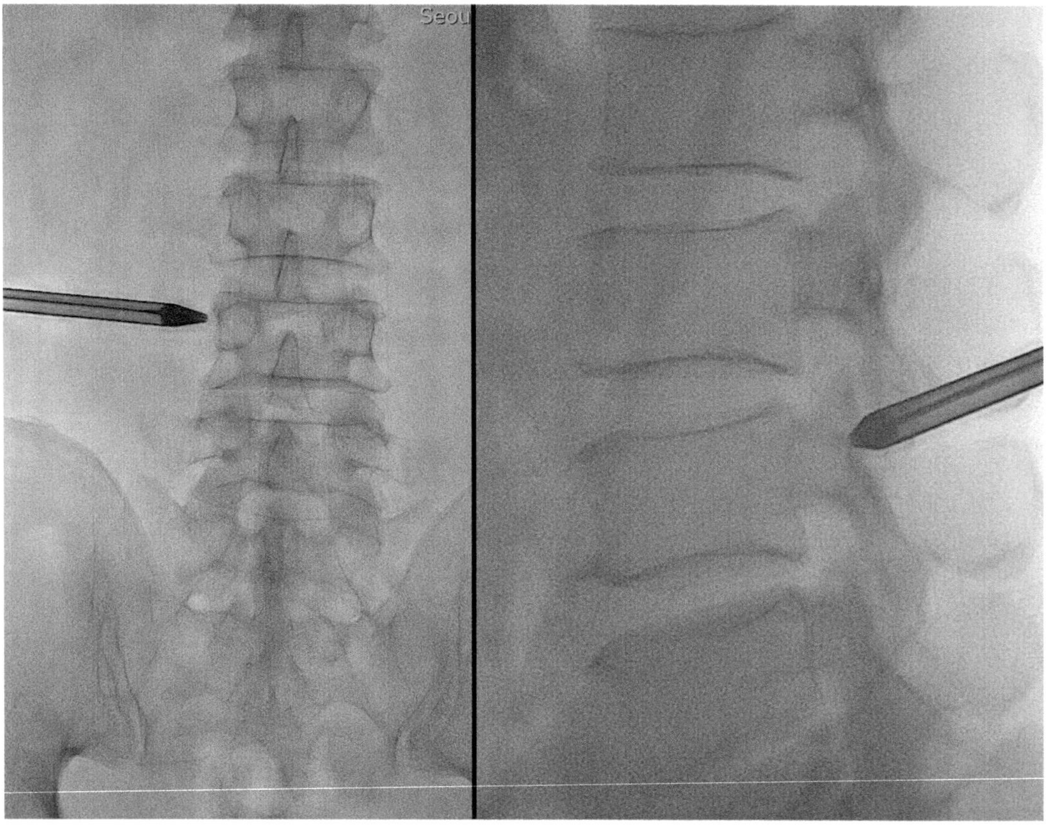

Fig. 2 A tapered, cannulated obturator is inserted along the guidewire and located in the lateral wall of the pedicle and confirmed with intraoperative fluoroscopy (AP and lateral views)

There is another technique with the use of trephine in this step. First, a trephine size of 3 mm is docked at the starting bony point as described above and is advanced without penetrating the medial pedicle wall under fluoroscopic guidance. Once a pilot hole is drilled through the pedicle, its trajectory is confirmed with C-arm fluoroscopy, and the tunnel is further widened with a larger trephine size of 5 mm. Then, the operator can dock the working cannula along the same trajectory and the endoscope is introduced into the cannula. The endoscopic burr is used to remove the medial pedicular wall under endoscopic visualization to enter the spinal canal.

6. Fragmentectomy

   When the disc is visualized, the bipolar RF probe can help shrink the fragment to be easily removed with flexible endoscopic forceps (Fig. 4). Afterward, the juxta-pedicular ventral epidural space is explored with an endoscopic nerve hook to fish for residual fragments. The initially displaced traversing nerve root is free and pulsatile. Epidural venous bleeding can be coagulated with the RF probe. Finally, the endoscope and working cannula are removed from the patient, and the wound is closed with a single skin suture.

All the crucial procedures of the surgery, as mentioned above, are described in the following video (Video 1).

How to Avoid Complications

1. Pedicle fracture

   The pedicle diameters determine the feasibility of the transpedicular approach and the risk of iatrogenic fracture. The width and cranial-

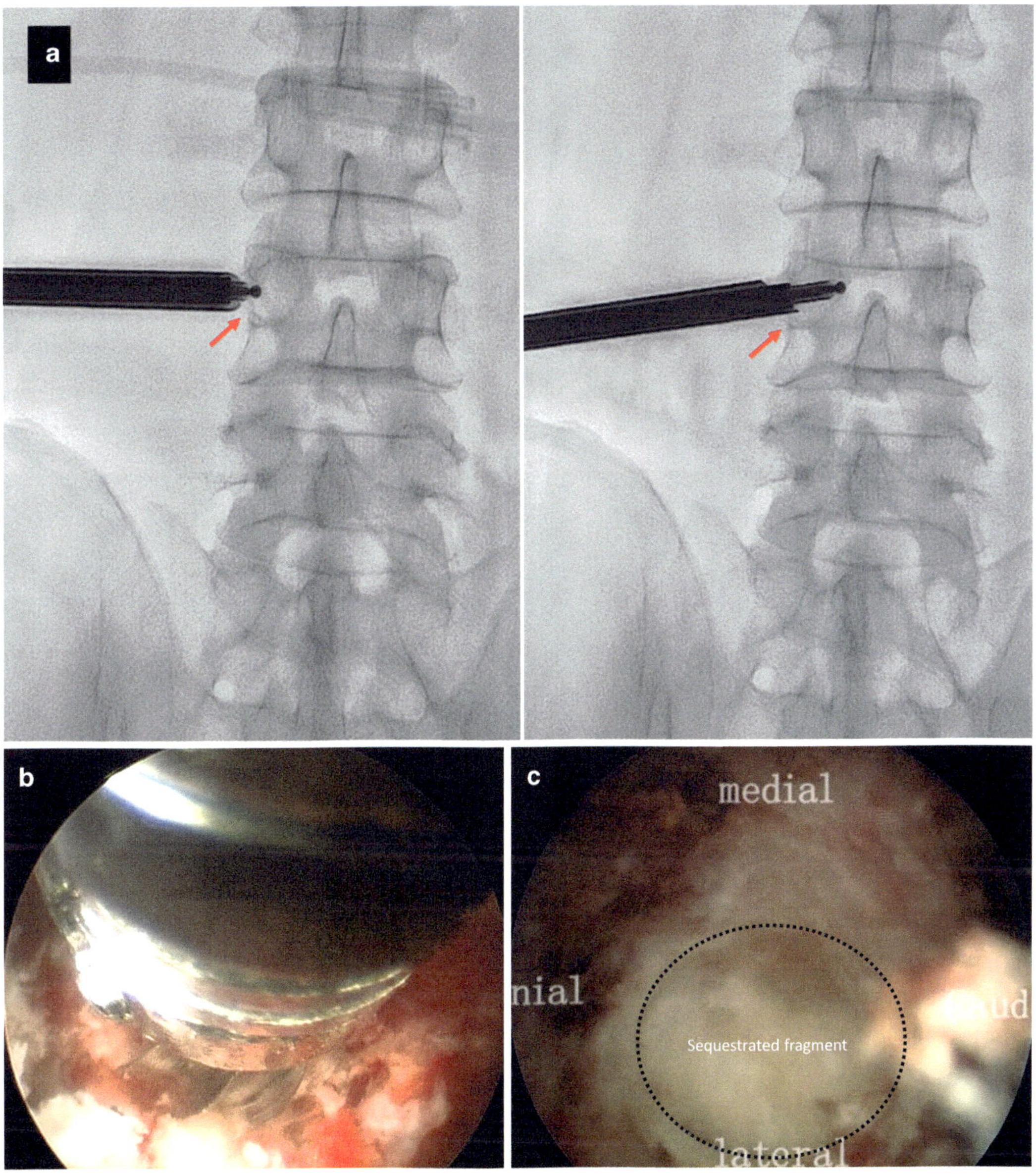

Fig. 3 The intraoperative fluoroscopic and endoscopic view during the creation of the transpedicular tunnel. (**a**) The tunnel through the pedicle is made with an endoscopic drill, from lateral to the medial wall (red arrows). Intermittent fluoroscopy can help with guiding the direction and depth of the endoscopic burr during creating the transpedicular tunnel. (**b**) Drilling the transpedicular tunnel with endoscopic burr. (**c**) A bone window is made at the medial pedicular wall (dotted line). The sequestrated disc fragment is identified through the bone window

caudal length of pedicle at the index level should be measured on preoperative CT images. The diameter of the bone corridor should not exceed 8 mm to preserve as much as pedicle mass and decrease the risk of iatrogenic fracture. Besides, the risk of fracture will gradually decrease with time due to the bone union of the transpedicular tunnel (Fig. 5). Severe osteoporosis is theoretically considered a risk factor of fracture. When the endoscope is inside the bone tunnel, movement of the instruments should be along the

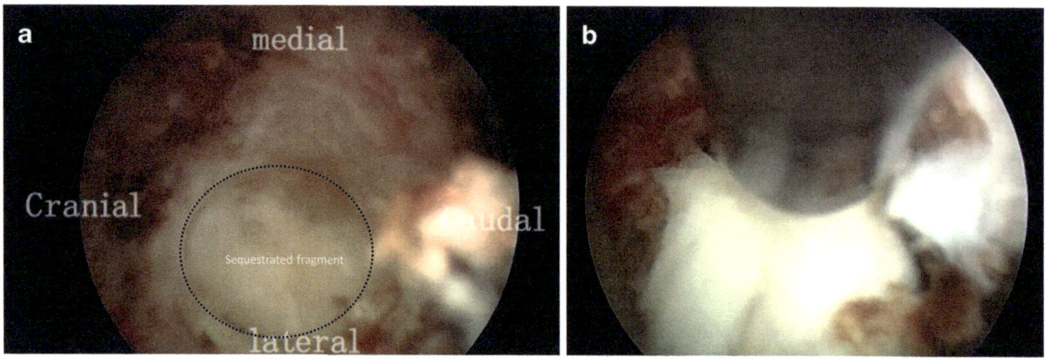

Fig. 4 The endoscopic forceps (black arrow on the AP view fluoroscopy) are used to remove the migrated fragment located medial to the pedicle

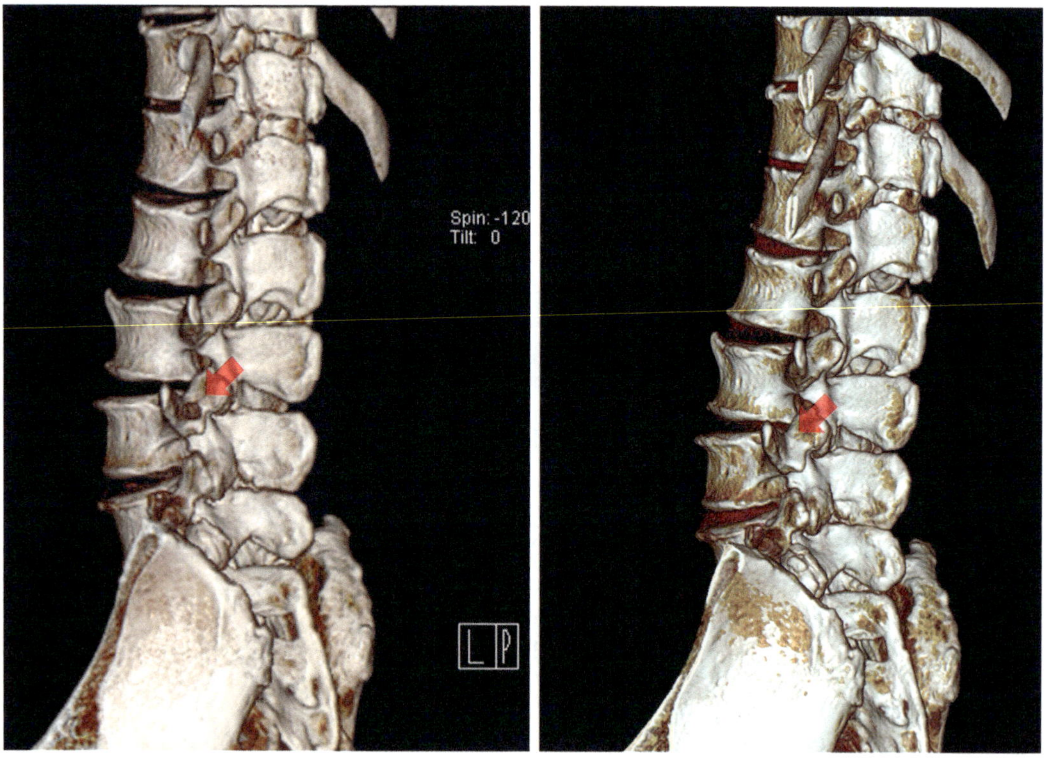

Fig. 5 The immediate postoperative (left) and the postoperative 37 months (right) follow-up CT reconstruction images showed the bone union of the transpedicular tunnel (red arrow)

trajectory forward and backward but not from side to side.

2. Epidural hematoma

   The bleeding sources during the procedure included cancerous bone of pedicle and epidural veins. Although it is efficient to make the tunnel with trephines, the use of an endoscopic burr under direct endoscopic visualization is highly encouraged. Bone bleeding while creating a tunnel through the pedicle with trephine can sometimes be significant and challenging to stop with the use of RF probe. The diamond tip of the endoscopic burr can be beneficial to stop bone bleeding due to thermal effect while drilling. Besides, increasing the pressure of continuous saline irrigation and hemostatic agents such as gelatin sponge or the Floseal hemostatic matrix might also help protect visualization and hemostasis. After removing the herniated disc, epidural bleeding should also be coagulated with bipolar RF probe meticulously to avoid epidural hematoma.

3. Residual fragment
   When the sequestrated disc is large and fragile fragment, the total removal of the disc may be difficult through the small surgical corridor. Curved hook and navigable forceps may help explore and grab the sequestrated disc fragment. The pulsatile expansion of the dural sac is one of the intraoperative findings after complete removal. Besides, intraoperative epidurography might help evaluate if a residual fragment is present.
4. Root injury
   With the transpedicular approach, the sequestrated fragment in the shoulder area is between traversing root and endoscopic instruments. Adequate control of bone bleeding can provide clear endoscopic visualization. It is safe to manipulate endoscopic instruments within an adequate range of working distances. The operator should avoid inserting forceps or drills too deep to injure the traversing root. Because the patient was conscious during the whole procedure, the surgeon should pay attention to possible root irritation signs reported by the patient intraoperatively.

Conclusion

The new technique of full-endoscopic transpedicular approach might be a potential alternative for surgical treatment of highly down-migrated disc herniation. It can decrease the risk of injury to the exiting root compared with the transforaminal approach. It also prevents the retraction of the nerve root, which is usually required in the interlaminar approach. However, careful evaluation of preoperative radiological images is essential for patient selection, planning the trajectory precisely, and preventing complications.

References

1. Choi G, et al. Percutaneous endoscopic approach for highly migrated intracanal disc herniations by foraminoplastic technique using rigid working channel endoscope. Spine (Phila Pa 1976). 2008;33(15):E508–15.
2. Yeom KS, Choi YS. Full endoscopic contralateral transforaminal discectomy for distally migrated lumbar disc herniation. J Orthop Sci. 2011;16(3):263–9.
3. Choi G, et al. Percutaneous endoscopic lumbar herniectomy for high-grade down-migrated L4-L5 disc through an L5-S1 interlaminar approach: a technical note. Minim Invasive Neurosurg. 2010;53(3):147–52.
4. Inomata Y, et al. Percutaneous endoscopic lumbar discectomy via adjacent interlaminar space for highly down-migrated lumbar disc herniation: a technical report. J Spine Surg. 2018;4(2):483–9.
5. Krzok G, et al. Transpedicular lumbar endoscopic surgery for highly migrated disk extrusions: preliminary series and surgical technique. World Neurosurg. 2016;95:299–303.
6. Krzok G, et al. Transpedicular endoscopic surgery for lumbar spinal synovial cyst-report of two cases. J Spine Surg. 2016;2(4):310–3.
7. Krzok G. Transpedicular endoscopic surgery for highly Downmigrated L5-S1 disc herniation. Case Rep Med. 2019;2019:5724342.
8. Uniyal P, Choi G, Khedkkar B. Percutaneous Transpedicular Lumbar Endoscopy: A Case Report. Int J Spine Surg. 2016;10:31.
9. Quillo-Olvera J, Akbary K, Kim JS. Percutaneous endoscopic transpedicular approach for high-grade down-migrated lumbar disc herniations. Acta Neurochir. 2018;160(8):1603–7.
10. Torun F, Tuna H, Buyukmumcu M, Caglar S, Baysefer A. The lumbar roots and pedicles: a morphometric analysis and anatomical features. J Clin Neurosci. 2008;15(8):895–9.

Biportal Endoscopic Approach (Biportal Endoscopic Lumbar Discectomy)

Nam Lee, Dong Hwa Heo, and Choon Keun Park

Introduction of Approach

Microdiscectomy is the gold standard surgical treatment for lumbar disc herniation refractory to conservative managements. Recently, various endoscopic approaches have been attempted for lumbar disc herniation. Among them, the technique of biportal endoscopic lumbar discectomy was based on microscopic surgery, and similar to microdiscectomy. Therefore, surgical anatomy and orientation of biportal endoscopic lumbar discectomy may be familiar to spine surgeon.

Biportal endoscopic surgery used two channels. First portal is endoscopic portal and the other is working portal [1–3]. General spine surgical instruments as well as endoscopic specialized instruments can be used through working portal (Fig. 1). Relative shorter learning curve is another advantage of biportal endoscopic lumbar surgery.

Indication and Contraindication

Indication of biportal endoscopic surgery is very similar with conventional lumbar microsurgery. All types of herniated lumbar disc (HLD) including protrusion, extrusion, sequestration type, and central, paracentral, bilateral disc herniation are indication of this procedure. In addition, recurrent lumbar disc herniation, calcified disc herniation, and cauda equina syndrome are also included in indication of this approach [1]. Foraminal and extraforaminal type HLD can be treated by paraspinal approach using biportal endoscopic surgery.

Anesthesia and Position

Surgeon's preference and cooperation with anesthesiologist are very important. The physician can select among epidural anesthesia, spinal anesthesia, and general anesthesia. Epidural anesthesia is a less invasive procedure among them, so the authors recommend epidural anesthesia. In addition, if a mild intravenous sedation is applied, the physician can operate in situation like general anesthesia.

Electronic Supplementary Material The online version of this chapter (https://doi.org/10.1007/978-981-15-8253-0_13) contains supplementary material, which is available to authorized users.

N. Lee
Department of Neurosurgery, Neurosurgery, Yonsei Cheok Hospital, Busan, South Korea

D. H. Heo (✉)
Department of Neurosurgery, Seoul Bumin Hospital, Seoul, Republic of Korea

C. K. Park
Department of Neurosurgery, Wiltse Memorial Hospital, Suwon, South Korea

H. S. Kim et al. (eds.), *Advanced Techniques of Endoscopic Lumbar Spine Surgery*,
https://doi.org/10.1007/978-981-15-8253-0_13

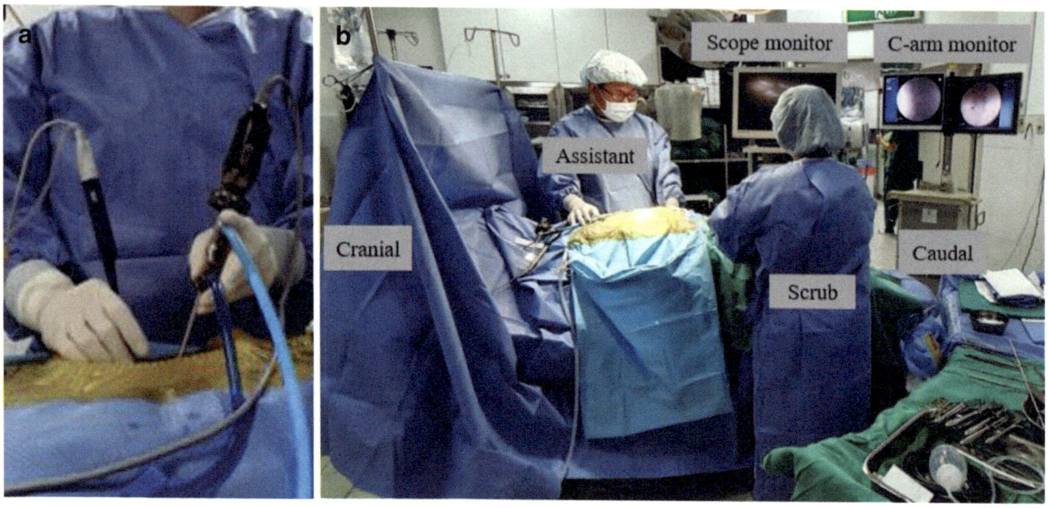

Fig. 1 Overview of biportal endoscopic lumbar discectomy (**a**). Setting of the operating room for biportal endoscopic surgery of left side approach (**b**)

The prone position on a Wilson frame is gold standard position (Fig. 1). A Wilson frame makes better surgical field because it induces distraction of the interlaminar space. C-arm fluoroscopy and a monitor for endoscopy were located at contralateral side to surgeon (Fig. 1).

Special Surgical Instruments (Figs. 2 and 3)

Serial dilators are essential to make portals (Fig. 2). Zero-degree endoscope is most commonly used in biportal endoscopic surgery. Basically, most of biportal endoscopic instruments were shorter than uniportal endoscopic surgical instruments (Fig. 2). Radiofrequency (RF) probe is very useful to control the intraoperative bleeding (Fig. 3). Various kinds of RF probes are available in biportal endoscopic surgery. The power of RF should be reduced when epidural space and dura were exposed. We prefer waterproof diamond drill for prevention and reduction of bone bleeding during operation (Fig. 3). All conventional surgical instruments are available in biportal endoscopic spine surgery.

Surgical Steps

1. **Mark the portal location.** Under fluoroscopic imaging, getting the true A-P image of target level is very important (Fig. 4a). And, we additionally check the locations of two portals using lateral C-arm fluoroscopic view. To make the incisions for portals, the physician must confirm two vertical lines: one is the midline and the other is medial pedicle line. Two portals were made under C-arm fluoroscopic guidance. Endoscopic portal was made at 1 cm cranially and the other working portal was made at 1 cm caudally from mid intervertebral disc space (Fig. 4a, b).
2. **Making "initial" working space (Video 1).** After confirming the locations for portals, make a skin incision using No. 10 blade. Penetrating the fascia clearly by blade is important at this point. One centimeter incision is sufficient for portals. Usually the instrument portal is made firstly. Insert the first serial dilator toward medially and cranially to touch the spinous-laminar junction of inferior laminar border (Fig. 5). After touching this point confirmed by fluoroscopic image, we must detach the muscle insertion

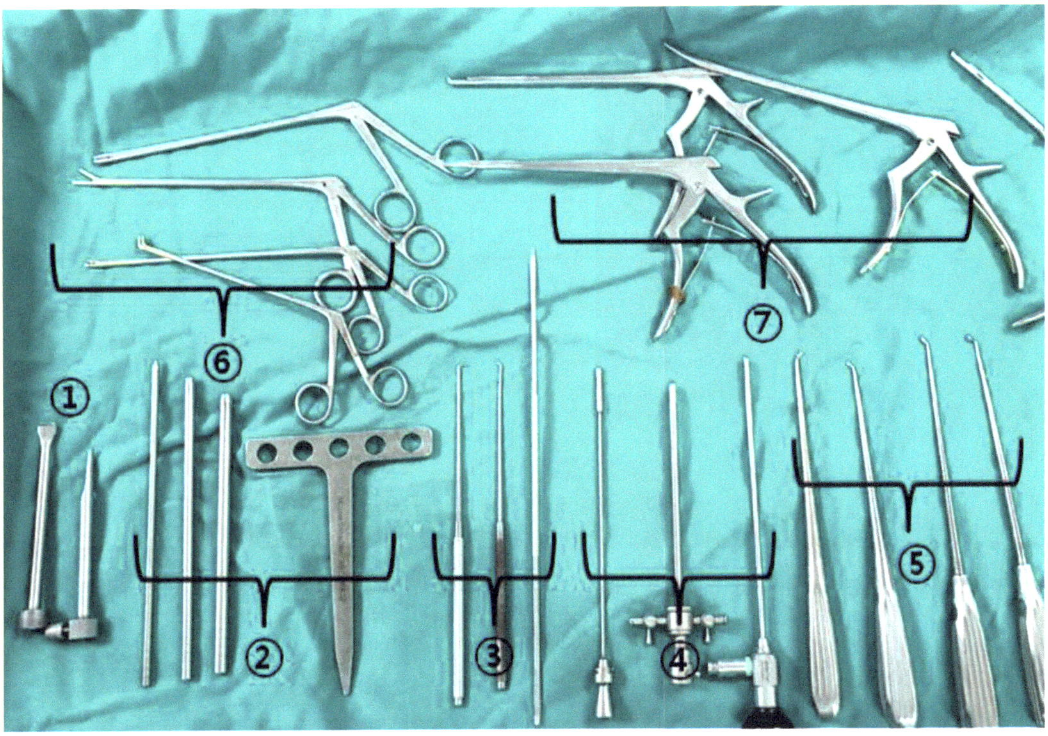

Fig. 2 (*1*) Endoscope retractor. (*2*) Serial dilators and muscle dissector. (*3*) Blunt hook—double-end probe. (*4*) Trocar for endoscope and 0 degree endoscope. (*5*) Various curved curettes. (*6*) Pituitary forceps. (*7*) Various Kerrison punches

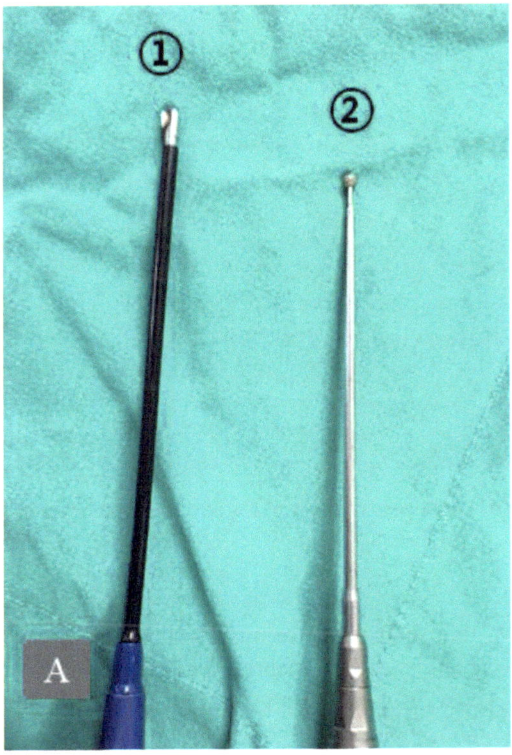

Fig. 3 (**a**): (*1*) Radiofrequency probe. (*2*) Small diameter of diamond burr

parts from laminar bone by scraping the surface of laminar bone (Fig. 5). In addition, we must feel the interlaminar space. Loss of the hardness feeling of laminar bone is the interlaminar space. After confirming this feeling, the next serial dilators or muscle dissector can be inserted through the portal. Next, endoscopic portal is made. First serial dilator or trocar for endoscope is a good tool for making endoscopic portal. We usually put in a working sheath or trocar at the working portal. The direction is medial and caudal from skin incision, and the target landing point is the same with the instrument portal. To make the initial working space successfully, two portals' distal endpoints must meet just on the laminar (Fig. 5a, b). After that, connect the 0 degree endoscope and open the water clamp. If the laminar surface is identified clearly by floating the muscle insertion parts dorsally from laminar bone, making the initial working space is finished.

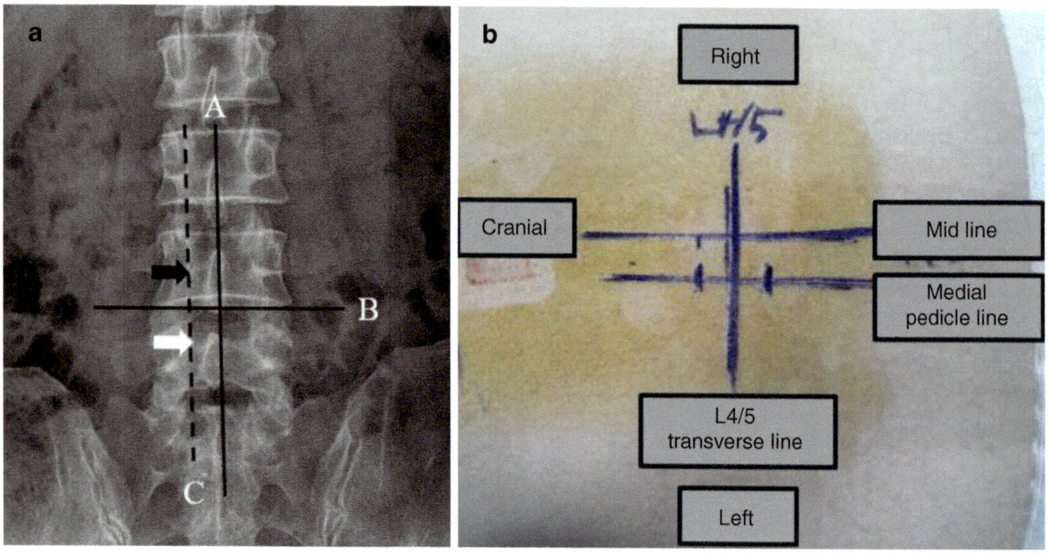

Fig. 4 Radiologic (**a**) and skin (**b**) marking for making two portals. Mid vertical line (**A**) and intervertebral disc transverse line at L45 (**B**). Medial pedicle line (**C**). Black arrow: cranial endoscopic portal (1 cm cranially from line **B**). White arrow: caudal instrument working portal (1 cm caudally from line **B**)

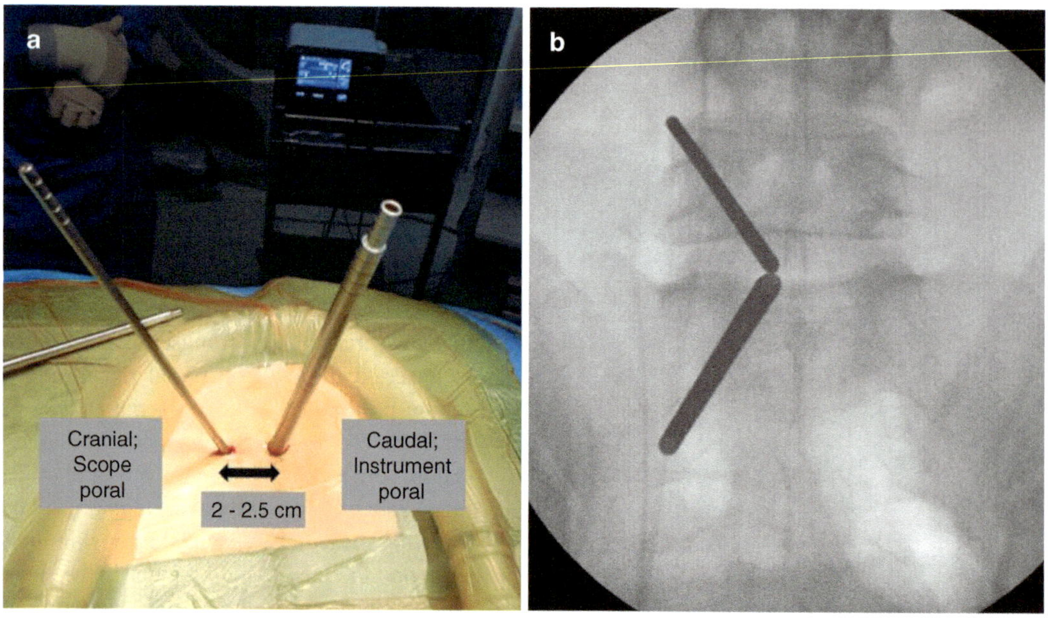

Fig. 5 (**a**) Two dilators are inserted to create the biportal. (**b**) Distal ends of the two dilators meet on the spinous-laminar junction

3. **Making "true" working space.** A partial hemilaminectomy is performed using electrical high-speed burr, Kerrison punch, or osteotome. The authors prefer high-speed burr with thin shaft. Because it is good for emission of bone dust and debris simultaneously. This work is started from spinous-laminar junction and removing the inferior portion of lamina

(Fig. 6a). This laminectomy should end up when the midline recess of the ligamentum flavum is exposed (Fig. 6b). It extends laterally until encountering the meeting point of inferior articular process of cephalad bone and superior articular process of caudal bone. The laminectomy makes the true working space for discectomy (Fig. 6c).

4. **Ipsilateral flavectomy.** The ligamentum flavum consists of a superficial layer and a deep layer. There is an interlayer slip of the ligamentum flavum that attaches to the superior border of caudal lamina. To accomplish total ipsilateral flavectomy, physician must identify the distal portion of ligamentum flavum (Fig. 6c). Now physician can identify all territories of the ipsilateral ligamentum flavum. The flavectomy is undergone from cranial to caudal, and medial to lateral. The distal portion of deep layer attaches to the anterosuperior surface of caudal lamina; to remove this area safely, authors prefer curette. Upward curved curette is very useful to detach the deep layer of ligament. A sweeping motion of the curette over the edge of the superior border of caudal lamina facilitates deep layer ligament detachment safely. Therefore, full ipsilateral flavectomy can be done just using conventional instruments such as hook, Kerrison punch, and pituitary forceps. After full layer ipsilateral flavectomy, we can clearly identify the epidural space including epidural fat tissue and dura mater (Fig. 6d).
5. **Exploration of epidural space.** The epidural fat tissue can act as a natural barrier for the prevention of postoperative adhesion. If

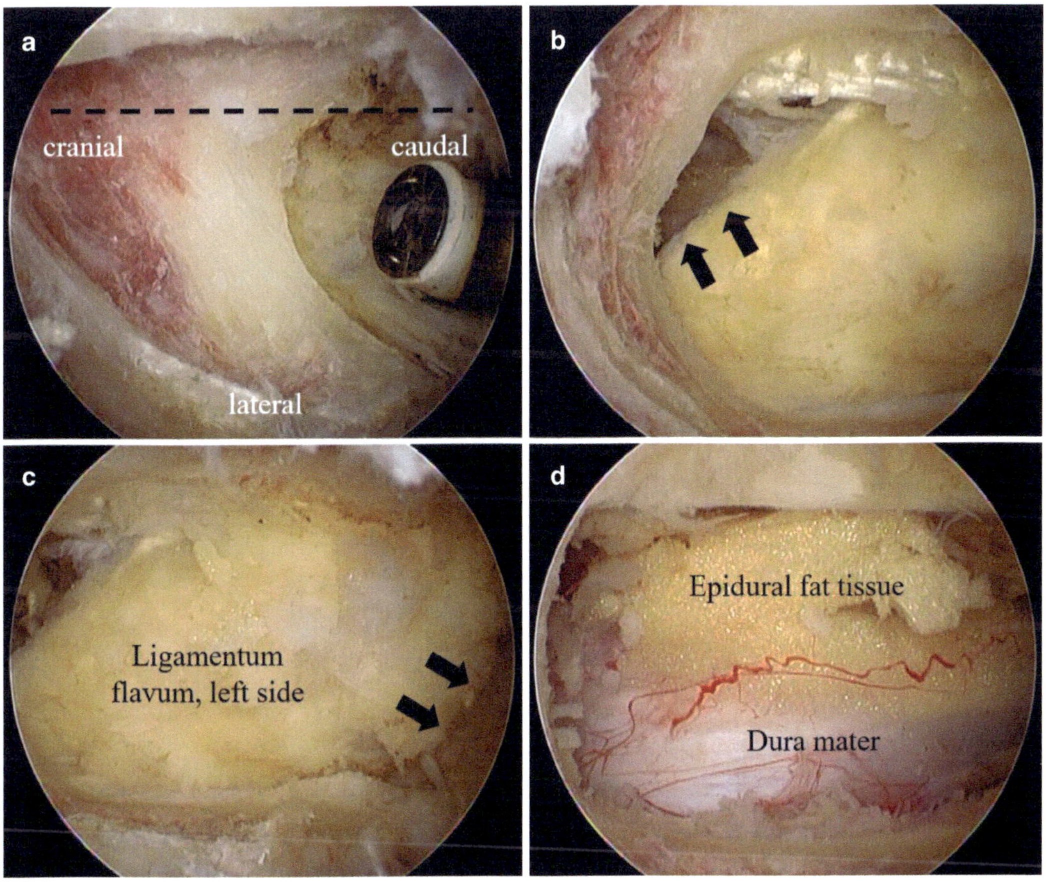

Fig. 6 (**a**) Left side approach view. Ipsilateral left side laminar was removed partially. (**b**) The endpoint of laminectomy cranial portion. Black arrows indicate proximal end of ipsilateral ligamentum flavum (LF). (**c**) The entire area of the ipsilateral LF is identified. Black arrows indicate distal end of ipsilateral LF. (**d**) After flavectomy, both epidural fat tissue and dura mater are confirmed. Also, the physician can see the epidural vessels

possible, epidural fat should be preserved as much as possible. However, the biportal endoscopic surgery is operated in water—the turbulence flow of water—and the fat tissue may disturb the clean operating field. In this situation, the authors recommend to remove the epidural fat tissue. The bleeding from epidural vessels can cause uncleaned operating field. Proper usage of radiofrequency (RF) is essential for controlling the epidural bleeding. Before manipulating the thecal sac, the medial wall of pedicle and lateral border of thecal sac should be identified using blunt hook. Once bloodless operating field is achieved, the compressed nerve root can be identified easily and the nerve root can be retracted medially using a blunt hook or dissector (Fig. 7a, b).

6. **Discectomy.** To do the discectomy safely, authors recommend the usage of nerve root retractor especially to the beginners. After retraction of nerve root medially, the extruded or sequestrated disc fragments are identified clearly (Fig. 7b). Using blunt hook or pituitary forceps, these fragments can be removed easily. In the case of sub-ligamentous fragments, application of RF on the thinned annulus can lead to an extraction of disc fragments. After initial decompression, subsequent discectomy is easier because the nerve root can be retracted more medially and smoothly, so physician can identify the posterior longitudinal ligament (PLL) which is located in midline (Fig. 7c, d). The surgeon can control the quantity of discectomy (Fig. 8). To achieve

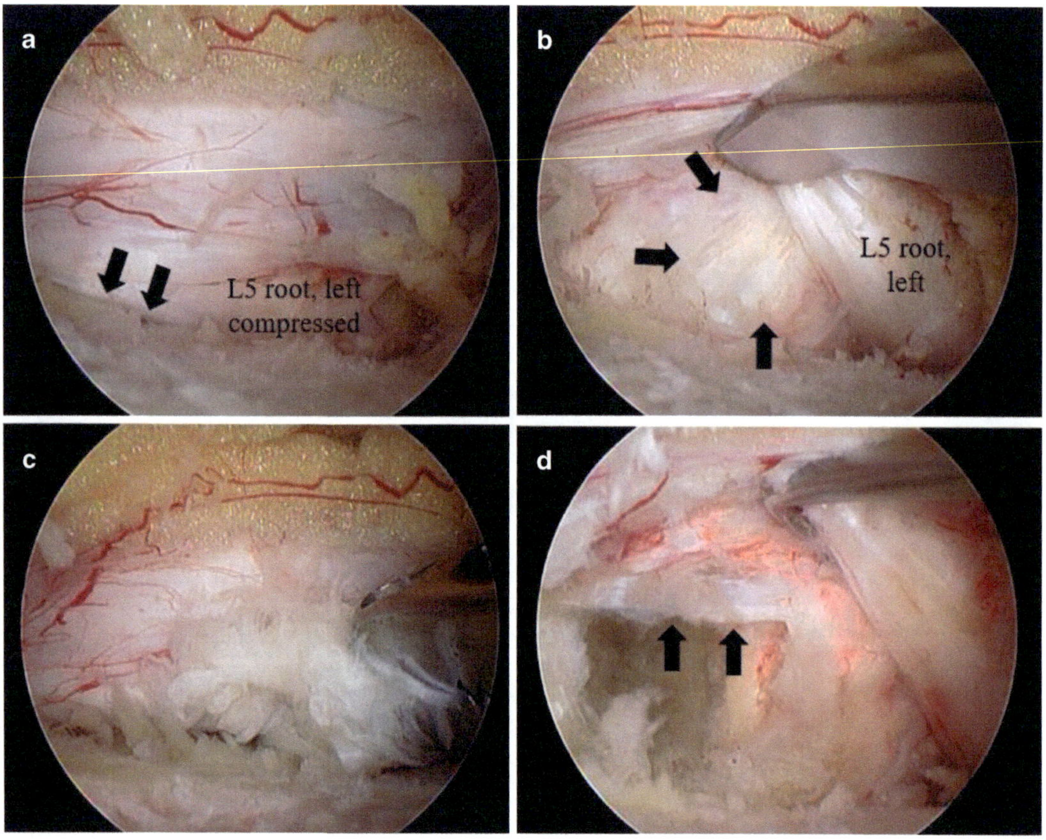

Fig. 7 (**a**) The compressed L5 root is identified. Black arrows indicate the shoulder portion on nerve root. (**b**) After retraction of compressed L5 root medially, extruded disc material is confirmed (black arrows). (**c**) The extruded disc material is removed by pituitary forceps. (**d**) After discectomy, the posterior longitudinal ligament is confirmed (black arrows)

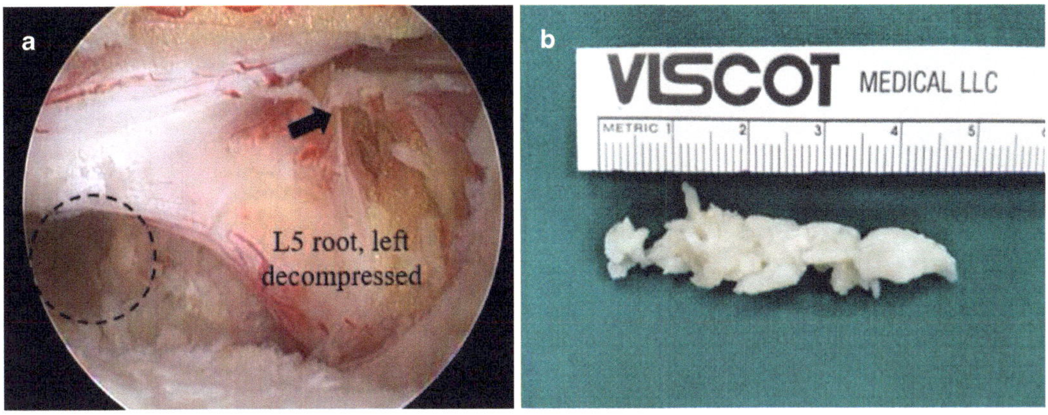

Fig. 8. (**a**) After sufficient discectomy, decompressed nerve is identified, and both shoulder and axillar parts of root are identified (dotted circle: discectomy site, black arrow: axillar part of nerve root). (**b**) The volume of removed intervertebral disc

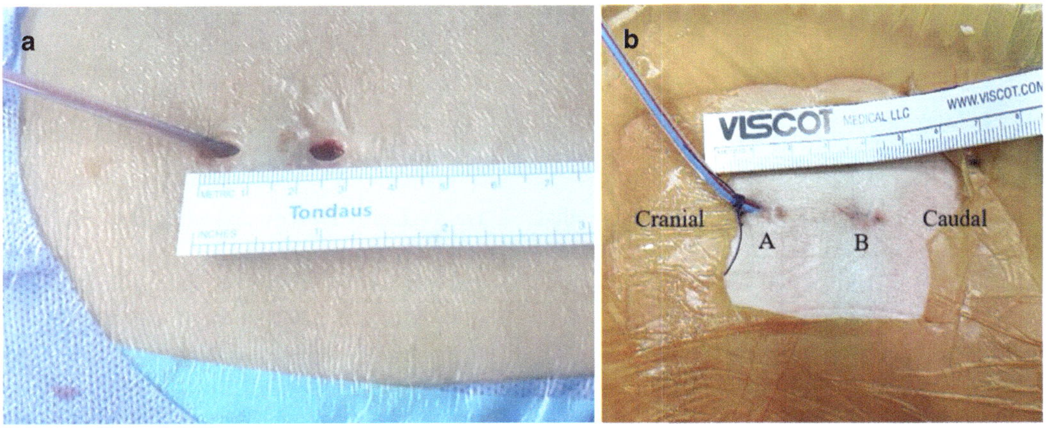

Fig. 9 Skin wound size of two portals. (**a**) Scope portal. (**b**) Working portal. A drainage is inserted

the sufficient discectomy, physician can add the annulotomy using No. 15 blade or Kerrison punch. Authors prefer the Kerrison punch to prevent unintended dura injury.

7. **Finish the procedure.** After adequate discectomy, the physician should inspect the operating field entirely. The remnant disc fragment or residual debris should be removed absolutely from the working space. Longer blunt hooks are used to explore the perineural space including shoulder and axillar portion of nerve root (Fig. 8). After biportal endoscopic discectomy, authors always put the drainage catheter over the dura mater (Fig. 9a). Although there is no prominent bleeding in the working space during operation, hidden epidural bleeding and muscular bleeding can be emerged after surgery. The fascial layer is closed with one-point absorbable suture and subcutaneous layer is also closed with absorbable suture too (Fig. 9). Finally, several pieces of sterilized tape are applied to skin closure.

Illustrated Cases

Case 1 (Video 2)

Forty-two-year-old male patient complained of severe lower back pain and left side radiating pain. The preoperative MRI images showed her-

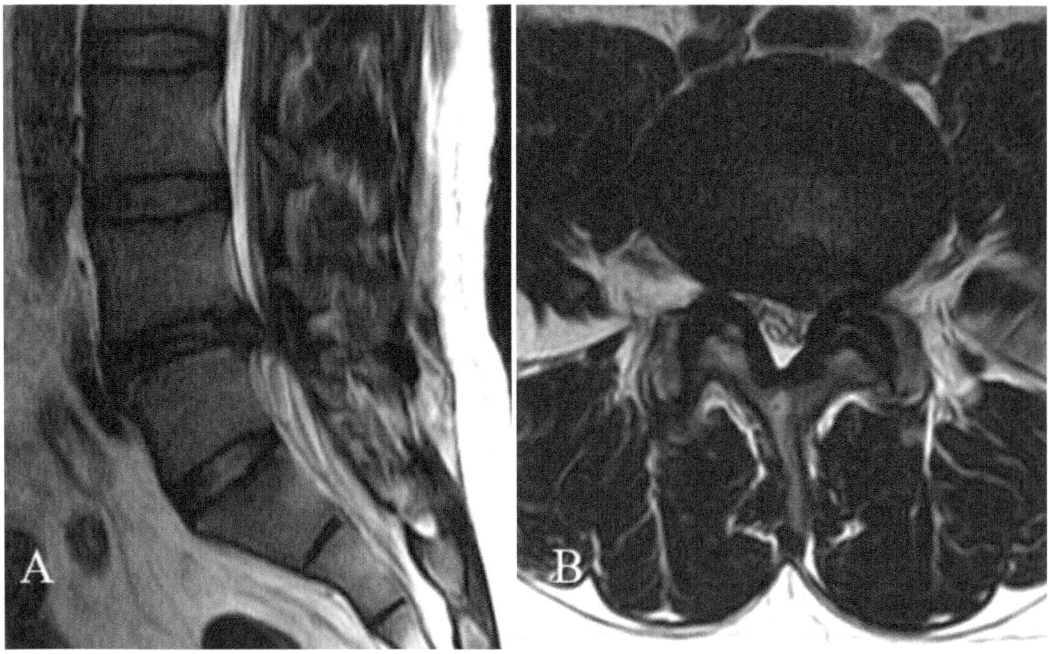

Fig. 10 (**a**) Preoperative MRI shows HLD L4/5 (sagittal view). (**b**) Axial view shows left side paracentral HLD at L4/5 intervertebral disc level

niated lumbar disc (HLD) L4/5 left side that compressed the L5 nerve root significantly (Fig. 10a, b). The author underwent biportal endoscopic discectomy surgery with left side approach (Fig. 7 and Video 1).

After decompression, the postoperative MRI (POD 1day) showed well-decompressed state at L4/5 level. There was no postoperative hematoma or prominent paraspinal muscle damage (Fig. 11a, b).

Case 2 (Foraminal HLD L5/S1, Right) (Figs. 12 and 13)
Fifty-four-year-old female patient complained of severe right side buttock pain and radiating pain. She showed L5 dermatome radiculopathy. Preoperative MRI images showed foraminal HLD L5/S1 right side that compressed the L5 dorsal root ganglion (DRG) (Fig. 12 a, b). The author performed biportal endoscopic decompression using right side paraspinal approach. Intraoperative endoscopic images during operation show sequential steps (Fig. 13). Postoperative MRI images (POD 1day) showed complete removal of HLD at L5/S1 level (Fig. 12c, d).

Case 3 (Highly Downward Migrated HLD L2/3, Left) (Figs. 14 and 15)
Sixty-two-year-old male patient complained of severe left side anterior thigh pain. His MRI showed highly downward migrated HLD L2/3 left side and ruptured disc material was located at L3 pedicle level (Fig. 14a, b). The author performed biportal endoscopic decompression using left side paramedian approach. Intraoperative endoscopic images show sequential steps (Fig. 15). The ruptured disc material disappeared completely in postoperative MRI images (POD 1day) (Fig. 14c, d).

Complication and Its Management

Most common complication is dura tear during flavectomy. This complication often happens in learning curve period [2]. Most common site of dura tear is lateral aspect of thecal sac or shoulder portion of traversing nerve root. This happens in the situation that there is not sufficient space or gap between deep layer of ligamentum flavum and dura mater. The flavectomy is per-

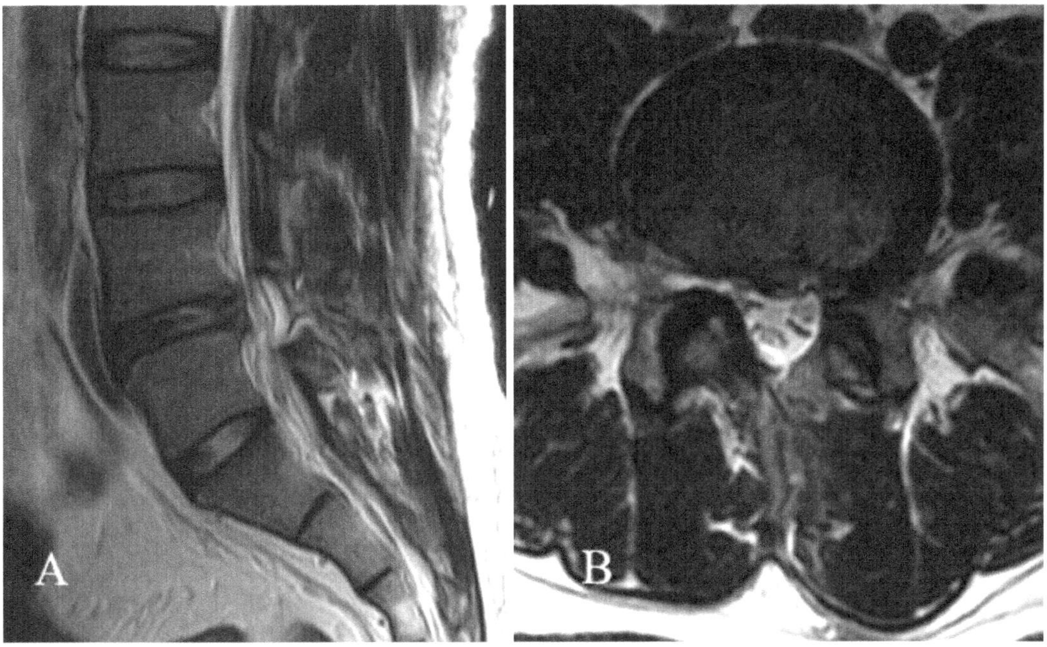

Fig. 11 (**a**) Postoperative MRI shows decompressed state at L4/5 (sagittal view). (**b**) Axial view shows well-decompressed lesion site at L4/5 intervertebral disc level. In addition, postoperative paraspinal muscle change is slight

formed mainly by Kerrison punch. The surgeon sometimes does not notice that the Kerrison punch trapped both ligament and dura mater. The dura mater locates just beneath the ligamentum flavum anatomically; if there is an adhesion between ligament and dura mater, the risk of dura defect may be increased. To reduce this complication, the surgeon should confirm the detachment of ligament from thecal sac using blunt hook or dissector especially in lateral aspect of ligament. If the size of dura defect is relatively small, simple dura packing is enough. If the size of dura defect is large and seems difficult to treat the defect, the surgeon should decide to convert to the open surgery promptly.

Postoperative epidural hematoma is another complication of posterior endoscopic approach. Meticulous bleeding control is necessary during operation. A drainage catheter was routinely inserted postoperatively for the prevention of epidural hematoma.

Discussion: Surgical Tip and Pitfall

Before starting of biportal endoscopic surgeries, the surgeon should have many experiences of microscopic spine surgery. The most significant advantage of this biportal endoscopic technique is that it can be applied to all types of lumbar disc herniation [4]. In order to successfully complete this approach, it is of most importance that the initial working space be created quickly. For beginners, this task is often insufficient, and this results in the poor vision of endoscopic operating field. The successful approach is that the cortical surface of the laminar bone is exposed immediately when water perfusion begins. Many beginners do not overcome this initial step, so they convert to the conventional open laminectomy. If you overcome this initial step, the rest of the biportal endoscopic surgery is similar conventional microdiscectomy, so the physician can performe this procedure well [5]. Furthermore, after acquiring discectomy using this technique, bilat-

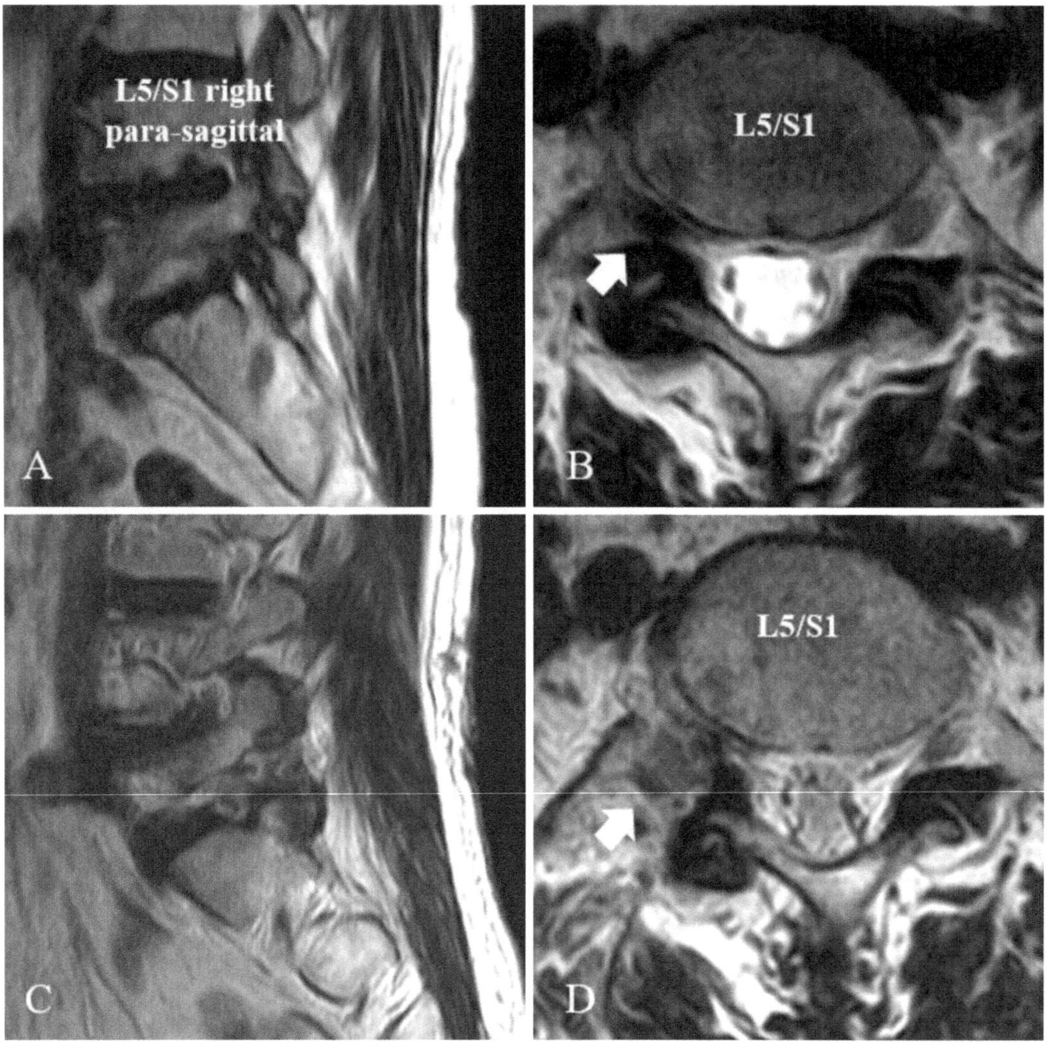

Fig. 12 Preoperative MRI images show foraminal HLD L5/S1 right side (**a** and **b**). Postoperative MRI images show complete removal of HLD at right foramen (**c** and **d**)

eral discectomy using unilateral laminotomy will be possible [6].

Most important factor to maintain the clean visual field during procedure is to keep the continuous water flow. The authors usually use a water irrigation pump set to 30 mmHg and keep this rate unless there is an unexpected event such as arterial bleeding or significant venous bleeding. In these situations, temporarily increasing water flow pressure can help to identify the bleeding site. In addition, bleeding site can be more difficult to identify when you pull back the endoscope, so it is easier to control the situation by placing the endoscope closer to the bleeding suspected site. It is very useful to use proper hemostatic materials such as Gelfoam® sponge, Floseal®, or bone wax. If bleeding is well controlled, the increased water flow pressure should be lowered back to the previous level. This is because if the in-flow pressure of the water is continuously increased in a situation where the outflow of the water is not smooth, the water may

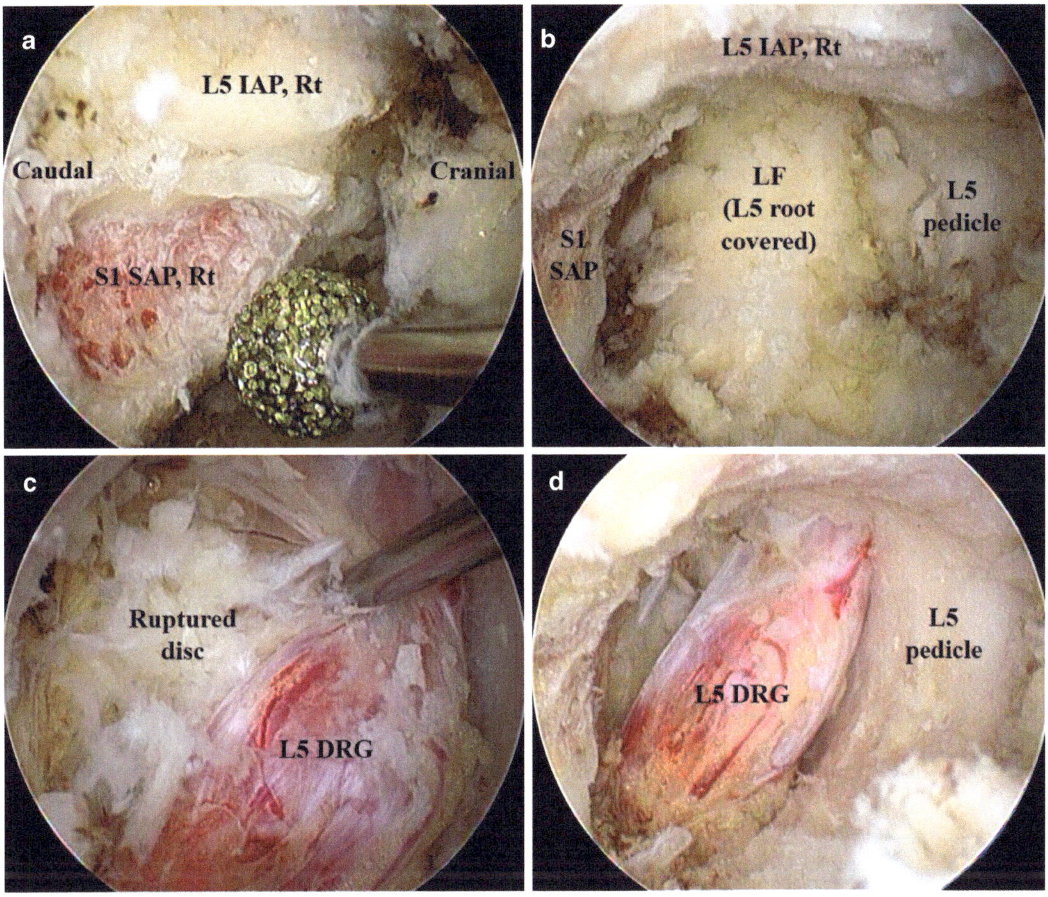

Fig. 13 Serial sequence images of foraminal decompression. (**a**) S1 superior articular process (SAP) removal is the first step of foraminal approach. L5 inferior articular process (IAP) was also identified clearly. (**b**) The image shows foraminal ligamentum flavum which covers the L5 root. (**c**) After flavectomy, compressed L5 DRG and ruptured disc material were confirmed. (**d**) The endpoint view of decompression, well-decompressed DRG was confirmed

penetrate into the paraspinal muscle or enter the spinal canal and press the dura mater. Therefore, the physician should make sure that the water is discharged well during procedure. Water penetrating into the paraspinal muscles can be seen by swelling of the skin on the surgical site.

Keeping the endoscopic orientation constantly is also a very important factor to complete this procedure successfully. One of the challenges for beginners is that endoscopic view is very different from conventional view. Endoscopic view is much closer to the target, making it difficult to maintain spinal anatomy orientation. In order to minimize this difficulty, it is recommended not to rotate the endoscope during surgery, but to maintain the patient's cranial-to-caudal and medial-to-lateral orientation. If the physician misses this orientation, he may perform surgery on normal areas other than the target lesion. If the orientation is uncertain or you encounter an unexpected anatomical structure, do not hesitate to check it with fluoroscopic imaging.

Finally, the height of the physician should be proper. If the height of the endoscopic surgery

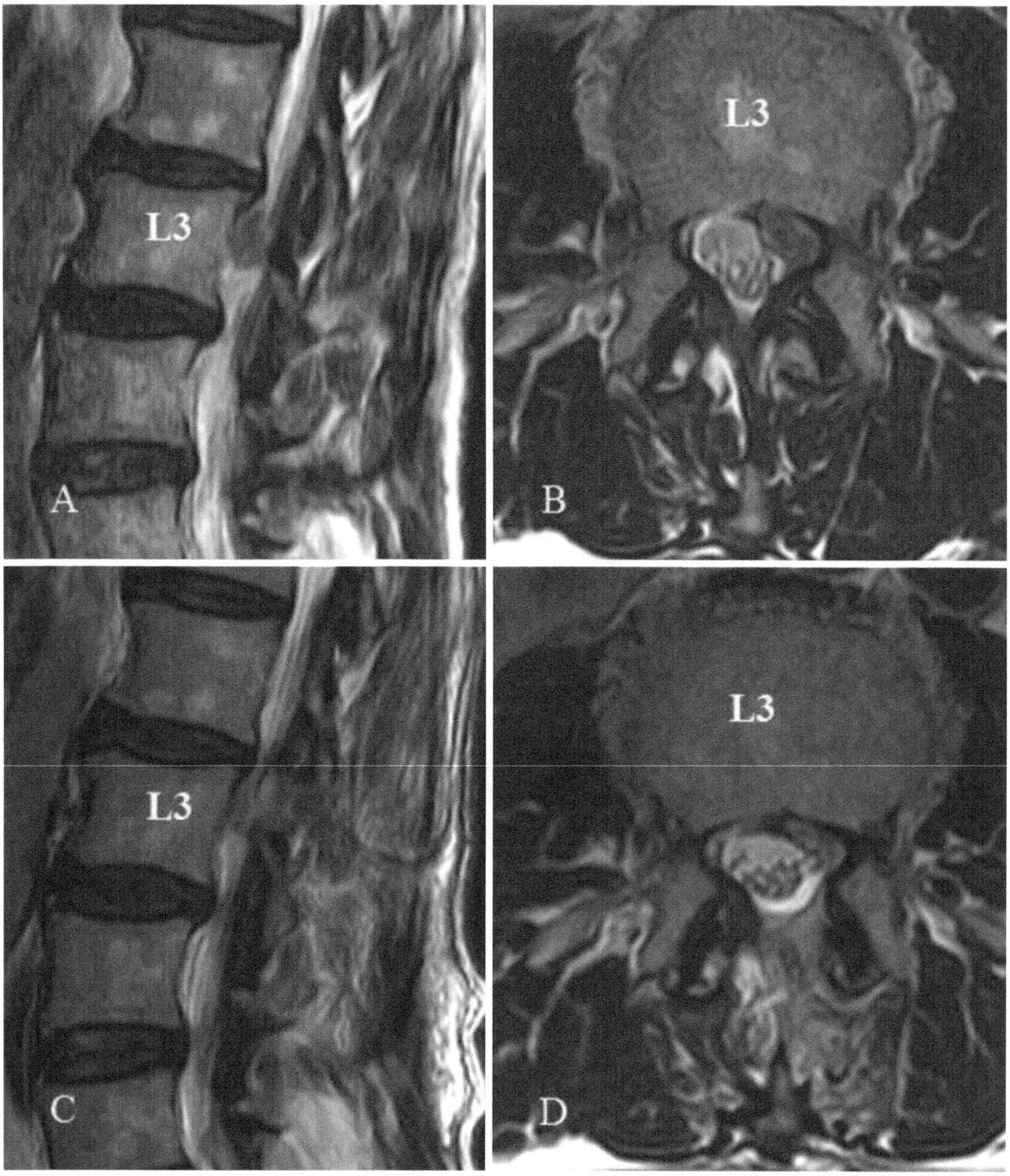

Fig. 14 Preoperative MRI images show highly downward migrated HLD L2/3 left side (**a** and **b**). Postoperative MRI images show complete removal of ruptured disc material (**c** and **d**)

field is too high, excessive force will be applied to both shoulder joints, causing both shoulder joints to fatigue easily. Therefore, if necessary, the height should be adjusted so that both shoulder joints of the physician can be comfortable using the appropriate steps.

Many good results have been published in areas that were difficult to treat with conventional endoscopic surgery, such as lumbar spinal stenosis or segmental instability [7–9].

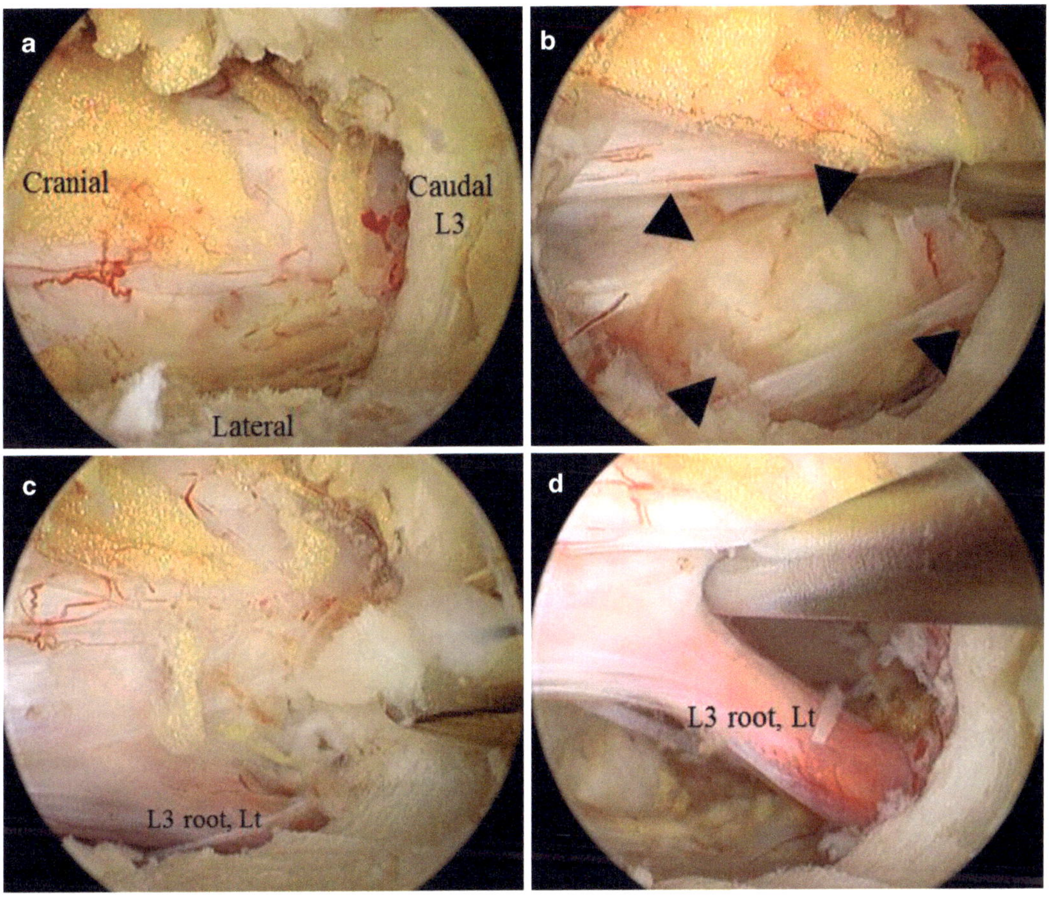

Fig. 15 Serial sequence images of L2/3 decompression. (**a**) After flavectomy, the epidural fat tissue and thecal sac were identified. (**b**) After retraction of L3 root medially, the downward migrated disc material was confirmed (black arrow heads). (**c**) The disc material was removed using pituitary forceps. (**d**) The endpoint view of decompression, well-decompressed L3 root was confirmed

References

1. Choi D-J, Jung J-T, Lee S-J, Kim Y-S, Jang H-J, Yoo B. Biportal endoscopic spinal surgery for recurrent lumbar disc herniations. Clin Orthop Surg. 2016;8:325–9.
2. Choi D-J, Choi C-M, Jung J-T, Lee S-J, Kim Y-S. Learning curve associated with complications in biportal endoscopic spinal surgery: challenges and strategies. Asian Spine J. 2016;10:624.
3. Heo DH, Lee DC, Park CK. Comparative analysis of three types of minimally invasive decompressive surgery for lumbar central stenosis: biportal endoscopy, uniportal endoscopy, and microsurgery. Neurosurg Focus. 2019;46:E9.
4. Heo DH, Kim JS, Park CW, Quillo-Olvera J, Park CK. Contralateral sublaminar endoscopic approach for removal of lumbar juxtafacet cysts using percutaneous biportal endoscopic surgery: technical report and preliminary results. World Neurosurg. 2019;122:474–9.
5. Eum JH, Heo DH, Son SK, Park CK. Percutaneous biportal endoscopic decompression for lumbar spinal stenosis: a technical note and preliminary clinical results. J Neurosurg: Spine. 2016;24:602–7.
6. Heo DH, Lee N, Park CW, Kim HS, Chung HJ. Endoscopic unilateral laminotomy with bilateral discectomy using biportal endoscopic approach: tech-

nical report and preliminary clinical results. World Neurosurg. 2020;137:31–7. https://doi.org/10.1016/j.wneu.2020.01.190.
7. Kim J-E, Choi D-J. Biportal Endoscopic transforaminal lumbar interbody fusion with arthroscopy. Clin Orthop Surg. 2018;10:248–52.
8. Ahn J-S, Lee H-J, Choi D-J, K-y L, S-j H. Extraforaminal approach of biportal endoscopic spinal surgery: a new endoscopic technique for transforaminal decompression and discectomy. J Neurosurg: Spine. 2018;28:492–8.
9. Heo DH, Quillo-Olvera J, Park CK. Can percutaneous biportal endoscopic surgery achieve enough canal decompression for degenerative lumbar stenosis? Prospective case–control study. World Neurosurg. 2018;120:e684–e9.

Part V

Endoscopic Lumbar Interbody Fusion

Endoscope-Assisted Oblique Lumbar Interbody Fusion

Jin-Sung Kim and Yadhu Kasetti Lokanath

Introduction (Key Point and Purpose) of Approach

Lumbar interbody fusion is an acceptable surgical intervention for various symptomatic pathological conditions of the lumbar spine varying from degenerative disc disease, discitis, pseudoarthrosis to degenerative spinal deformity. As spine surgery evolved, different techniques were designed in order to lessen the complication and improve outcome rates. With growing enthusiasm in spine surgery, the need of developing a technique which uses a natural corridor in a less invasive way but without compromising the final outcome was necessary. Intervertebral disc (IVD) space can be approached from anterior, posterior and from lateral side, each approach having its own merits and demerits. Lateral lumbar interbody fusion (LLIF) includes trans-psoas and anterior to psoas/pre-psoas approach. Trans psoas can be either direct lateral interbody fusion (DLIF) or extreme lumbar interbody fusion (XLIF), and pre-psoas or anterior to psoas approach is referred to as oblique lateral interbody fusion (OLIF). Minimally invasive (MI) LLIF has gained popularity because of several advantages such as minimal blood loss, minimal tissue dissection, larger and wider footprint of implant and increased load bearing capacity on cortical bone finally achieving more lordosis of lumbar spine and fusion rates [1, 2]. OLIF, a variant of LLIF which is a bone and muscle preserving MI technique, uses the natural corridor between great vessels and anterior border of the psoas muscle to approach the disc space and minimizing approach-related complications (Fig. 1) [3, 4]. OLIF approach is reported to decrease the incidence of neurologic injury than DLIF and has become popular technique among spine surgeons [5]. OLIF is also considered an alternative approach to Anterior lumbar interbody fusion (ALIF), as the latter is associated with iliac vessel and peritoneal injury [6–8]. Though OLIF has gained popularity in the recent past, Fraser et al. in 1992 initially described comprehensive retroperitoneal muscle splitting dissection along fibres of external oblique but sparing of the internal oblique and transversus abdominis muscle to access mid-lumbar and lumbosacral spine [4]. Numerous modifications were carried out in 1997 by Mayer which are now standardized and used by several groups as a modernistic present-day OLIF approach [9], and in 2012, Silvestre et al. publicized the term OLIF [10]. The modifi-

J.-S. Kim (✉)
Department of Neurosurgery, Seoul St. Mary's Hospital, The Catholic University of Korea, Seoul, South Korea

Y. K. Lokanath
Spine Centre, Department of Neurosurgery, Seoul St. Mary's Hospital, College of Medicine, The Catholic University of Korea, Seoul, South Korea

Department of Neurosurgery, Aster RV hospital, Bangalore, Karnataka, India

H. S. Kim et al. (eds.), *Advanced Techniques of Endoscopic Lumbar Spine Surgery*,
https://doi.org/10.1007/978-981-15-8253-0_14

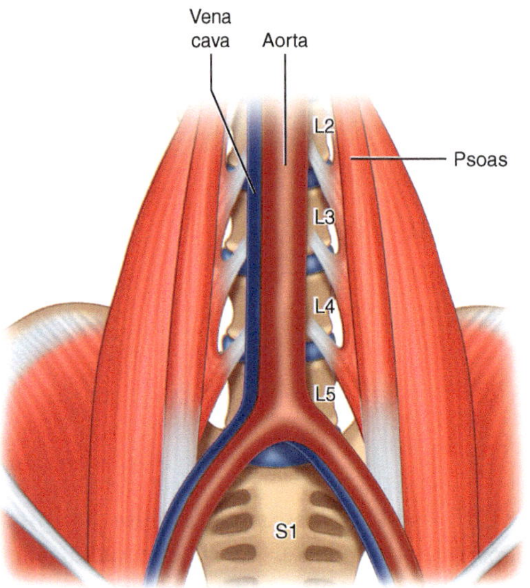

Fig. 1 Artist depiction of the pre-psoas corridor. Vena cava is on right side, psoas muscle on left. The disc spaces are highlighted in yellow. (Courtesy of Anthony M. DiGiorgio, DO, MHA, New Orleans, LA)

cation of Mayer's OLIF technique with the use of a tubular system was carried out by Hynes [11, 12]. Irrespective of the technique used, the goal should be adequate decompression and good interbody fusion. OLIF indirectly decompresses the canal by a large interbody cage [11, 13]. Although OLIF achieves indirect decompression by an interbody cage, there is always a concern about direct complete decompression in cases of central and foraminal lumbar disc herniation. In these situations, indirect decompression will not be adequate and direct decompression is required which can be accomplished using an endoscope referred to as endoscope-assisted OLIF. Using the same or different OLIF trajectory endoscopic system can be introduced to precisely approach the intracanal or contralateral foraminal lesion, thus achieving direct decompression [14, 16]. Endoscope can be used from T12 to S1 with regard to cranial and caudal level requiring added technical manoeuvres like ribs resection and ligation of vessel, with the help of specialized instruments and retractor system without any additional posterior procedure [15]. Endoscope enhances visualization of operative surgical area avoiding injury to neural and vascular structure, assists to visualize the hidden areas accordingly adding to uncomplicated successful surgery [16] and even aids in endplate preparation under vision fulfilling goals of both direct and indirect decompression.

Indication

1. Instability/canal stenosis with upward or downward migration of ruptured disc fragment.
2. Lumbar segmental instability with dural compression by a central herniated lumbar disc.
3. Degenerative lumbar spondylolisthesis with right foraminal or central disc herniation.
4. Central stenosis with right foraminal or central disc herniation.
5. Adjacent segment disease with disc herniation.

Type of Herniated Nucleus Pulposus (HNP) accessible by Endoscope

- Non-migrated HNP.
- Migrated HNP.
- Recurrent HNP.
- High canal compromised HNP. Central and foraminal HNP.

Contraindication

1. Visceral disease—difficult access.
2. Previous history of retroperitoneal surgery.
3. Abdominal aortic disease.
4. Severe facet hypertrophy and lateral recess stenosis (Grade 3).

Anaesthesia and Position

General anaesthesia is preferred choice as the patient is in lateral position and initial interbody work is performed in decubitus position on a radiolucent operating table and turned prone for percutaneous pedicle screw fixation.

(a) Lateral decubitus position on a radiolucent operating table (Fig. 2).
  - The choice of laterality, left or right up depends upon surgeon's preference, operative indication and laterality of scoliosis.
  - Preferred is right decubitus position as the space between the psoas muscle and iliac vessels is spacious and wider on the left side [13].
  - Liver on right side makes difficult access and keeps the surgeon towards the aorta rather than the fragile inferior vena cava [13].
  - Approaching from the side of concavity is sometimes favoured in scoliosis to minimize the number of incisions needed [13].

(b) Head to be well supported with padding or placed on ahead ring.
(c) Arms are positioned and supported with a padded elbow support or an arm sling or using armrest.
(d) Roller or a padded device is placed under the patient's waist to support the spine, along the chest wall, below the axilla to prevent brachial plexus injury.
(e) Hip is positioned just below the point of 'table break'.
(f) Pillow is placed between the knees and legs.
(g) Proper strapping of patient at level of shoulder and waist.
(h) Flexion of lower limbs (depends on left/right lateral position—flexion of the top leg allows relaxation of the ipsilateral psoas and lumbar

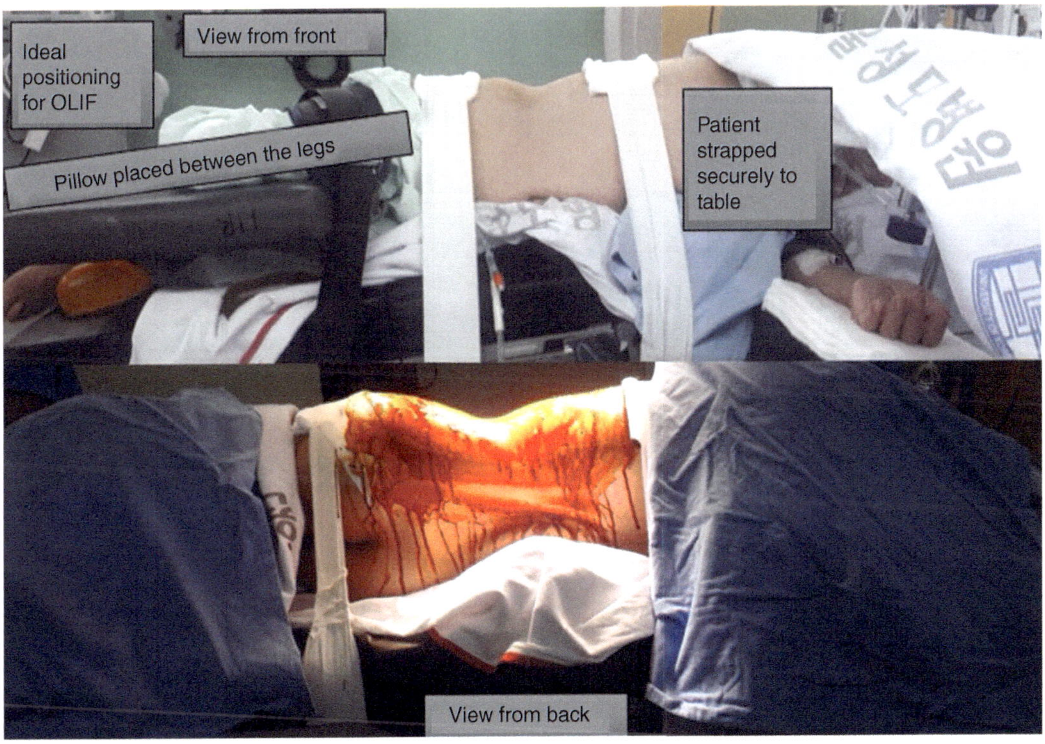

Fig. 2 Patient positioning

plexus, thus reducing traction during the procedure).

(i) Once patient is fully secured, operative table is placed in reverse Trendelenburg as this facilitates to bring the spine parallel to the floor.

Special Surgical Instruments

- OLIF retractor system.
- Endoscopy unit—bevelled working cannula, 30° endoscope, working cannula 7 mm.
- Radiofrequency probe (Fig. 3a).
- Semi-flexible/straight forceps (Fig. 3b).
- Angled hook (Fig. 3c).
- Tip-control burr (Fig. 3d).
- In general, an endoscope with a working channel and two irrigation channels used for full-endoscopic lumbar discectomy is preferred.

Surgical Steps (Illustration)

Once the patient is placed in lateral position and secured to operating table, sequential operative steps are described below.

1. Skin incision (Fig. 4).
   (a) Once the patient is positioned, true AP and lateral fluoroscopic images are taken.
   (b) Anterior vertebral line and borders of disc space are marked under X-ray guidance.
   (c) An oblique or vertical incision of about 3–4 cm is made 5 cm in front midportion of desired level.
   (d) The surgeon performs the procedure standing in front of the patient.
2. Muscle dissection.
   (a) Exposure of skin and subcutaneous fascia will aid in the visualization of the fascia of external oblique.

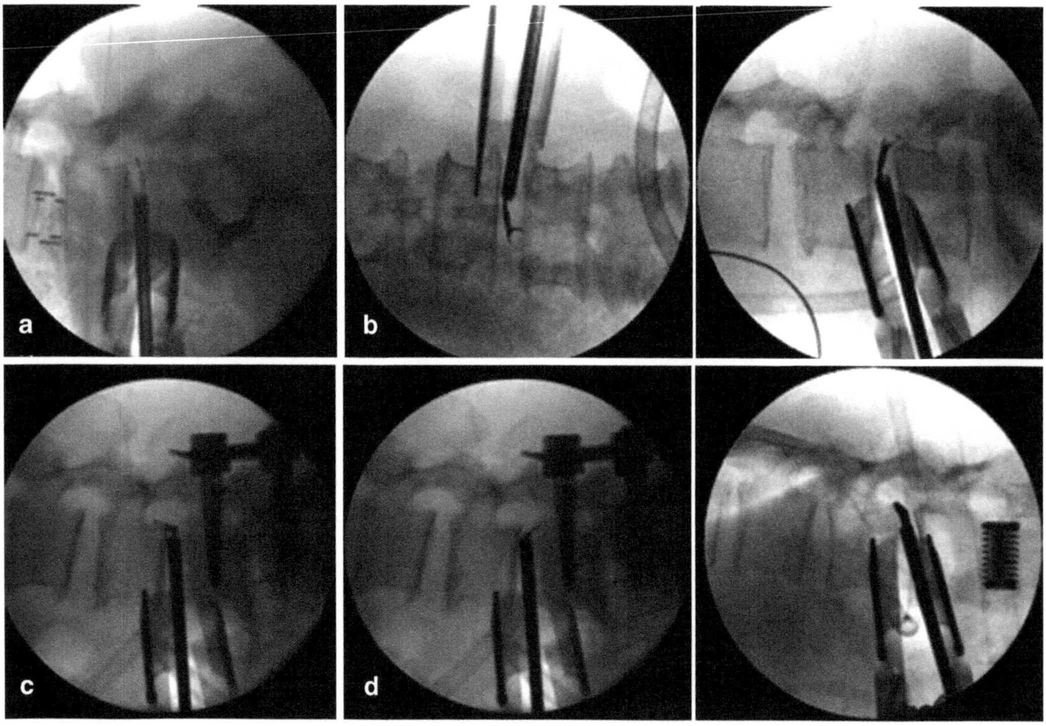

Fig. 3 Instrument used in endoscopic OLIF. (**a**) Radiofrequency probe. (**b**) Semi-flexible/straight forceps. (**c**) Angled hook. (**d**) Tip-control burr

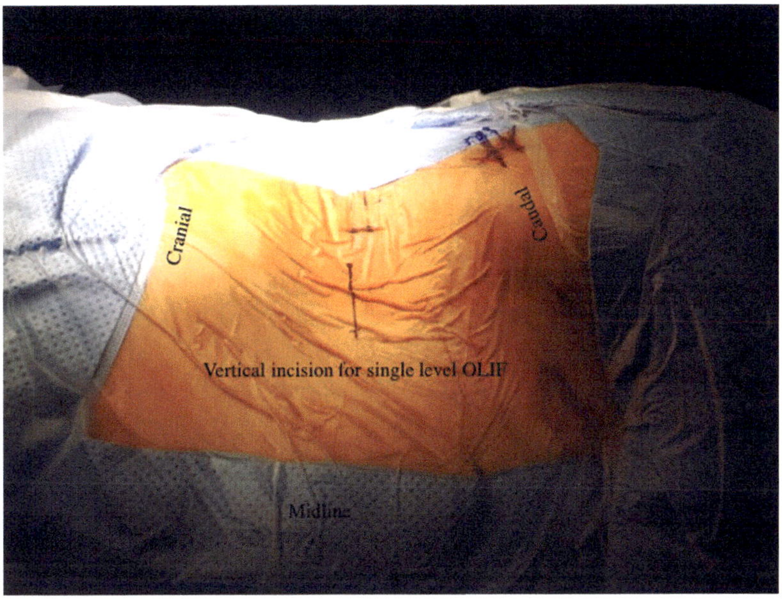

Fig. 4 Image showing incision for a single-level OLIF

(b) Initially, the fascia over the muscle fibres is opened with electrocautery, and muscles are split in direction of fibres.
(c) Sequential dissection of the abdominal wall muscles (external oblique, internal oblique and transversus abdominis muscle) is performed using the muscle splitting technique.
(d) Iliohypogastric or ilioinguinal nerves may be encountered beneath the internal oblique muscle which needs identification, preservation by a meticulous dissection and mobilization.
(e) After transversalis fascia (aponeurotic membrane between the inner surface of the transversus abdominis muscle and the parietal peritoneum) is encountered, the direction of force from the index finger is directed posteriorly and obliquely towards the iliac crest and posterior spine, preventing entry into the peritoneal cavity.
(f) Blunt instrument is used to sweep fascia, a sense giving away is left on entering retroperitoneal space.
(g) If two-level fusion is planned, the same skin incision can be used in a different path or the same access can be used for two level (surgeon's preference).

3. Retroperitoneal dissection.
   (a) After exposure of transversalis fascia, the fascia bluntly swiped using index finger to access the retroperitoneal fat.
   (b) Retroperitoneal fat is readily visible as yellowish spongy structure underneath the fascia and should be swept in all directions to ensure the peritoneum is not adherent to the fascia.
   (c) The ureter is generally retracted along with this retroperitoneal fat.
   (d) Use the index finger to guide along the quadratus muscle directing finger medially to palpate the transverse process.
   (e) Slide the index finger down to the psoas muscle.
4. Identifying the psoas borders and dissection.
   (a) After exposing and mobilizing retroperitoneal fatty tissue and peritoneum, blunt finger dissection using the index finger is recommended.
   (b) Next step is identifying the anterior border of the psoas muscle and confirming it by palpation using the index finger.

(c) Gentle mobilisation of peritoneum in all direction cranial and caudal , ventral and dorsal cranial and caudal, ventral and dorsal (back-and-forth and up-and-down movements) to adequately mobilize the peritoneal contents anteriorly including the ureter that is loosely attached to the peritoneum, and the retroperitoneal fat anteriorly, anterior psoas border and intervertebral space is felt and palpated (Fig. 5).

5. Exposure of disc space and psoas mobilization.

(a) Ideally non-touch psoas technique which will minimize injury to nerves within psoas and psoas muscle itself.

(b) Motor nerves typically are found in the posterior one-third of the psoas muscle as demonstrated in cadaveric studies [17].

(c) Psoas mobilsation if required should be performed anteriorly in upper lumbar levels and at L4-L5 segmental artery runs can directly run across disc space which should be observed during OLIF [18].

6. Initial needle placement.

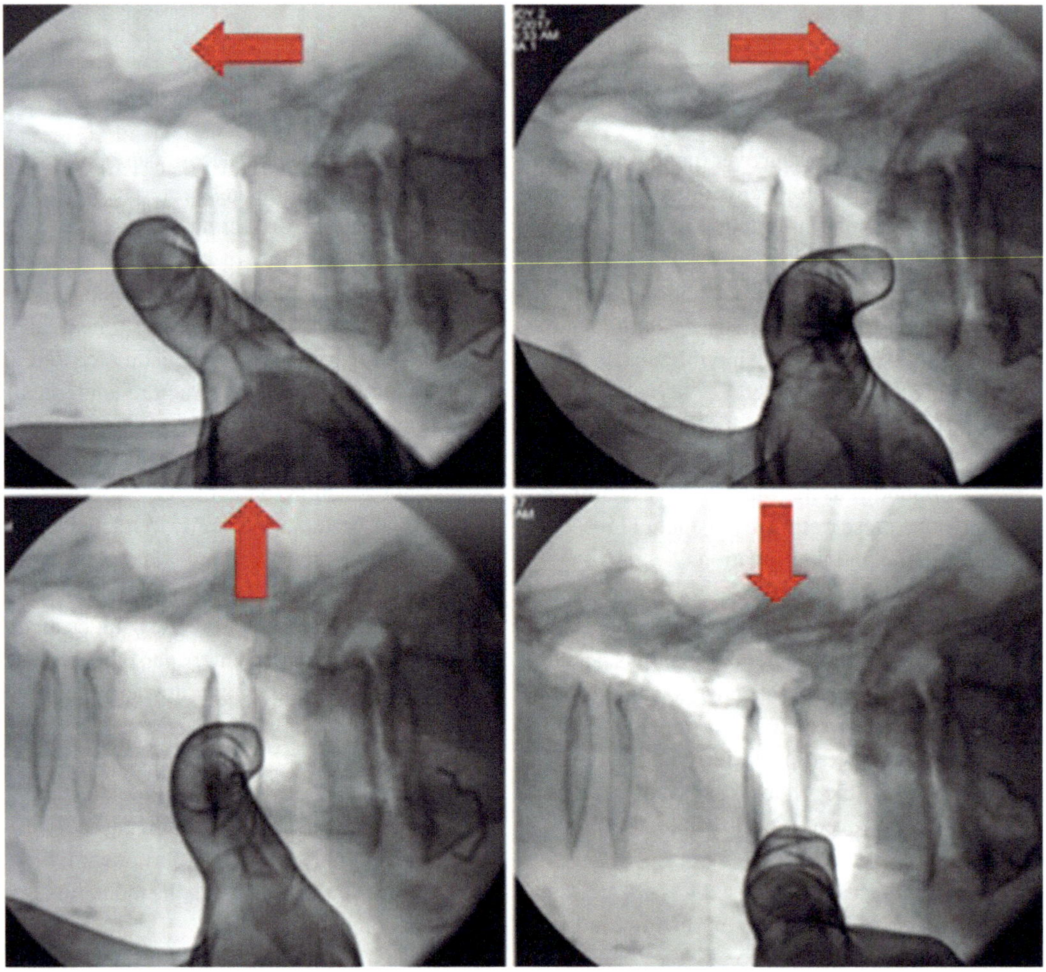

Fig. 5 Intraoperative fluoroscopic images depicting the posterior mobilization of the anterior belly of the psoas muscle through the use of cardinal index finger movements. Red colour arrows point to the direction of motion of index figure for mobilization

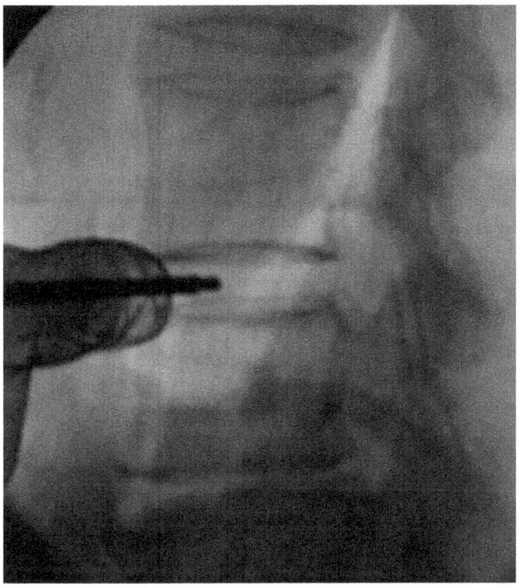

Fig. 6 Manoeuvre performed using index finger as a protection of the initial needle during its insertion as seen on lateral fluoroscopic image

(a) Initial guide wire is placed at anterior one-third to anterior half of the disc space [13].
(b) The tip of the needle should be protected underneath using the index finger while passing through OLIF trajectory to disc space to avoid injury to vascular structure (Fig. 6).
(c) After confirming the index level and site of annulus puncture under fluoroscopy, serial dilatation can be performed.

7. Docking.
   (a) Serial dilatation can be performed after confirmation of guide wire poisition on xay; serial dilatation can be made; a 22 mm diameter retractor of appropriate length can be glided over the final dilator and anchored to table mounted arm and fixed securely.
   (b) Stability pin should be inserted with caution on upper edge of lower vertebral body at L1-L2 and L2-L3 , and on the lower edge of upper vertebral body at L3-L4 and L4-L5 [18].
   (c) Blades of retractor are opened to expose the disc space and centred over anterior half of the disc space; blades should be parallel with the disc space which will aid in easier discectomy and endplate preparation.
   (d) Should be taken so that the blades of retractor should not damage the psoas muscle.
8. Annulotomy and discectomy.
   (a) Box annulotomy.
   (b) Annulus must be incised at least 18 mm in length or full length of available area [19].
   (c) Discectomy is performed using disc forceps, pituitary rongeurs, curettes and rasps.
   (d) Cobb elevator is inserted and rotated across to relaese contralateral ann Contralateral annulus release performed with help of cobb elevator with rotational manoeuvre; tip of cobb elavator should not cross beyond 3 to 4 mm the lateral border of vertebral body [19].
   (e) All steps to be performed under fluoroscopic guidance.
9. Endplate preparation.
   (a) Endplate is prepared with curettes, shaver and long pituitary forceps under C-arm fluoroscopic guidance. We always check adequacy of endplate preparation by injecting contrast into IVD space (Fig. 7).
   (b) Adequacy of endplate preparation can be confirmed using endoscope.
   (c) Orthogonal manoeuvre, points to a 90° angle that is formed with the instruments when placed perpendicularly to the sagittal plane of the vertebral body and there is a 90° angle correction of the instruments [20]. which is necessary during interbody cage placement.
10. Additional discectomy—hidden fragments.

    Endoscope can be inserted through the same retractor system or an additional incision of approximately 1 cm in length depending upon the target disc pathology (Figs. 8 and 9).

    (a) Endoscope can be used to see the presence of any remnant disc material and

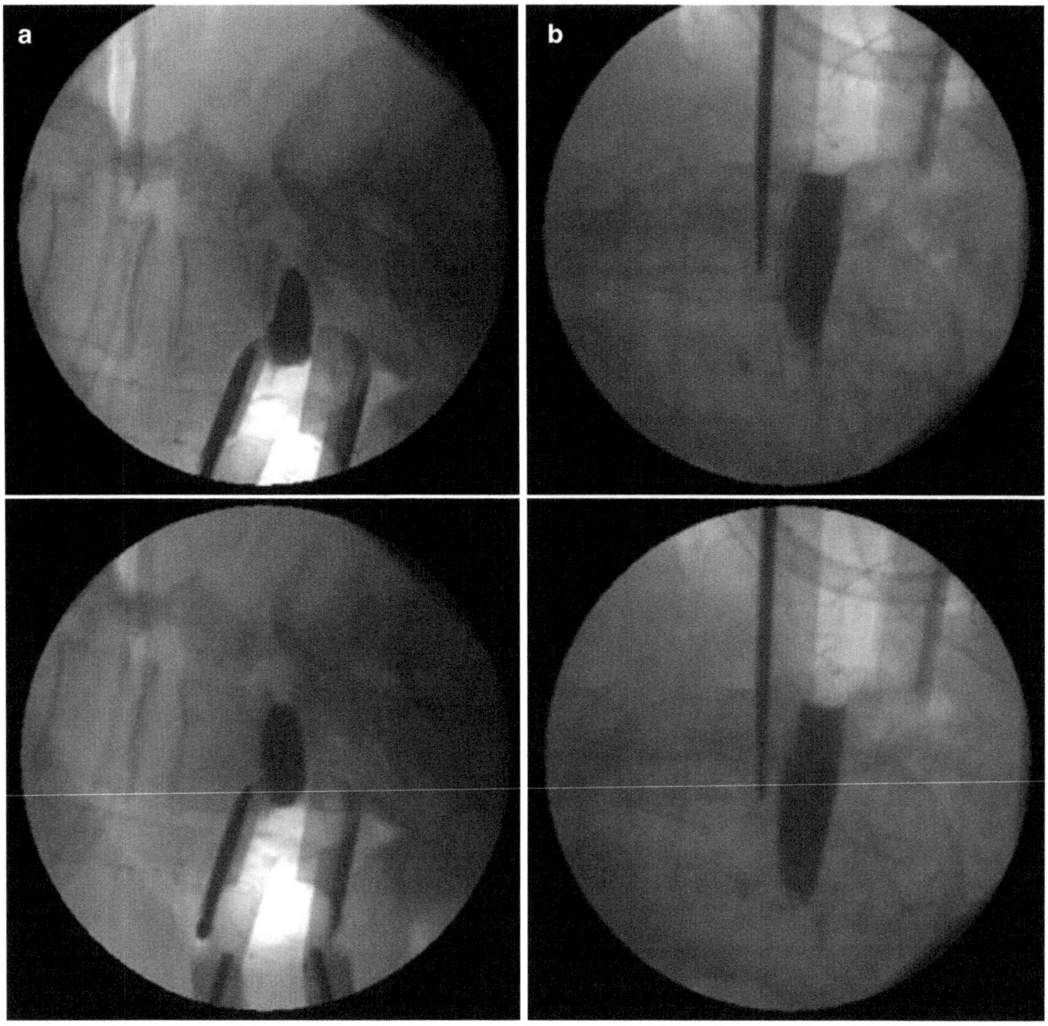

Fig. 7 Images showing endplates after injection contrast agent. (**a**) Inadequately prepared endplates. (**b**) Fluoroscopic images after adequate preparation

assess endplate preparation. Cartilaginous endplates can be prepared using curettes and shaver under direct endoscopic guidance (Fig. 10).

(b) Paracentral disc—paracentral disc can be removed by levering technique with the help of angled and semi-flexible forceps under direct vision using an endoscope (Fig. 11).

(c) Retained or missed disc fragment—in a few situations, there may be missed or sometimes possibility of some fragments being left behind. With the help of an endoscope and other access instruments, retained or missed disc fragments can be removed under endoscopic vision. The ventral part of the dura can be identified and can confirm good pulsation of the dura after the Valsalva manoeuvre, which is the end point of decompression. At this point, surgeons can evaluate whether a ventral discectomy is sufficient or not [15].

(d) Migrated disc fragment—migrated disc fragment can be removed with the assistance of a specialized angled hook or tip-

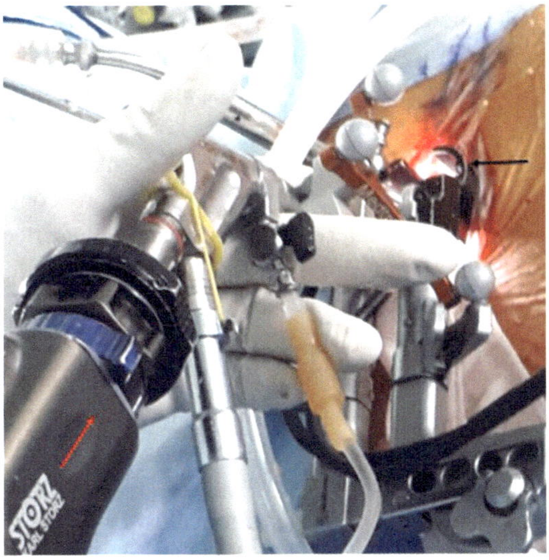

Fig. 8 Intraoperative image showing endoscope (red arrow) in the tubular OLIF retractor (black arrow)

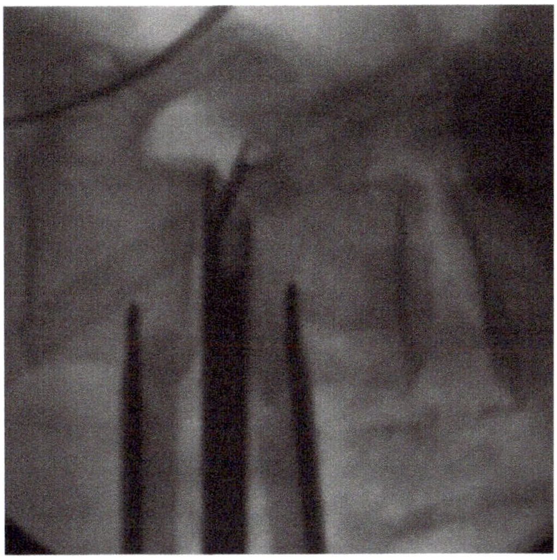

Fig. 9 Endoscope inserted through the OLIF retractor

Fig. 10 Intraoperative endoscopic view of remnant disc material after initial endplate preparation

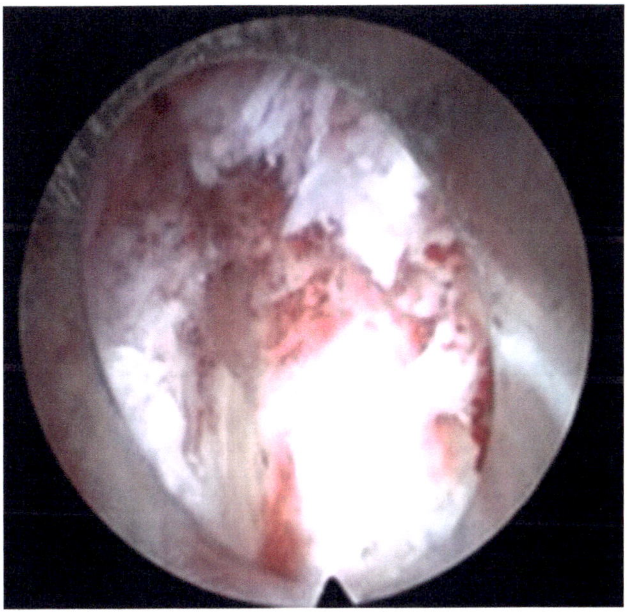

control burr (Fig. 12a), migrated disc fragment can be grasped through the annular defect by angled hook and endoscopic forceps (Fig. 12b, c) [15].

(e) Contralateral foramen—contralateral neural foramen exploration, removal of foraminal ruptured disc particles and posterior longitudinal ligament (PLL) resection for exploration of epidural space can be done if required [21].

(f) Central disc herniation—the central disc herniation can be decompressed using semi-flexible endoscopic forceps under direct endoscopic visualization till PLL or ventral side of the dura mater is recognized [22].

(g) Foraminal disc herniation—the foramen can be explored using endoscope and angled instruments and ruptured disc material can be removed under vision [22].

Upon completion of discectomy, radiofrequency coagulator can be used for annular sealing. The end point of endoscopic ventral decompression would be floating ventral dura with the Valsalva manoeuvre under saline irrigation.

11. Implant trail and cage insertion—after sufficient discectomy and endplate preparation, sequential trail implant spacer is used to open up and distract the space until adequate disc space and foraminal heigth is obtained which is confirmed on fluoroscopy. Appropriate sized interbody cage with required lordotic angle spanning the entire length of cortex (cortex to cortex) (Fig. 13) based on surgeon preference is inserted in orthogonal manoeuvre under fluoroscopic guidance. Interbody cage should be inserted between the anterior and middle thirds of the IVD space on the lateral view, and centrally place on the anteroposterior view [27]. Advantage of Endoscopic OLIF is no need of additional posterior decompression but always anterior construct should be supported with posterior pedicle screw fixation. MI-OLIF can be safely performed without neuromonitoring [11].

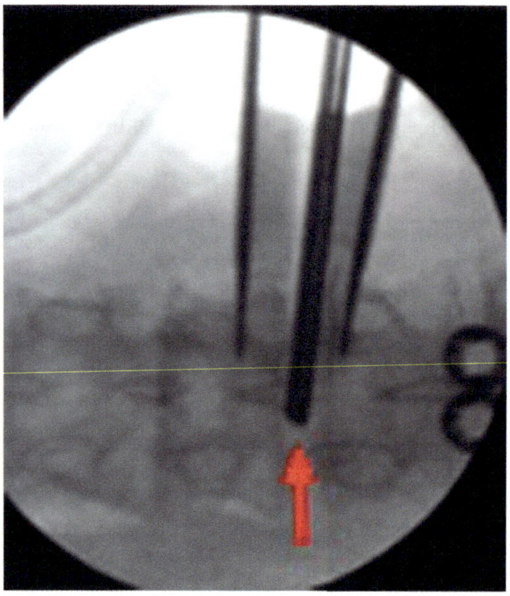

Fig. 11 Intraoperative fluoroscopic C-arm AP image showing an endoscope was introduced through a tubular retractor that was used for the OLIF procedure. The tip of the endoscope was located at the right paracentral area in AP view (red arrow)

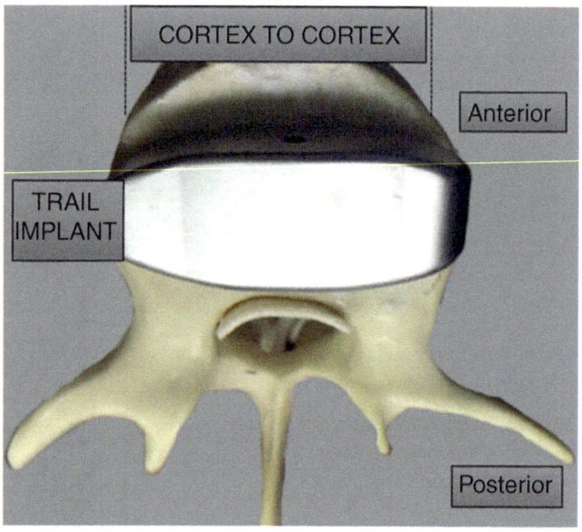

Fig. 13 Reconstructed image showing ideal implant position (cortex to cortex and anterior third of disc space)

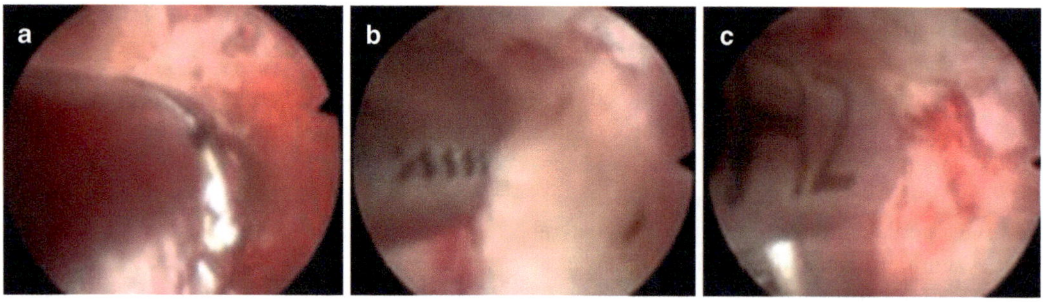

Fig. 12 Endoscopic images. (**a**) Bony edge of the vertebral body removed by tip-control burr. (**b**, **c**) Following this, an upward migrated disc fragment was removed using the endoscopic forceps and right-angled hook

Illustrated Case

53 year old female patient, wheel chair bound with history of open lumbar fusion at L3-L4 and L5-L6 prsented with progressive weakness of lower limbs with voiding difficultly and saddle anaestheia with multiple comorbid conditions. Neurological examination revealved hip flexion 3/5, knee extension 3/5, ankle dorsiflexion 3/5, great toe dorsiflexion 2/5, ankle plantar flexion 4/5 in both lower limbs with sensory hypoesthesia around 50 % involving all the dermatome.

Imaging showed interbody fusion at L3–L4 and L5–L6 with L2–L3 degenerative disc disease with huge left paracentral disc fragment compressing neural elements. The patient underwent L2–L3 OLIF with removal of left paracentral disc fragment using endoscope assistance supplemented with posterior pedicle screw fixation without need of any additional posteriordecompression (Figs. 14 and 15).

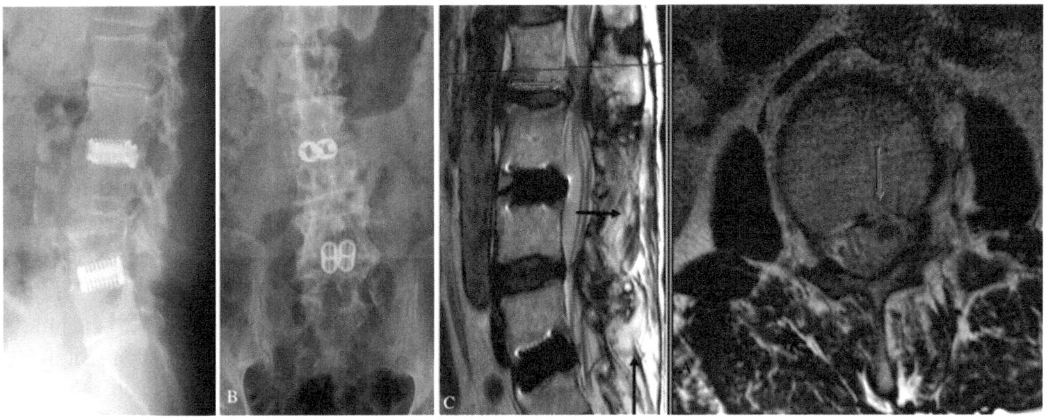

Fig. 14 Preoperative (**a** and **b**) showing AP/lateral X-ray images with L3–L4, L5–L6 interbody cage with reduced disc height at L2–L3 with mild degenerative scoliosis. (**c**) Sagittal T2 showing paraspinal muscle atrophy (black arrows) with L2–L3 extruded disc with upward migration (red arrow). (**d**) Axial T2 image showing huge left paracentral disc causing compression on thecal sac and nerve root

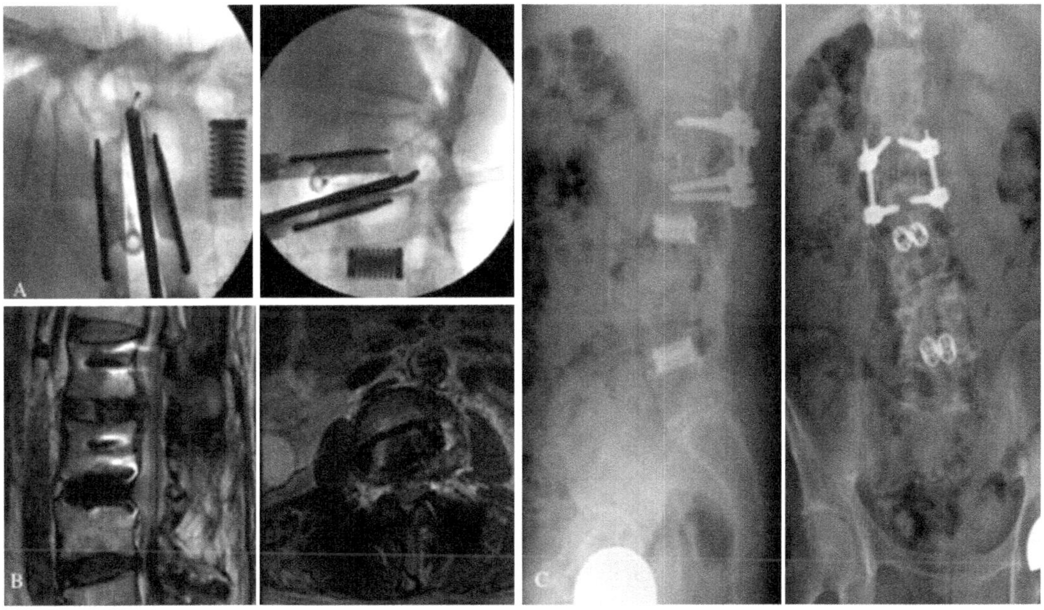

Fig. 15 (**a**) Intraoperative fluoroscopic image showing endoscopic semi-flexible probe used to remove paracentral disc herniation. (**b**) Postoperative sagittal and axial MRI showing an interbody cage at L2–L3 with disc height restoration. (**c**) Immediate postoperative AP/lateral X-ray showing L2–L3 interbody cage with pedicle screw at L2 and L3 with stand-alone cage at L3–L4 and L5–L6

Complication and its Management

Complications include injury to the lumbar plexus leading to postoperative sensory and motor symptoms, vascular complication, dural tears, ureteral injury and cage and wound site-related complications.

To describe the entire demography of complication is not the scope of this chapter.

Incisional site pain in 2.2% and sympathetic chain injury and vascular injuries are reported in 1.7% of cases [10], vascular laceration and dural tears comprising 3.9% and transientileus, retroperitoneal hematoma, urinary tract infection, wound infection and worsening of radiculopathy in 17.6% of cases [22]. The largest clinical series on OLIF reported several possible complications like sensory nerve injury, psoas weakness, vertebral body fracture, motor nerve injury, anterior longitudinal ligament rupture, surgical site infection, pleural laceration, segmental artery injury, peritoneum laceration, cage malpositioning, retroperitoneal hematoma, ureteral injury, abdominal wall hernia, ileus, major vascular injury and posterior conversion [23].

Complication prevention in any surgical procedure needs adequate surgical planning. The strategy to avoid complications can be classified as preoperative planning and intraoperative avoidance techniques.

Choosing the Right Operative Strategy

1. Preoperative planning.
   (a) Imaging.
   - MRI and CT are the imaging modality of choice, preferably in right lateral decubitus position for accuracy in preoperative planning [23].
   - Imaging should provide the position and course of lumbar arterial and venous vessels, as well as their posterior and lateral migration on the contralateral side of the approach [24].
   - Evaluation of preoperative images-analysing the position of vascular structure to operative level, psoas muscle morphology its thickness and relation to surrounding neural structures, the operative corridor between anterior border of left psoas and left lateral border of vascular structure depending upon levels (aorta and iliac artery).

   (b) Positioning.
   - The ideal position would be right lateral decubitus position for approach from left side.
   - The patient should be firmly secured to operative adhesive tapes to avoid any undue movement of the patient during the surgical procedure.
   - Mild flexion of the left hip to relax the psoas muscle [26].
   - Operative table should be mildly flexed, because when the patient in lateral position over a flexed table and time lapsed in this position is directly proportional to postoperative neuropraxia [23].
   - Fluoroscopic images should be squared-parallel endplates and centred spinous process.
   - Inaccurate fluoroscopic images can lead to wrongly placed incision or might require a noncosmetic bigger incision [20].
2. Intraoperative planning.
   (c) Muscular dissection.
   (d) Muscular dissection should be performed along direction of muscle fibres [20].
   - Use of bipolar cautery should be minimized in the intramuscular plane.
   - Avoid excessive muscular dissection and meticulous muscular closure of abdominal wall to prevent dysaesthesias and abdominal wall paresis after the procedure [26, 27].

   (e) Meticulous and Safe retroperitoneal dissection will aid in exposure of the disc space and prevent injury to retroperitoneal structures and inadvertent opening of peritoneum.

(f) Mobilization of psoas.
  - In order to avoid injury to the genitofemoral nerve (which runs on the anterolateral surface of the psoas muscle), lumbar plexus and psoas muscle, meticulous dissection of the anterior belly of the psoas muscle should be performed that does not go beyond the median coronal plane [26, 28–30].
  - Lessen the retraction time of the psoas muscle against the transverse process as prolonged retraction time may injury lumbar plexus [29, 30].

(g) Retractor assembly should be placed under direct vision because of potential risk to the ureter, sympathetic chain or vascular structures [26].

(h) Avoiding vascular injury.
  - Vascular insult happens during anterior mobilization of great vessels and placement of stability pin for securing the retractor.
  - Vascular injury during mobilization can be avoided through the use of a detailed preoperative assessment through imaging and with a minimal medial exposure [25].
  - Stability pin has to be inserted proximal to the endplates as we have discussed in the surgical technique above [20].
  - Precaution to be taken upon fixation of the tubular retractor at the L4–L5 space and if possible to avoid the fixation of stability pin on L5 which can prevent laceration to the iliolumbar vein [18].
  - Use of preoperative MRI should prognosticate localization of vessels [20].

(i) Avoiding ureteral injury.

  The following steps would minimize ureteral injury:
  - Complete dissection and retraction of retroperitoneal fatty tissue before starting the discectomy [31].
  - Survey of intervertebral disc through tubular retractor [31].
  - Anterior mobilization of the ureter with blunt and soft dissection [31].
  - Postoperative fever, abdominal pain and distension, vomiting and leucocytosis on blood investigations would favour a possibility of ureteric injury in view of any adverse intraoperative event [32, 33].

(j) Sympathetic chain injury.
  - Sympathetic chain is placed in anterior third of vertebral body, placing tubular retractor posterior to the sympathetic chain and thus diminishing its manipulation and avoiding injury [20].

(k) Endplate and contralateral nerve injury.
  - Avoid overzealous endplate preparation; this can lead to cage subsidence.
  - Contralateral release with Cobb should be performed under cautions; all steps should be performed under fluoroscopic guidance with blunt surgical tools to avoid a contralateral psoas muscle and lumbar plexus injury [12].

(l) Spinal canal injury.
  - OLIF offer indirect compression, and any attempt for direct decompression through conventional discectomy is not suggested as it carries risk of spinal canal irruption [14, 15].

(m) Avoiding dural tears.
  - To avoid dural and contralateral nerve root injury, the surgeon must know the OLIF trajectory angle and cage tilt angle based on images and anatomy [34].
  - Intraoperative C-arm images should be frequently checked, especially at the stage of contralateral annular release [34].

(n) Saline irrigation.
  - Endoscopic assistance always requires fluid medium. Normal saline is routinely used. Saline irrigation not only helps in proper visualization of the operative area, as there is a continuous

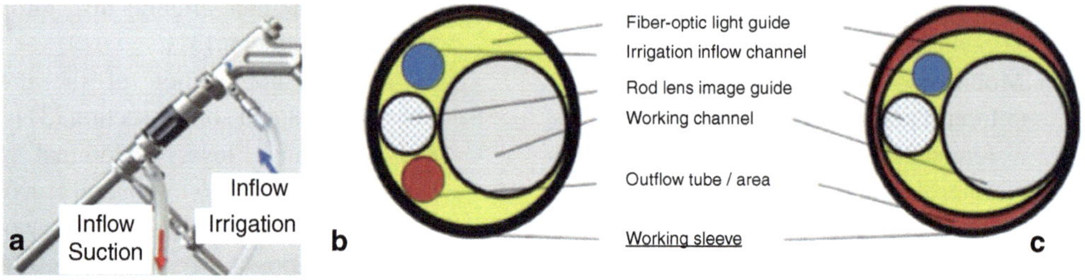

Fig. 16 (**a**) Endoscopic showing inflow and outflow irrigation set. Full-endoscopic systems showing various channels of endoscope, (**b**) inflow and outflow through separate channels in the endoscope, (**c**) inflow through irrigation channel, large outflow channel in the space between oval endoscope cross section and round working sleeve

flow of fluid medium risk of infection is very minimal. Considering intraoperative fluid accumulation due to saline irrigation in retroperitoneum the present generation full endoscope system has inflow and outflow channels which prevents a critical pressure increase in the spinal canal and prevents fluid accumulation (Fig. 16) [35, 36].

Brief Discussion

Key Points

Benefits of Endoscopic OLIF

Endoscopic-assisted OLIF explores the ventral portion of the spinal canal, epidural space and central canal and permits removal of ruptured disc particles at the foramen and also endplate exploration [15], achieving both direct and indirect decompression. Though ALIF can achieve both direct and indirect decompression, access-related complication, need of vascular surgeon assistance in the initial learning curve and other complications like abdominal visceral injury, retrograde ejaculation and vascular injury are the drawbacks. Posterior fusion procedure can achieve direct decompression with facetectomy, laminectomy and discectomy, but drawbacks include risk of substantial bleeding, epidural adhesion, posterior Muscle and ligamentous injury contributing to postoperative back pain and use of a small-sized cage. On the other hand, LLIF, including DLIF and OLIF, preserves ligamentous structures and posterior anatomical structures (including the lamina, facet and posterior spinal muscles). Decreased blood loss is an additional benefit merit of endoscopically assisted OLIF compared with that seen with the posterior approach [14]. Endoscope-assisted OLIF has some limitations; surgeons are trained to approach the herniated IVD from posterior; in a given situation, the patient is placed in lateral position and orientation of spinal canal and foramen accordingly changes. The surgeon has to keep this in mind while using an endoscope in OLIF. Other limiting factors include accessing the contralateral foramen [37] and difficult scenario like removal of posterior osteophytes, migrated discs and calcified discs. But with the advent of newer and advanced spinal endoscopic devices, these limitations can be avoided [14].

To summarize, OLIF is a relatively safe tool that can achieve powerful indirect decompression with ligamentotaxis, better restoration of disc height in case of collapsed disc space achieving enough lordosis and better fusion rates because of wider footprint of an interbody cage with no injury to muscles, facets and posterior ligamentous structure. When supplemented with endoscope, endoscope-assisted OLIF achieves direct compression by removing ruptured disc fragments with added advantage of accessing the contralateral disc herniation through a same incision and ipsilateral disc herniation need a separate incision because working angle and different trajectory is needed and finally even bone spur at corner of vertebral body can be removed using endoscopic burr. Endoscopic OLIF can achieve 360° circumferential full decompression and fusion without any additional laminectomy.

References

1. Pimenta L, Turner AWL, Dooley ZA, Parikh RD, Peterson MD. Biomechanics of lateral interbody spacers: Going wider for going stiffer. Sci World J. 2012; https://doi.org/10.1100/2012/38181.
2. Castro L, Oliveira R, Amaral L. Marchi, and L. Pimenta. Is the lateral transpsoas approach feasible for the treatment of adult degenerative scoliosis? Clin Orthop Relat Res. 2014;472(6):1776–83.
3. Wolfla CE, Maiman DJ, Coufal FJ, Wallace JR. Retroperitoneal lateral lumbar interbody fusion with titanium threaded fusion cages. J Neurosurg Spine. 2002;96:50–5.
4. Fraser RD, Gogan WJ. A modified muscle- splitting approach to the lumbosacral spine. Spine (Phila Pa 1976). 1992;17:943–8.
5. Jeffrey Katzell MD. Endoscopic foraminal decompression preceding oblique lateral lumbar interbody fusion to decrease the incidence of post-operative dysaesthesia. Int J Spine Surg. 2014;8:Article 19. doi: 10.14444/1019
6. Phan K, Thayaparan GK, Mobbs RJ. Anterior lumbar interbody fusion versus transforaminal lumbar interbody fusion – systematic review and meta-analysis. Br J Neurosurg. 2015;29:705–11.
7. Rao PJ, Ghent F, Phan K, et al. Stand-alone anterior lumbar interbody fusion for treatment of degenerative spondylolisthesis. J Clin Neurosci. 2015;22:1619–24.
8. Rao PJ, Loganathan A, Yeung V, et al. Outcomes of anterior lumbar interbody fusion surgery based on indication: a prospective study. Neurosurgery. 2015;76:7–23. [discussion 23–4]
9. Mayer HM. A new microsurgical technique for minimally invasive anterior lumbar interbody fusion. Spine (Phila Pa 1976). 1997;22:691–9. [discussion 700]
10. Silvestre C, Mac-Thiong JM, Hilmi R, et al. Complications and morbidities of mini-open anterior retroperitoneal lumbar interbody fusion: oblique lumbar interbody fusion in 179 patients. Asian Spine J. 2012;6:89–97.
11. Hynes RA, Otsuki B, Kimura H, Takemoto M, Matsuda S. Effect of indirect neural decompression through oblique lateral interbody fusion for degenerative lumbar disease. Spine. 2015;40(3):E175–82.
12. Abe K, Orita S, Mannoji C, Motegi H, Aramomi M, Ishikawa T, Kotani T, Akazawa T, et al. Perioperative complications in 155 patients who underwent oblique lateral interbody fusion surgery: perspectives and indications from a retrospective, multicenter survey. Spine (Phila Pa 1976). 2017;42(1):55–62. https://doi.org/10.1097/BRS.0000000000001650.
13. Sardhara J, Singh S, et al. Neuro-navigation assisted pre-psoas minimally invasive oblique lumbar interbody fusion (MI-OLIF): New roads and impediments. Neurol India. 2019;67:803 012.
14. Heo DH, Kim JS, et al. Clinical and radiological outcomes of spinal endoscopic discectomy–assisted oblique lumbar interbody fusion: preliminary results. Neurosurg Focus. 2017;43(2):E13.
15. Kim J-S, Seong J-H, et al. Endoscope-assisted oblique lumbar interbody fusion for the treatment of cauda equina syndrome: a technical note : Eur Spine J. Ann Transl Med. 2018;6(6):101. https://doi.org/10.1007/s00586-016-4902-9.
16. Kyoh Y. Minimally invasive endoscopic-assisted lateral lumbar interbody fusion: technical report and preliminary results. Neurospine. 2019;16(1):72–81. https://doi.org/10.14245/ns.1938024.012.
17. Moro T, Kikuchi S, Konno S, et al. An anatomic study of the lumbar plexus with respect to retroperitoneal endoscopic surgery. Spine (Phila Pa 1976). 2003;28(5):423–8. discussion 427-8
18. Orita SB, Inage K, Sainoh T, et al. Lower lumbar segmental arteries can intersect over the intervertebral disc in the oblique lateral interbody fusion approach with a risk for arterial injury: Radiological analysis of lumbar segmental arteries by using magnetic resonance imaging. Spine (Phila Pa 1976). 2017;42(3):135–42. https://doi.org/10.1097/BRS.0000000000001700.
19. Orita S, Inage K, Furuya T, Koda M, Aoki Y. Oblique Lateral Interbody Fusion (OLIF): Indications and techniques :operative technique in orthopaedics. 2017:1048–6666. https://doi.org/10.1053/j.oto.2017.09.004.
20. Quillo-Olvera J, Lin GX, Jo HJ, Kim JS. Complications on minimally invasive oblique lumbar interbody fusion at L2-L5 levels: a review of the literature and surgical strategies. Ann Transl Med. 2018;6(6):101. https://doi.org/10.21037/atm.2018.01.22.
21. Seong J-H, Kim J-SL. Endoscopic Spine Surgery:Chapter 26. In: Laparoscope- and Endoscope-Assisted Oblique Lumbar Interbody Fusion. 2nd ed. (ISBN 978-1-62623-264-8).
22. Kaiser MG, Haid RW Jr, Subach BR, et al. Comparison of the mini-open versus laparoscopic approach for anterior lumbar interbody fusion: a retrospective review. Neurosurgery. 2002;51:97–103. discussion 103-5
23. Molinares DM, Davis TT, Fung DA. Retroperitoneal oblique corridor to the L2-S1 intervertebral discs: an MRI study. J Neurosurg Spine. 2016;24(2):248–55. https://doi.org/10.3171/2015.3.
24. Regev GJ, Kim CW. Safety and the anatomy of the retroperitoneal lateral corridor with respect to the minimally invasive lateral lumbar intervertebral fusion approach. Neurosurg Clin N Am. 2014;25:211–8.

25. Hynes RA. Oblique lateral approach to the lumbar spine (L2-L5). In: Watkins III RG, Watkins IV RG, editors. Surgical approaches to the spine. New York: Springer; 2015. p. 223–34.
26. Liu L, Liang Y, Zhang H, et al. Imaging anatomical research on the operative windows of oblique lumbar interbody fusion. PLoS One. 2016;11:e0163452.
27. Korenkov M, Rixen D, Paul A, et al. Combined abdominal wall paresis and incisional hernia after laparoscopic cholecystectomy. Surg Endosc. 1999;13:268–9.
28. Mehren C, Mayer HM, Zandanell C, et al. The oblique anterolateral approach to the lumbar spine provides access to the lumbar spine with few early complications. Clin Orthop Relat Res. 2016;474:2020–7.
29. Gragnaniello C, Seex K. Anterior to psoas (ATP) fusion of the lumbar spine: evolution of a technique facilitated by changes in equipment. J Spine Surg. 2016;2:256–65.
30. Gragnaniello C, Seex KA. Anterior to psoas fusion of the lumbar spine. Neurosurg Focus. 2013;35:Video 13.
31. Kanno K, Ohtori S, Orita S, Yamauchi K, Eguchi Y, Aoki Y, et al. Miniopen oblique lateral L5-S1 interbody fusion: a report of 2 cases. Case Rep Orthop. 2014:603531. https://doi.org/10.1155/2014/603531. PMID: 25400963
32. Fujibayashi S, Otsuki B, Kimura H, et al. Preoperative assessment of the ureter with dual-phase contrast- enhanced computed tomography for lateral lumbar interbody fusion procedures. J Orthop Sci. 2017;22:420–4.
33. Lee HJ, Kim JS, Ryu KS, et al. Ureter injury as a complication of oblique lumbar interbody fusion. World Neurosurg. 2017, 102:693.e7–693.e14.
34. Chang JC, Kim J-S, Jo H. Ventral Dural Injury After Oblique Lumbar Interbody Fusion. World Neurosurg. 2016; https://doi.org/10.1016/j.wneu.2016.11.028.
35. Richard Wolf GmbH. Endoscopic spine work unit. s.l.:s.n. 2017
36. Richard Wolf GmbH. Several product pictures. s.l.:s.n. 2017
37. Heo DH, Choi WS, Park CK, Kim JS. Minimally invasive oblique lumbar interbody fusion with spinal endoscope assistance: technical note. World Neurosurg. 2016;96:530–6.

Endoscopic LIF (Uniportal); Endoscopic TLIF; FELIF (Full Endoscopic Lumbar Interbody Fusion)

Myung Soo Youn

Introduction (Key Point and Purpose) of Approach

There are numerous spinal fusion techniques in lumbar interbody fusion (LIF), including ALIF, PLIF, TLIF, DLIF, and OLIF by open discectomy. With the advancement of endoscopic surgery, several percutaneous endoscopic fusion techniques have been reported [1, 2]. However, these techniques have shown limitations, especially in the insertion of the established rigid bullet-shaped cage. In general, the established bullet-shaped cage is too large and rigid to pass through the endoscopic working channel. So, the author has made some modifications in the following instruments (reamer, cage holding rod, and funnel-shaped device for bone graft) in endoscopic situation, all surgical procedures for the endoscopic fusion were able to be monitored through endoscopic view [3]. This approach is based on the TLIF approach.

Indication and Contraindication

1. Indication.
   (a) Lumbar foraminal stenosis with segmental instability.
   (b) Lumbar disc herniation with segmental instability.
   (c) Mild spondylolisthesis (less than Meyerding grade II).
2. Contraindication.
   (a) Severe disc space narrowing: due to limitations of the endoscopic procedure.
   (b) Severe spondylolisthesis (more than Meyerding grade III): due to limitations of the reduction of listhesis.
   (c) Any disease that could adversely affect bone quality may be unable to undergo a fusion surgery.

Anesthesia and Position

Generally, endoscopic TLIF is performed under general anesthesia or epidural anesthesia. But endoscopic TLIF can be performed under local anesthesia with conscious sedation. We can reduce the risks related with general anesthesia and check the real-time feedback from the patient by local anesthesia. Therefore, endoscopic TLIF is useful especially with the elderly or medically compromised patients.

As a premedication for conscious sedation, midazolam (0.05 mg/kg) is injected intramuscularly 30 min before surgery. Dexmedetomidine (1 mcg/kg during 10 min for loading dose and 0.2–0.7 mcg/kg/h for maintenance dose) is intravenously administered during operation time. The

M. S. Youn (✉)
Department of Orthopedic Surgery, Busan Keun Hospital, Busan, South Korea

H. S. Kim et al. (eds.), *Advanced Techniques of Endoscopic Lumbar Spine Surgery*,
https://doi.org/10.1007/978-981-15-8253-0_15

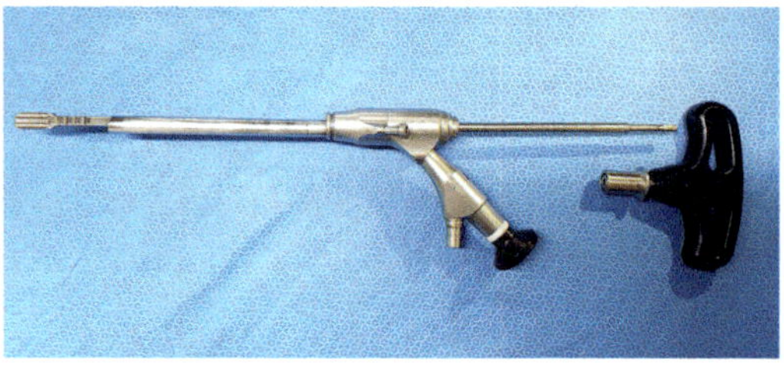

Fig. 1 Modified locking handle mechanism to distal part of reamer

patient was placed in the prone position on a radiolucent table. The skin entry point was located at the lateral edge of paravertebral back muscle (about 8–13 cm lateral to the midline, depending on the patient's waist circumference).

Special Surgical Instruments

Several custom-made instruments are essential in performing endoscopic TLIF, because the conventional reamer used for open discectomy could not pass through the working channel of the endoscope. We improved the locking handle mechanism at the distal part of the reamer (Fig. 1) and working cannula (16–20 mm of diameter) (Fig. 2). The PEEK TLIF cage (11–14 mm of height, 38 mm of length, bullet shaped) is mounted on the cage holding rod after the rod was inserted into the working channel (Fig. 3a, b). Allograft is placed into the anterior disc space through a funnel-shaped bone graft device (Fig. 4).

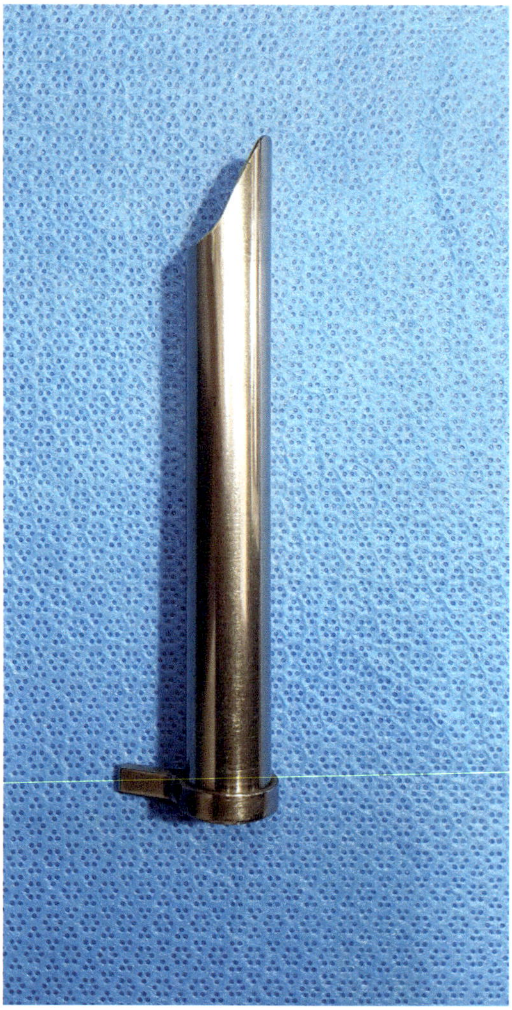

Fig. 2 Custom made sheath to pass the rigid bullet shaped cage

Surgical Steps: Summarized with Video File (Video 1)

The best indication of endoscopic TLIF (FELIF) is the case with unilateral foraminal stenosis and instability. Sometimes foraminal stenosis may be combined with central stenosis. So, endoscopic TLIF can be performed either by itself or combined with posterior decompression.

1. Endoscopic partial facetectomy (EPF) of superior articular process (SAP)

   We have to set the target point of initial needling on the surface of the facet joint. A tapered obturator is inserted over the guide wire to not intervertebral foramen but the facet joint; this step will prevent damage of the exiting nerve root avoiding direct contact with it. After the working cannula and endoscope are inserted, the surgeon can see the surface of the facet joint via endoscopic visualization. Once the facet joint is identified, osteotomy on superior half of SAP can be completed. The partial removal of SAP is an essential step to carry out endoscopic TLIF, because it provides us with enough space and clear epiduroscopic view (Fig. 5a, b).

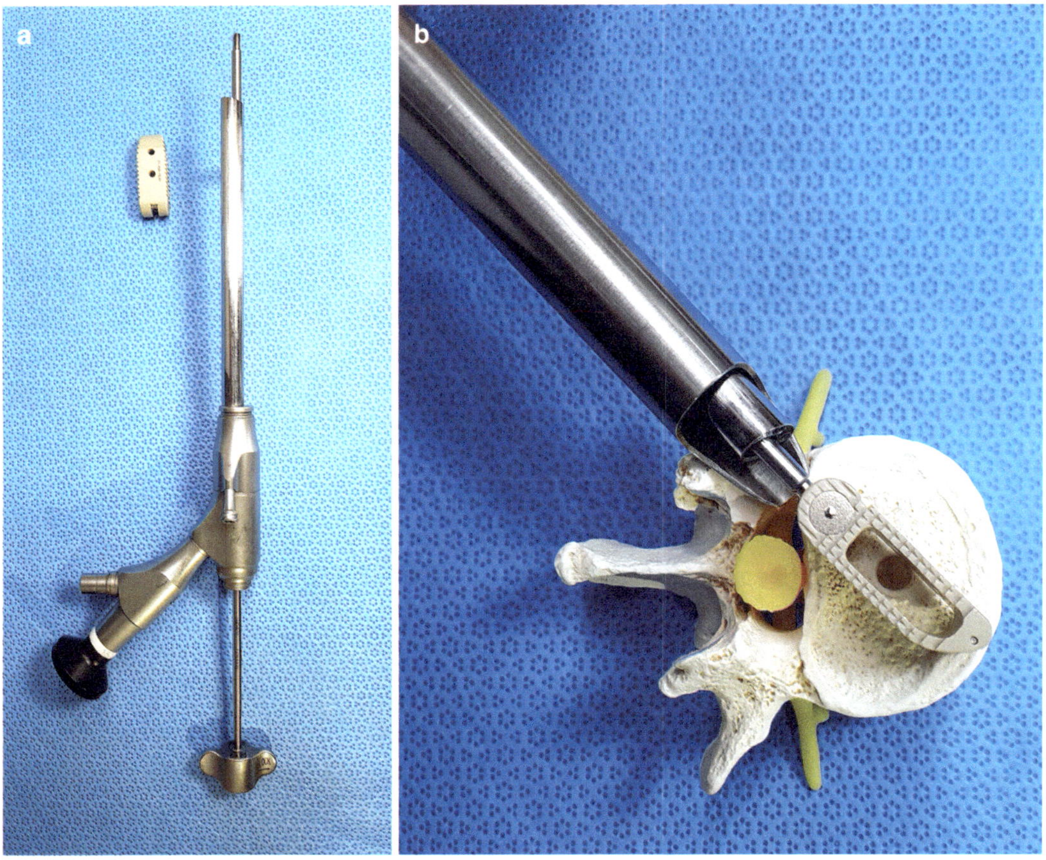

Fig. 3 Placement of PEEK cage under full endoscopic and fluoroscopic guidance

2. Endplate preparation

   After direct decompression with removal of SAP, endoscopic reamer is inserted to the disc space under fluoroscopic and endoscopic guidance (Fig. 6a–c). The reamer is expanded and rotated in the disc space with endoscopic visualization. The things that we have to remove are disc material and cartilage inside the disc space. Because the conventional small endoscope can be inserted into the disc space, we can remove disc material and cartilage from the intact subchondral bone. So, we can improve the accuracy of the endplate preparation with endoscopic guidance (Fig. 7).
3. Bone graft, cage insertion, and percutaneous screw fixation

After the disc space preparation, allograft is placed into the anterior disc space through a funnel-shaped bone graft device. The PEEK TLIF cage can be inserted by the cage holding rod under fluoroscopic and full endoscopic view. Percutaneous pedicle screws are then placed using an anteroposterior fluoroscopic technique with Jamshidi needles. These tracts are injected with 20 cc of bupivacaine (Exparel, diluted 1:2–40 mL total volume) under pressure into the posterior musculature dived evenly between the four screw insertion tracts, especially in local anesthesia.

Illustrated Case or Cases

Case

A 65-year-old female complained of the symptom with both leg radiating pain for 1 year. She has a history of a performed L4/5/S1 fusion surgery 7 years ago (Fig. 8a–c). Her symptoms were not controlled with conservative treatment

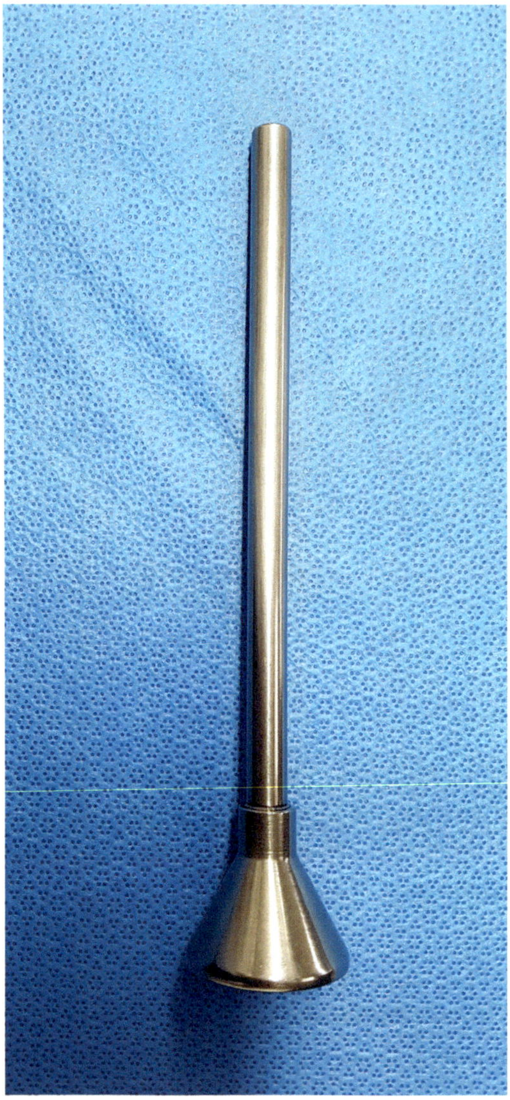

Fig. 4 Custom made funnel shaped bone graft device

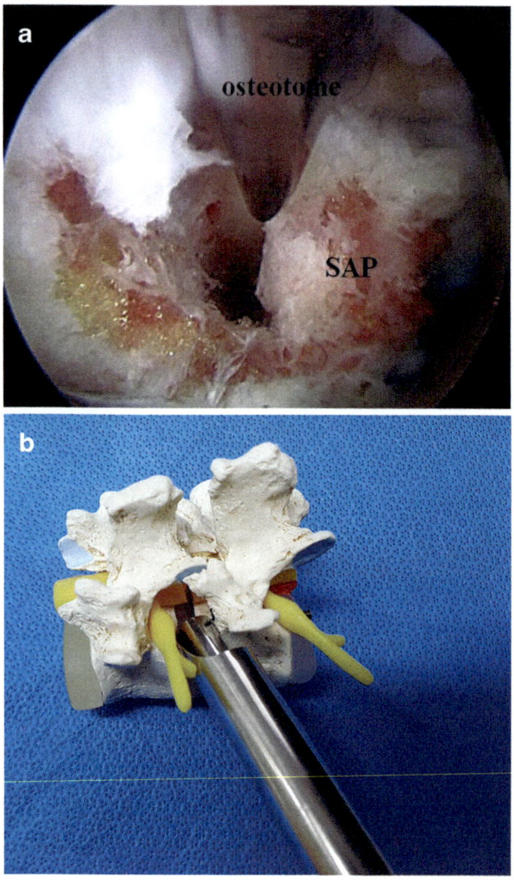

Fig. 5 (**a**) Once the joint is identified via endoscopic view, osteotomy of superior articular process is performed by using endoscopic osteotome. (**b**) After the partial resection of superior articular process on sawbone

for 6 months. We can see the severe foraminal stenosis on both sides of the MRI view (Fig. 9a, b). Endoscopic decompression and cage insertion were performed (Fig. 10a–c). Previous screws were removed and new screws were fixed percutaneously (Fig. 11a, b).

Limitation, Complication, and its Management

1. Neural tissue injury

   There are possibilities of either exiting nerve root or dural injuries during the insertion of a working sheath or cage. Therefore, the initial target should be on the facet joint. During a cage insertion, clear endoscopic view and proper placement of a working cannula are essential for the prevention of neural tissue injuries.

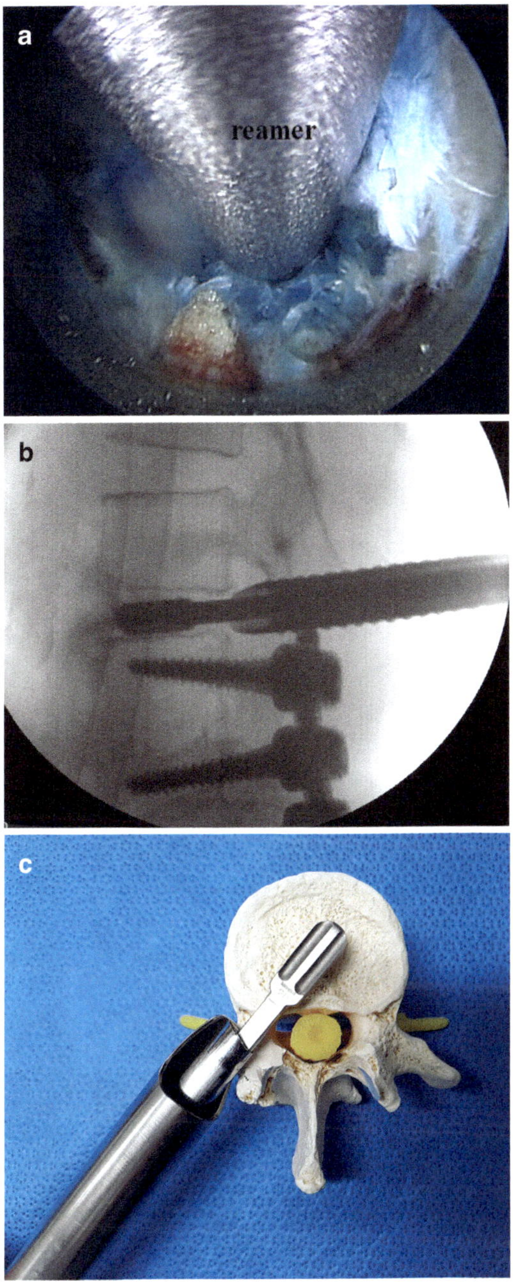

Fig. 6 (**a**, **b**) Custom-made endoscopic reamer is inserted to disc space under endoscopic and fluoroscopic guidance. (**c**) Axial demonstrated image on saw bone

2. Dural tear

   A dural tear may happen during the cage insertion. A small-sized dural tear may be controlled with several sealants or direct repair with endoscopic help. In most cases, open conversion surgery is needed to repair of dural tear.

3. Limited indication

   Endoscopic TLIF is a minimally invasive technique that has the same approach route with TLIF surgery through the unilateral facet joint. In cases with high-grade spondylolisthesis, the reduction of slippage may be impossible because of contralateral intact facet joint. In patients with disc space narrowing or a very narrow Kambin's triangle, it may be difficult to achieve sufficient disc preparation for a safe cage insertion. Therefore, it is important to select proper case with appropriate indication before surgery.

4. Limited interbody fusion

   Judging by the part of the bone union, the union rate of endoscopic TLIF is unclear and not yet established. It may be good in respect of clear vision and precise endplate preparation for the increased union potential. It may be difficult to have interbody fusion if not enough autograft is available or if a fusion cage is not sufficient because of limited working space.

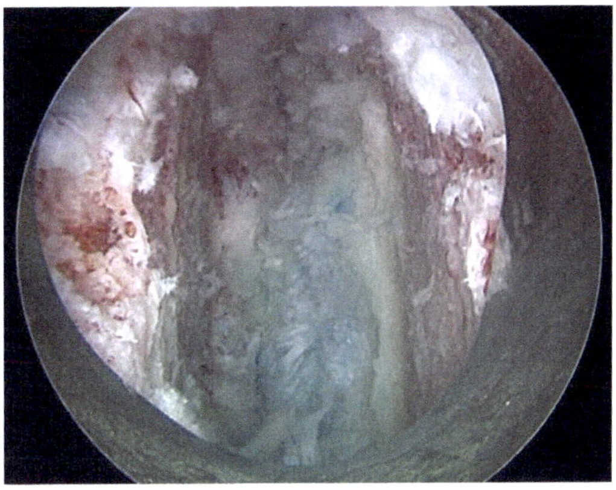

Fig. 7 Endoscopic view of the vertebral endplate after preparation for fusion showing the intact cortical bone

Surgical Tip and Pitfall

Transforaminal lumbar interbody fusion (TLIF) is considered a standard lumbar fusion technique, providing effective decompression of the neural

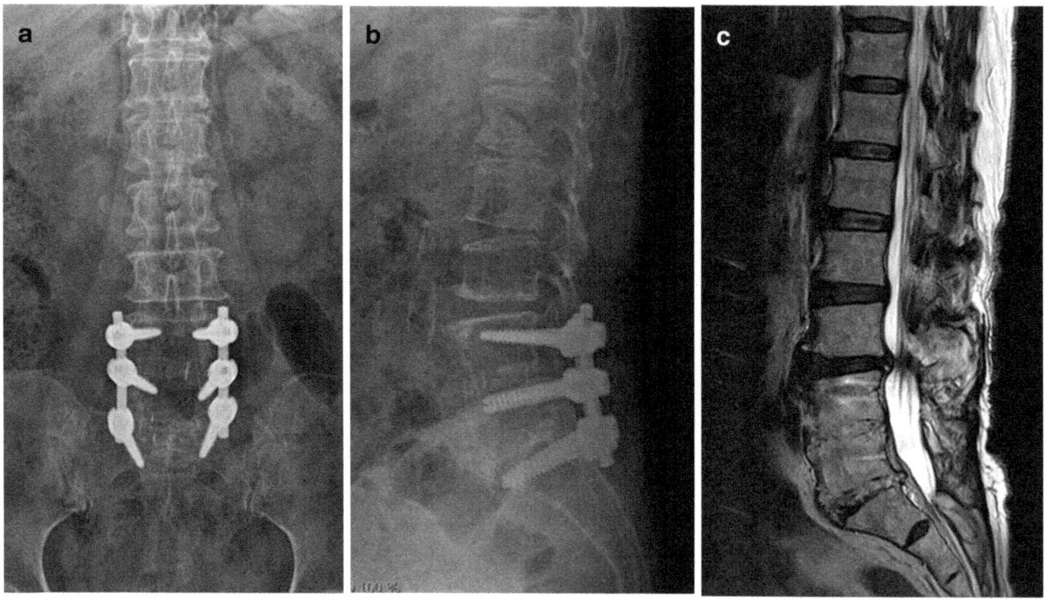

Fig. 8 A 65-year-old female has performed L4/5/S1 fusion surgery previously. Plain film shows well fused state on L4/5/S1 level. We can see the stenotic lesion on L3/4 segment on MRI view

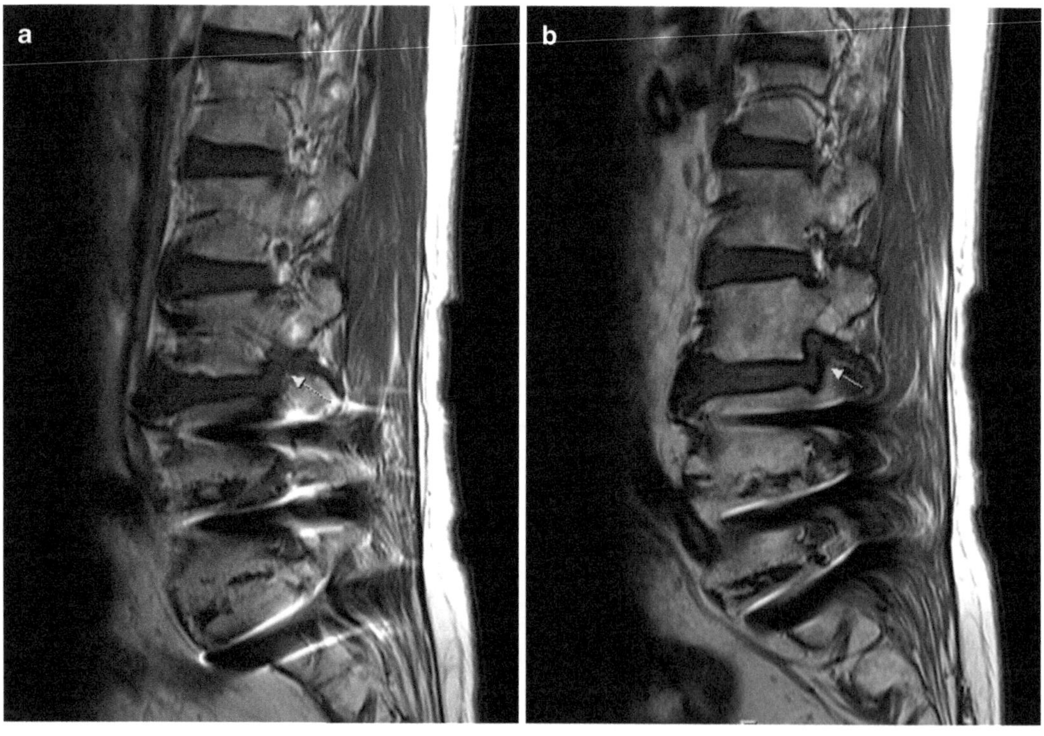

Fig. 9 MRI views shows severe foraminal stenosis without fat signal on both sides. Endoscopic LIF has advantage especially in the treatment of the case with foraminal stenosis

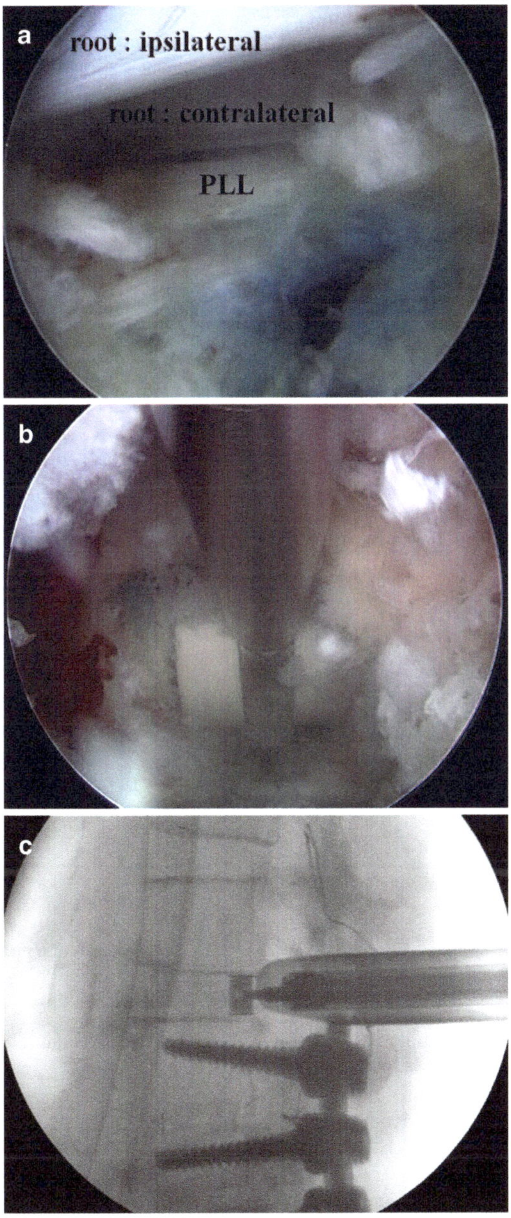

Fig. 10 We can decompress on the ventral side of both nerve roots by uniportal endoscopic technique. And, we can insert cage safely under endoscopic guidance

tissue while avoiding neural injury [4–6]. With the advancement of the endoscopic instruments and techniques, endoscopic TLIF has been widely performed nowadays. There are some differences between endoscopic TLIF and MIS TLIF techniques [7].

1. The skin incision of endoscopic TLIF is smaller but there is no evidence that it has less muscle trauma than MIS TLIF.
2. Sometimes, the endoscopic TLIF can be performed under local anesthesia with conscious sedation, which is a unique benefit of this technique.
3. In general, endplate preparation by reamer and curette in open discectomy surgery is performed in blind step. Therefore, subchondral bone may be damaged during this step. This may result in subsidence of the cage on follow-up exams. Endplate preparation during endoscopic TLIF confirms the adequacy of the visual preparation, rather than relying on palpation with instruments.
4. There is no established optimal instrumentation technique that has accomplished solid fusion or stabilization of the vertebral segment in endoscopic TLIF.

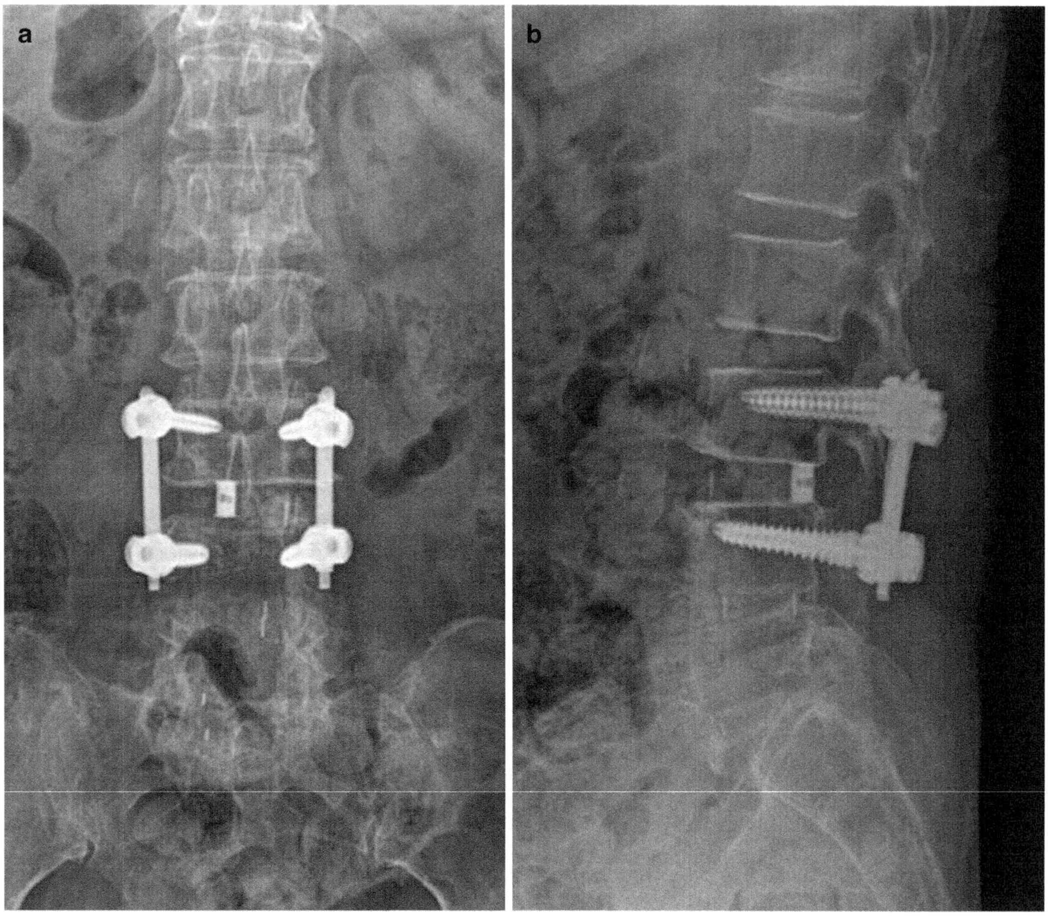

Fig. 11 Postoperative plain radiographs : previous screws were removed and new screws were fixed with percutaneous technique

References

1. Osman SG. Endoscopic transforaminal decompression, interbody fusion, and percutaneous screw implantation of the lumbar spine: a case series report. Int J Spine Sur. 2012;1(6):157–66.
2. Wang MY, Grossman J. Endoscopic minimally invasive transforaminal interbody fusion without general anesthesia: initial clinical experience with 1-year follow-up. Neurosurg Focus. 2016;40(2):E13.
3. Youn MS, Shin JK, Goh TS, et al. Full endoscopic lumbar interbody fusion (FELIF): technical note. Eur Spine J. 2018;27(8):1949–55.
4. Rosenberg WS, Mummaneni PV. Transforaminal lumbar interbody fusion: technique, complications, and early results. Neurosurgery. 2001;48(3):569–74. discussion 574-575
5. Hee HT, Castro FP Jr, Majd ME, et al. Anterior/posterior lumbar fusion versus transforaminal lumbar interbody fusion: analysis of complications and predictive factors. J Spinal Disord. 2001;14(6):533–40.
6. Moskowitz A. Transforaminal lumbar interbody fusion. Orthop Clin North Am. 2002;33(2):359–66.
7. Ahn Y, Youn MS, Heo DH. Endoscopic transforaminal lumbar interbody fusion: a comprehensive review. Expert Rev Med Devices. 2019;16(5):373–80.

Biportal Endoscopic Transforaminal Lumbar Interbody Fusion

Dong Hwa Heo, Man Kyu Park, and Jin Hwa Eum

Introduction

Various types of lumbar fusion surgeries were performed for lumbar degenerative disease such as instability, spondylolysis, and spondylolisthesis. Minimally invasive lumbar fusion surgeries have advantages such as preservation of normal structures and facilitation of recovery after surgery [1–3].

Recently, endoscopic lumbar interbody fusion surgeries have been attempted for lumbar degenerative disease [1]. Especially, biportal endoscopic lumbar interbody fusion surgeries can perform direct neural decompression of central and foraminal stenosis (Fig. 1a) [3–5] as well as complete endplate preparation under high magnified endoscopic vision [2, 6]. Basically, the technique of biportal endoscopic transforaminal lumbar interbody fusion (TLIF) is the same as minimally invasive TLIF using tubular retractor systems. Compared to conventional or minimally invasive TLIF, biportal endoscopic TLIF might have benefit of endplate preparation and reduction of postoperative wound pain [2, 6].

Electronic Supplementary Material The online version of this chapter (https://doi.org/10.1007/978-981-15-8253-0_16) contains supplementary material, which is available to authorized users.

D. H. Heo
Department of Neurosurgery, Seoul Bumin Hospital, Seoul, South Korea

M. K. Park (✉)
Spine Center, Neurosurgery, Parkweonwook Hospital, Busan, South Korea

J. H. Eum
Spine Center, Neurosurgery, Medrex hospital, Seoul, South Korea

Indication and Contraindication

Basically, indications of biportal endoscopic TLIF were the same as minimally invasive TLIF using tubular retractor systems [2, 6].

- Indication.
  - Lumbar instability.
  - Degenerative spondylolisthesis.
  - Isthmic spondylolisthesis.
  - Recurrent lumbar disc herniation after discectomy.
  - Lumbar central and foraminal stenosis.
- Relative Contraindication.
  - High-grade lumbar spondylolisthesis.
- Contraindication.
  - Infectious spinal disease.
  - Tumorous condition.

Anesthesia and Position

General endotracheal anesthesia was preferred. Epidural anesthesia with sedation was another option of single level fusion. Prone position was

H. S. Kim et al. (eds.), *Advanced Techniques of Endoscopic Lumbar Spine Surgery*,
https://doi.org/10.1007/978-981-15-8253-0_16

necessary for this fusion procedure for subsequent percutaneous pedicle screw fixation after insertion of an interbody cage.

Special Surgical Instruments

Specialized tool kit set was necessary for biportal endoscopic TLIF. Angled dissectors and Penfield dissector were useful for endoscopic guided endplate preparation. We used angled endplate curettes for contralateral endplate preparation. Radiofrequency (RF) probes were necessary for dissection of soft tissue and bleeding control. Specialized dura retractor was necessary for insertion of interbody fusion cages (Fig. 1a, b). Although a single straight long TLIF cage was usually used in biportal endoscopic TLIF, two short interbody fusion cages can be inserted via unilateral biportal endoscopic approaches.

Surgical Steps (Videos 1 and 2)

1. Making two portals: Waterproof surgical drape was used for this operation. Generally, two skin incisions were made over the ipsilateral pedicle areas. If fusion surgery of L4–5 was performed, unilateral two skin incisions were made on L4 and L5 pedicle areas for decompression and a cage insertion ipsilaterally (Fig. 2). Direction of surgical approach depended on dominant symptomatic side. Serial dilators were inserted at working channel. And a working sheath was inserted at working portal for well drainage of irrigation fluid.
2. Neural decompression: Firstly, we should expose ipsilateral laminar and facet joint capsule using RF probes. Ipsilateral laminotomy of the lower part of cranial lamina and the upper part of caudal lamina was done using Kerrison punches and endoscopic drill. And an ipsilateral inferior articular process was removed using drill and osteotomes. Bone working was preferred to use Kerrison punches or osteotome rather than drill for collecting bone graft. Ipsilateral ligamentum flavum was easily removed after bony decompression. After decompression of ipsilateral lateral recess with traversing nerve root, contralateral ligamentum flavum was removed under endoscopic guidance. If the patient has central stenosis with bilateral radicular pain, contralateral ligamentum flavum should be removed until complete

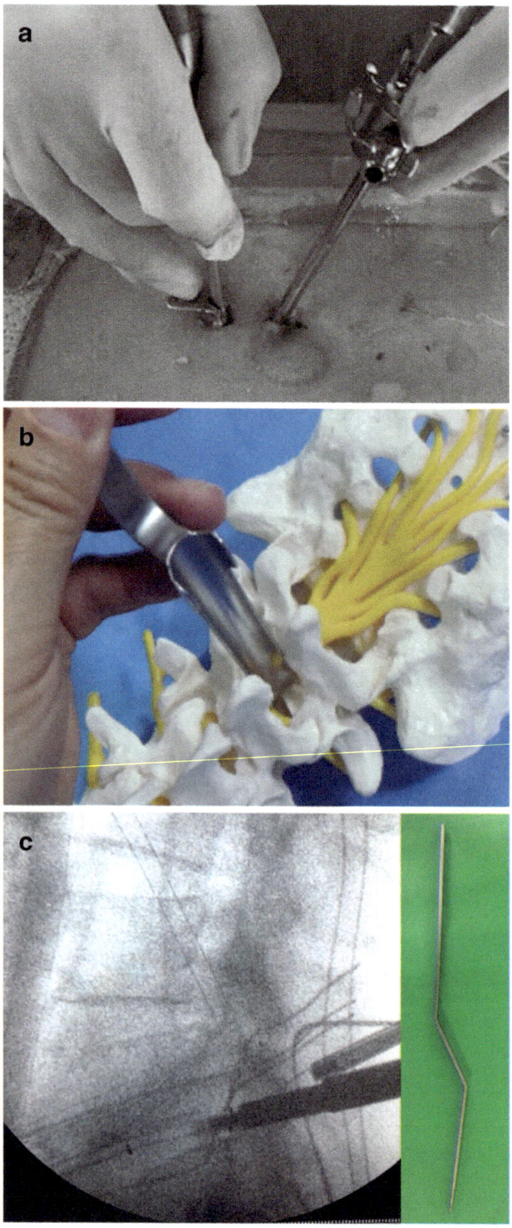

Fig. 1 Overview of biportal endoscopic lumbar interbody fusion (**a**). Specialized dura retractors (**b** and **c**). Specialized dura retractor was used during a TLIF cage insertion

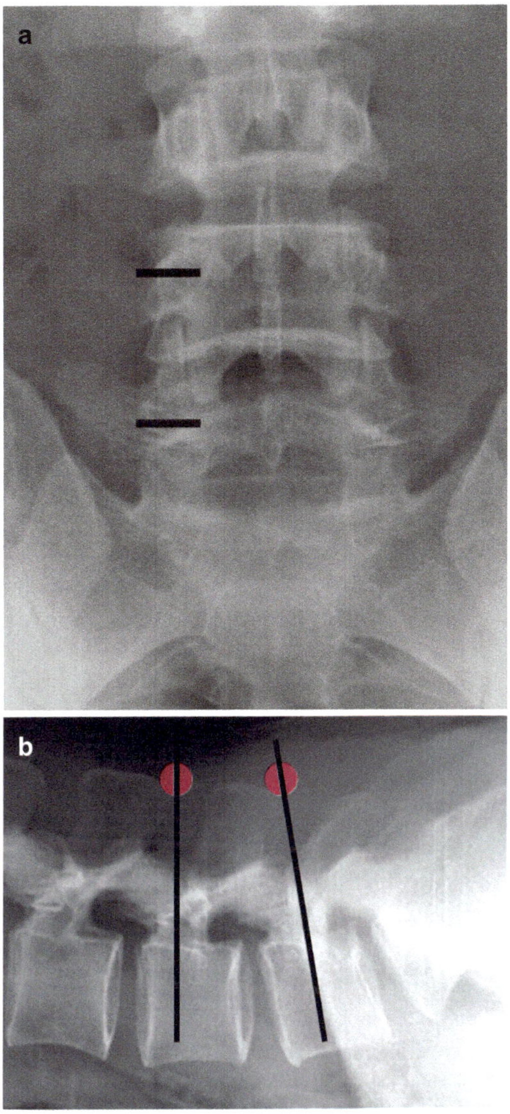

Fig. 2 Skin incision points of making two portals for biportal endoscopic TLIF. Usually, two channels were made over ipsilateral pedicle area, and these two skin incisions were also used for pedicle screw insertion. Anteroposterior view (**a**); lateral view (**b**)

decompression of contralateral traversing nerve root. Medial part of ipsilateral superior articular process was removed for a large size cage insertion. If the patient has concomitant foraminal stenosis or foraminal disc herniation, ipsilateral superior articular process was completely removed for exiting nerve root decompression. Autologous bone chips which were taken from laminar and facet bone were used for fusion material.

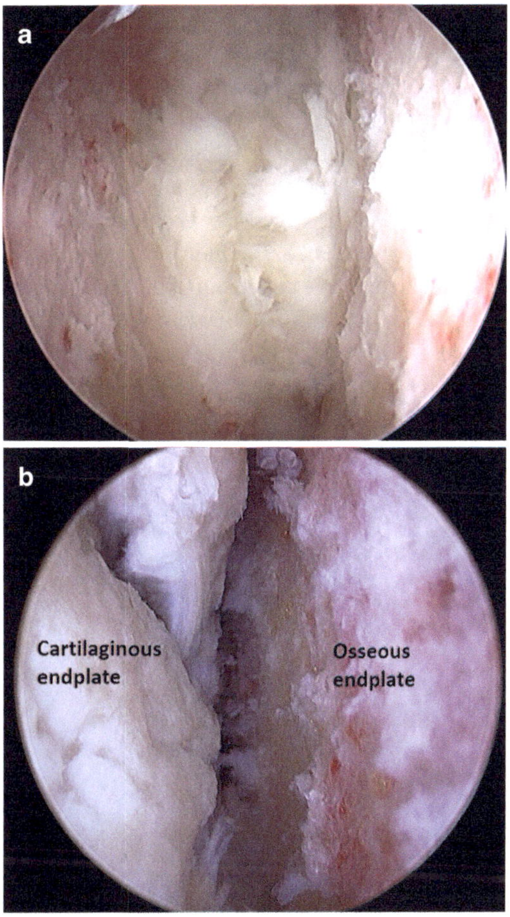

Fig. 3 Endoscopic view of endplate preparation. Cartilaginous endplate was completely separated from osseous endplate (**a**). Final endoscopic view of endplate preparation (**b**)

3. Disc removal and endplate preparation (Video 1): Annulus fibrosus was incised by RF probe or blunt knife. Nucleus pulposus materials were removed using various sizes of straight pituitary forceps or angled pituitary forceps. We usually dissect and separate the cartilaginous endplate from the osseous endplate using angled dissectors or using angled dissectors under magnified endoscopi vision. The cartilaginous endplate can be completely removed from osseous endplate without any injury of osseous endplate under magnified endoscopic view (Fig. 3).
4. Insertion of fusion materials and cage: Fusion materials such as allograft of autologous bone

were inserted using specialized making funnel before a cage insertion (Fig. 4). A large volume of fusion materials can be putted in the interbody space using a funnel under C-arm fluoroscopic guidance. Dura was retracted by specialized making retractors. A large size common TLIF cage was inserted after dura retraction under C-arm fluoroscopic guidance. An inserted cage can be repositioned using an impactor under C-arm fluoroscopic and endoscopic guidance. A drainage catheter was finally inserted for the prevention of postoperative epidural hematoma.

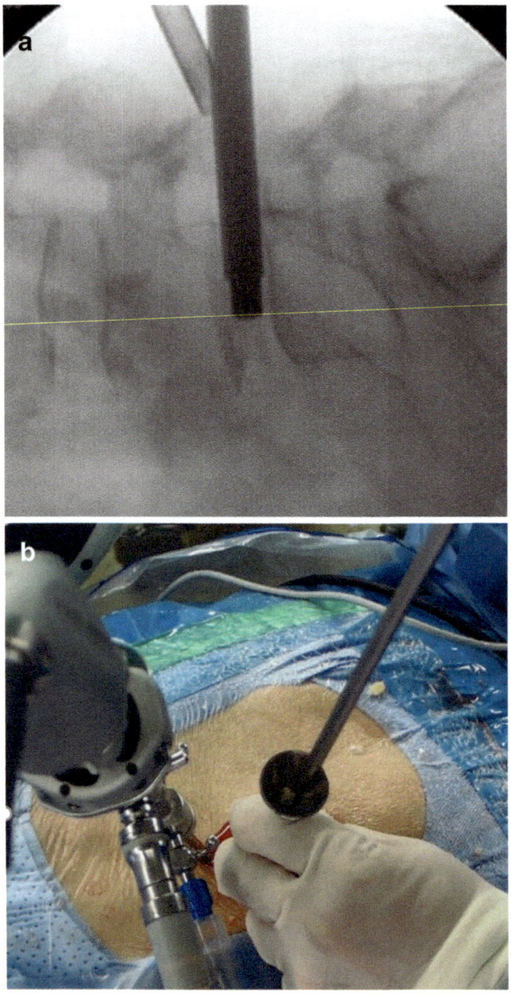

Fig. 4 Insertion of fusion materials into intervertebral space using a funnel. (**a**) C-arm fluoroscopic view and (**b**) overview of insertion of fusion materials using a specialized funnel

5. Percutaneous pedicle screw insertion: After a cage insertion, pedicle screws were inserted percutaneously under C-arm fluoroscopic guidance. Two skin incisions of two portals were also used for ipsilateral pedicle screws insertion. Contralateral pedicle screws were inserted using additional small skin incisions.

Illustrated Case or Cases

1. A 57-year-old female patient complained of neurological intermittent claudication and left radicular buttock and leg pain. Simple X-ray shows disc space narrowing of L5–S1 (Fig. 5). Preoperative MR images show lateral recess stenosis with left side foraminal stenosis at L5–S1 area. We performed the biportal endoscopic TLIF by left sided approach (Fig. 5). Intraoperative images reveal complete decompression of left L5 and S1 nerve roots. Cartilaginous endplate was removed from osseous endplate without injury. Postoperative MRI T2-weighted images show well-decompressive status of left lateral recess and foraminal area of L5–S1 (Fig. 5). Symptoms of this patient were significantly improved after surgery.
2. A 76-year-old male patient presented radicular pain of both legs and neurological intermittent claudication. X-ray and MR images show degenerative spondylolisthesis with stenosis at L4–5 area (Fig. 6). We performed biportal endoscopic TLIF and percutaneous pedicle screw fixation at L4–5. Postoperative X-ray and MR images show well reduction of spondylolisthesis and complete neural decompression of L4–5 (Fig. 6). Postoperatively, radicular pain was resolved.

Complication and its Management

Although bleeding points were small and tiny, bleeding should be controlled during surgery, whenever bleeding points were detected. Becuase intraoperative bleeding blurred the filed of endoscopic vision. Sometimes endoscopic fusion procedures cannot proceed and were converted to microsurgery due to blurred vision by diffuse bleeding.

Dural tear occurred during surgery like microsurgery. Small dura tear can be treated by TachoSil application. Large dural defect should be sutured under microscopic view. Massive use of RF may induce dermal injury to neural structures. When the dura was exposed, the power of RF should be reduced and used intermittently.

Prolonged operation time may increase epidural pressure by irrigation fluid and morbidities of general anesthesia. This endoscopic fusion surgery should be attempted after many experiences of endoscopic discectomy and decompressive procedures.

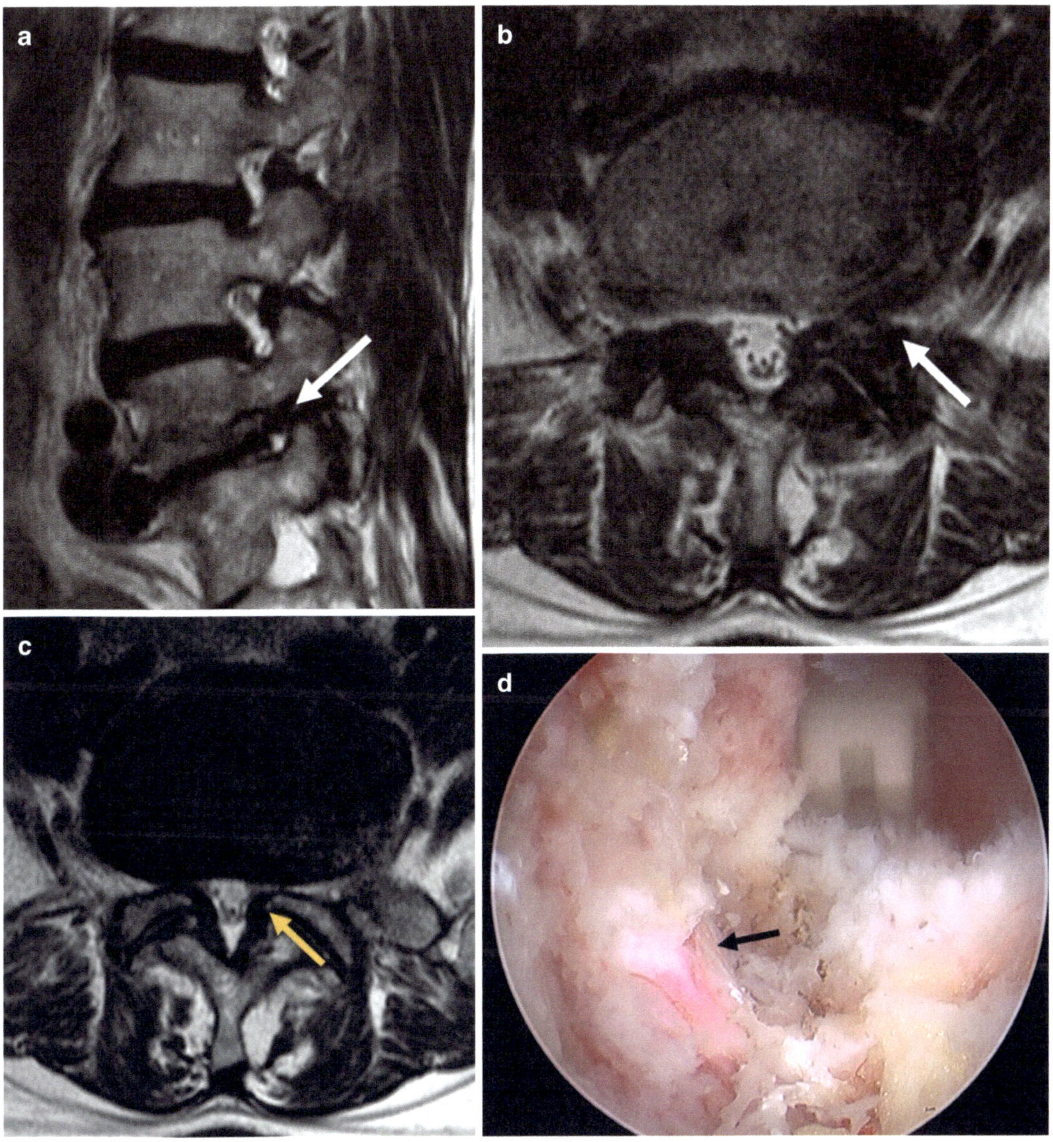

Fig. 5 A 57-year-old female patient presented with left leg pain with claudication. Preoperative MR images showed left sided foraminal stenosis (**a** and **b**, arrows) with lateral recess stenosis (**c**, yellow arrow). Intraoperative endoscopic images revealed complete decompression of left side L5 exiting nerve root (**d**) and S1 traversing nerve root (**e**). Narrowed intervertebral disc space of L5-S1 (**f**) was widen after biportal endoscopic TLIF (**g**). Postoperative MR images showed decompression of foraminal stenosis (**h** and **i**) and lateral recess stenosis (**j**) of left L5–S1

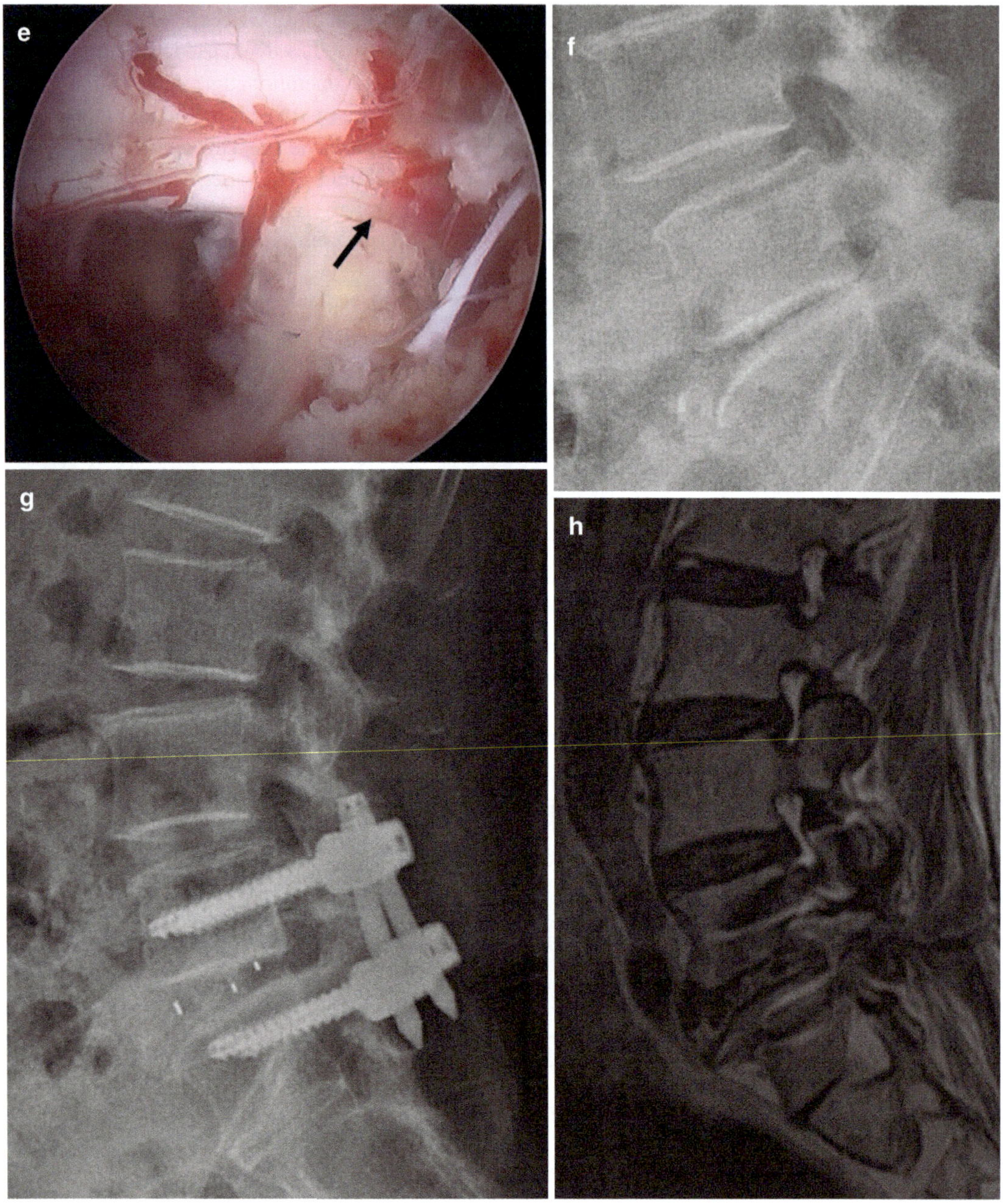

Fig. 5 (continued)

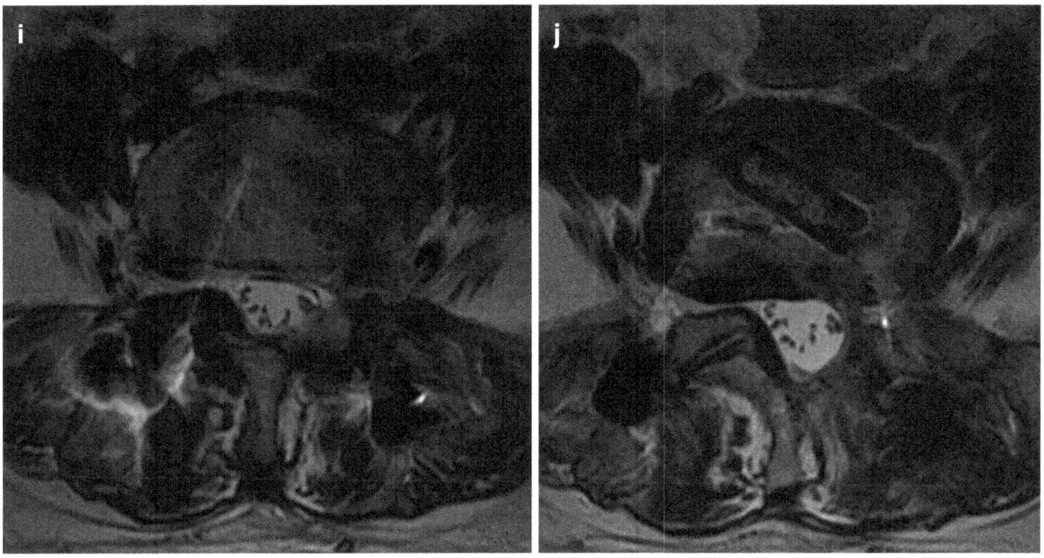

Fig. 5 (continued)

Brief Discussion (Surgical Tip and Pitfall)

Basically, this endoscopic technique is similar to minimally invasive TLIF using tubular retractor systems. Therefore, we can achieve direct neural decompression of central canal as well as exiting and traversing nerve roots [5, 7]. Endoscopic endplate preparation is another great advantage of biportal endoscopic lumbar interbody fusion surgery [3, 6, 7]. Endplate preparation without endplate injury was important for fusion and prevention of cage subsidence. Biportal endoscopic endplate preparation may prevent the injury of osseous endplate and incomplete removal of cartilaginous endplate. We need to find the dissection space between osseous endplate and cartilaginous endplate using small diameter of shavers, curved dissectors, and diamond drill. If you find the interspace between cartilaginous and osseous endplates, you can separate cartilaginous endplate from osseous endplate using dissectors. Although there were some limitations of contralateral endplate preparation, curve endplate curettes and 30° endoscope may help perform contralateral endplate preparation.

Specialized nerve retractors were necessary for safe insertion of a large size TLIF cage, because endoscopic vision was narrow during a cage insertion. Moreover, we recommended C-arm fluoroscopic monitoring during a TLIF cage insertion. A TLIF cage was deeply inserted and repositioned from sagittal to coronal angle for prevention of pullout of cage and making lumbar segmental lordosis.

We suggested that expandable TLIF cages may be useful in endoscopic lumbar interbody fusion surgery in aspects of making lordosis, safe insertion of cage without dural injury, and disc height restoration.

Recently, the concept of enhanced recovery after surgery (ERAS) has been attempted and applied in spine surgery [8]. ERAS program can accelerate early recovery and prevent postoperative complications after major surgery [8]. Endoscopic fusion procedures including biportal endoscopic approaches may be important to ERAS of major spine surgery [2]. If biportal endoscopic fusion surgeries are performed with ERAS protocol, postoperative pain and complications were significantly decreased compared to conventional lumbar fusion operation.

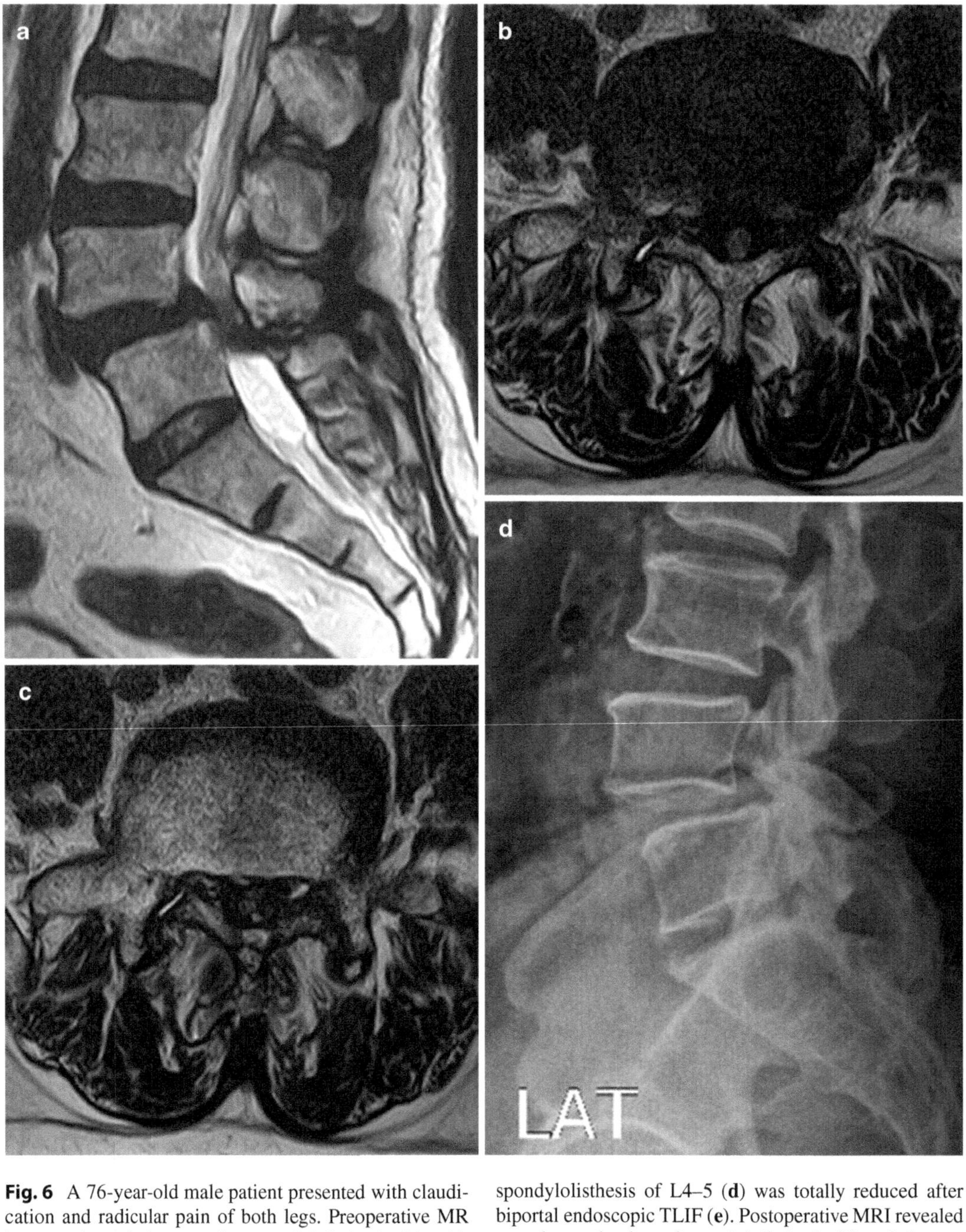

Fig. 6 A 76-year-old male patient presented with claudication and radicular pain of both legs. Preoperative MR images showed degenerative spondylolisthesis (**a**) with severe central stenosis (**b** and **c**) of L4–5. Preoperative spondylolisthesis of L4–5 (**d**) was totally reduced after biportal endoscopic TLIF (**e**). Postoperative MRI revealed complete reduction of spondylolisthesis (F) and decompression of central stenosis of L4–5 (**g** and **h**)

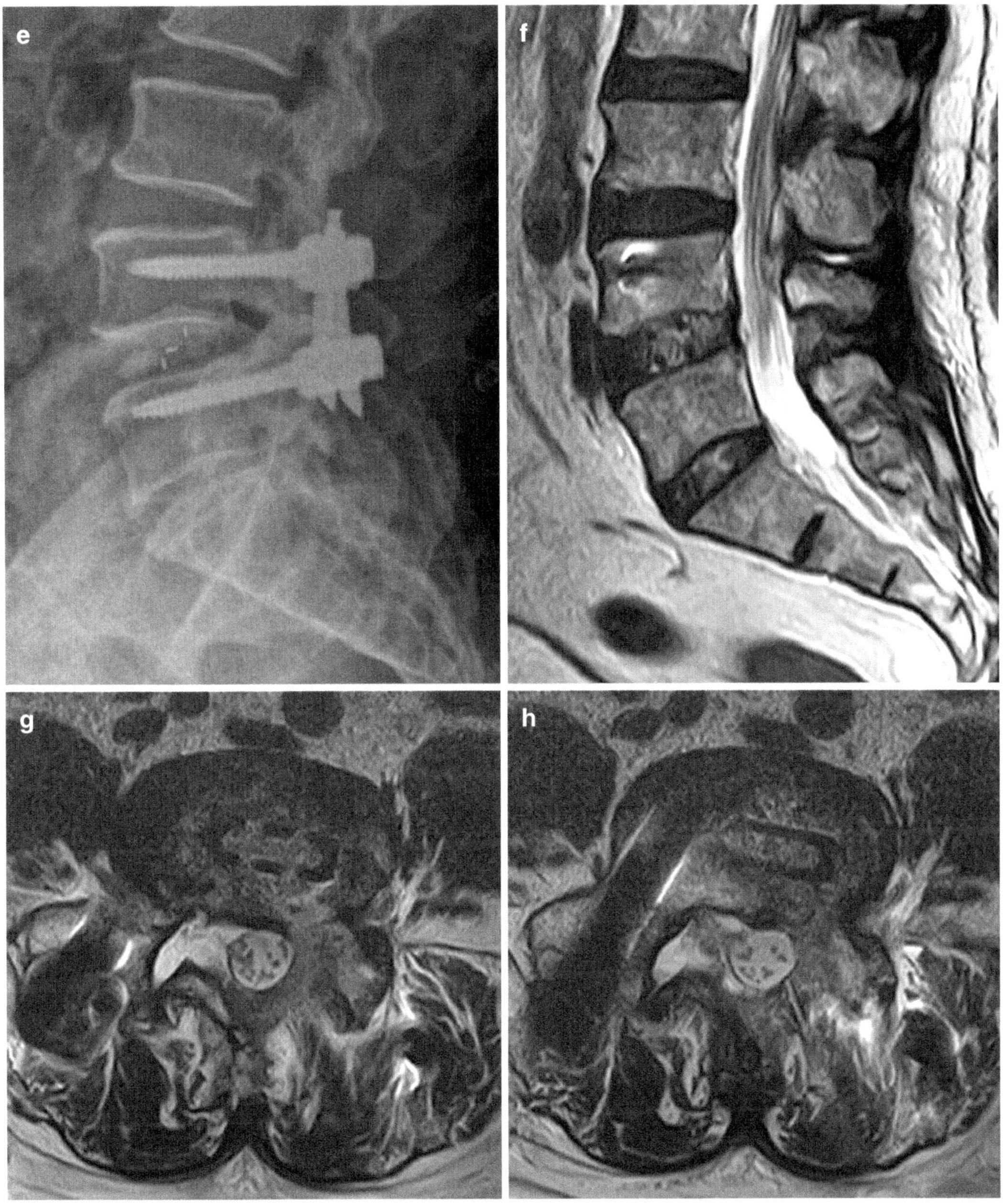

Fig. 6 (continued)

References

1. Ahn Y, Youn MS, Heo DH. Endoscopic transforaminal lumbar interbody fusion: a comprehensive review. Expert Rev Med Devices. May 2019;16(5):373–80.
2. Heo DH, Park CK. Clinical results of percutaneous biportal endoscopic lumbar interbody fusion with application of enhanced recovery after surgery. Neurosurg Focus. 2019;46(4):E18.
3. Park M, Park S, Son S, Park W, Choi S. Clinical and radiological outcomes of unilateral biportal endoscopic lumbar interbody fusion (ULIF) compared with conventional posterior lumbar interbody fusion (PLIF): 1-year follow-up. Neurosurg Rev. 2019;42(3):753–61.
4. Lin GX, Huang P, Kotheeranurak V, et al. A systematic review of unilateral Biportal endoscopic spinal surgery: preliminary clinical results and complications. World Neurosurg. May 2019;125:425–32.
5. Heo DH, Lee DC, Park CK. Comparative analysis of three types of minimally invasive decompressive surgery for lumbar central stenosis: biportal endoscopy, uniportal endoscopy, and microsurgery. Neurosurg Focus. 2019;46(5):E9.
6. Heo DH, Son SK, Eum JH, Park CK. Fully endoscopic lumbar interbody fusion using a percutaneous unilateral biportal endoscopic technique: technical note and preliminary clinical results. Neurosurg Focus. 2017;43(2):E8.
7. Heo DH, Park CK. Clinical results of percutaneous biportal endoscopic lumbar interbody fusion with application of enhanced recovery after surgery. Neurosurg Focus. 2019;46(4):E18.
8. Brusko GD, Kolcun JPG, Heger JA, et al. Reductions in length of stay, narcotics use, and pain following implementation of an enhanced recovery after surgery program for 1- to 3-level lumbar fusion surgery. Neurosurg Focus. 2019;46(4):E4.

GPSR Compliance

The European Union's (EU) General Product Safety Regulation (GPSR) is a set of rules that requires consumer products to be safe and our obligations to ensure this.

If you have any concerns about our products, you can contact us on ProductSafety@springernature.com

In case Publisher is established outside the EU, the EU authorized representative is:

Springer Nature Customer Service Center GmbH
Europaplatz 3
69115 Heidelberg, Germany

Batch number: 10732801

Printed by Printforce, the Netherlands